Ruta Nonacs, MD, PhD

A Deeper Shade of Blue

A Woman's
Guide to Recognizing
and Treating Depression in
Her Childbearing Years

Simon & Schuster Paperbacks
New York London Toronto Sydney

SIMON & SCHUSTER PAPERBACKS
1230 Avenue of the Americas
New York, NY 10020

First Simon & Schuster trade paperback edition August 2007

SIMON & SCHUSTER PAPERBACKS and colophon are registered trademarks
of Simon & Schuster, Inc.

This publication contains the opinions and ideas of its author. It is intended to provide helpful and informative material on the subjects addressed in the publication. It is sold with the
understanding that the author and publisher are not engaged in rendering medical, health, or
any other kind of personal professional services in the book. The reader should consult his or
her medical, health, or other competent professional before adopting any of the suggestions
in this book or drawing inferences from it.

The author and publisher specifically disclaim all responsibility for any liability, loss, or
risk, personal or otherwise, which is incurred as a consequence, directly or indirectly, of the
use and application of any of the contents of this book.

For information about special discounts for bulk purchases,
please contact Simon & Schuster Special Sales at
1-800-456-6798 or business@simonandschuster.com.

Designed by Karolina Harris

Manufactured in the United States of America

10 9 8 7 6 5 4 3 2 1

The Library of Congress has cataloged the hardcover edition as follows:
    Nonacs, Ruta.
A deeper shade of blue : a woman's guide to recognizing and treating depression in her
    childbearing years / Ruta Nonacs.
        p.   cm.
Includes bibliographical references (p.)
    1. Women—Mental health.   2. Women—Psychology.   3. Motherhood—Psychological
aspects.   4. Mental illness in pregnancy.   5. Postpartum depression.   I. Title.

RC451.4.W6N66   2006
616.85'270082—dc22   200604502

ISBN-13: 978-0-7432-5473-1
ISBN-10:   0-7432-5473-2
ISBN-13: 978-0-7432-5475-5 (pbk)
ISBN-10:   0-7432-5475-9 (pbk)

Acknowledgments

This book has been a project spanning many years, and many people have helped me along the way. First of all, I would like to thank my husband, Steven Schlozman; without his love, encouragement, patience, and thoughtful insights, I would not have been able to complete this book. And I could not have succeeded without the love and support of my parents, Drs. Mirdza Neiders and Edgars Nonacs. I am grateful to the many people who helped to transform my enthusiasm for my work into a tangible project: Mary Albon, Eric Nonacs, Diane Cardwell, Dr. Vivien Schlozman, Dr. Daniel Schlozman, Dr. Suzanne Bender, Dr. Julie Newman, Dr. Alicia Powell, Dr. Karen Carlson, and Dr. Bonnie Oye.

Long a lover of books, I never imagined that I would be able to write one, and I am grateful to those people who have helped me to make this dream a reality. Dr. Victor Doyno, Dr. Theodore Stern, and Ellie Hackett all helped me to develop my skills as a writer. I am grateful to my agent, Gail Ross, whose enthusiasm and expertise were so important in the earliest stages of launching this project. My editor, Sydny Miner, gently guided me through the process of writing this book, and I have appreciated her gracious support and encouragement and her unwavering enthusiasm for this project.

I am especially grateful to Dr. Lee Cohen; his experience, enthusiasm, and ardent dedication to the patients he cares for have shaped my development as a physician. I am indebted to my colleagues at the Center for Women's Mental Health at the Massachusetts General Hospital: Dr. Hadine Joffe, Dr. Helen Kim, Dr. Adele Viguera, Dr. Claudio Soares, Dr. Laura Petrillo, Dr. Kimberly Pearson, Dr. Julia Coleman, Ellen Feldman, and Fredda Zuckerman. They have helped to create a rich and supportive environment, and without their experience and wisdom, I would not have been able to pursue this project.

Finally, I am grateful to the many women and their families who have shared their experiences with me. It has been a privilege as their physician to care for them, and I hope their experiences can help other women who read this book.

For my daughters, Sofia and Naomi

Contents

Foreword

The last decade has brought great advances in our understanding of depression and the ways to treat this serious illness. Nonetheless, a majority of patients who suffer from depression do not get appropriately diagnosed or treated. These individuals suffer the significant consequences of untreated mood disturbance. In addition, the impact of depression on others, including partners, friends, and family members who surround those suffering from this illness, is too often underestimated. Despite the consistent finding from well-conducted studies that depression is more common in women than in men and that it is particularly common during the childbearing years, it has really only been during the last fifteen years that attention has been paid to treatment of depression in women during critical times such as pregnancy, the postpartum period, and the interval following miscarriage.

A *Deeper Shade of Blue* takes great steps to provide us with a clear road map to a more complete understanding of depression during the childbearing years, its recognition and treatment, and indeed the extent to which it is treatable. The information found here will empower those who require treatment to work with those who can provide it.

We have yet to completely understand what underlies women's vulnerability to depression during critical times in their reproductive years. Meanwhile, too few sources of information on what is presently known have been available thus far. The Internet has vast potential, and yet it can sometimes incompletely inform or even misinform us when we search it for answers. Nor should we have to rely on magazines for discussion of a problem as serious as depression. In A *Deeper Shade of Blue*, readers will find full explanations regarding a wide range of mood disorders that appear to be linked in some fashion to female reproductive biology. For example, they will find a discussion of PMS, and particularly the more severe form of PMS known as premenstrual dysphoric disorder (PMDD), which used to be a pejorative term but has evolved over the last decade into a more clearly understood problem of mood. They will read a demystifying description of infertility treatments and an honest discussion of the range of experiences associated with pregnancy loss, for which there is not only helpful information but encouragement to follow a woman's own intuitive feelings, rather than an expectation to "move on" after so significant a loss. They will read straightforward descriptions of what women actually experience during pregnancy, from normal mood swings to clinically significant depression in need of professional evaluation and treatment.

Postpartum depression remains one of the most common complications in modern obstetrics, and yet it remains largely undetected and frequently untreated. Just as the general range of feelings experienced by postpartum women varies widely—ambivalence, joy, confusion—postpartum depression may be very different for the single mom, the older mom, the mom managing a fussier baby, the mom caring for a newborn in an unfamiliar culture with a level of support different from her native one.

From PMS, to depression during pregnancy, to postpartum mood disorders, women need to be able to distinguish what is normal from what is more serious and in need of definitive treatment. Perhaps the most critical message of this book is that a failure to recognize and treat depression during the childbearing years cannot be an option. With the publication of *A Deeper Shade of Blue*, women are given a valuable resource that offers them a way to better understand depression as they collaborate with family, friends, and care providers in the process of treatment and recovery.

Lee S. Cohen, MD
Boston, Massachusetts
February 2006

Part One

Introduction

Chapter 1

A Neglected Problem

Depression During the Childbearing Years

Despite the intense efforts of the medical community and the media to publicize the problem of depression and to educate the public, depression remains both confusing and controversial. For many, depression can be a serious and potentially life-threatening problem. The tragedy surrounding Andrea Yates and the death of her five children in 2000 stands as a testament to the devastating effects of mental illness. Depression, however, refers to a wide-ranging spectrum of problems. For those familiar with depression, this is a potentially life-ravaging illness, yet the word *depression* has entered into our daily lexicon and is often used to describe any unpleasant mood or feeling. And far too commonly, depression is portrayed as a malady of the self-obsessed—a sign of self-indulgence or an excuse for laziness or bad behavior.

Over the past decade, many have worked to correct these misperceptions, yet, according to a recent survey conducted by the National Mental Health Association, Americans are more likely to view depression as a sign of personal weakness than as an illness. Depression, however, is not simply a symptom of a weak character or an exaggerated response to the stresses of daily living. It is a real and potentially devastating illness. While it may vary tremendously from person to person in terms of its severity and its spectrum of symptoms, depression, when left untreated, is an illness that threatens a person's capacity to function effectively and to derive pleasure from life.

Although depression affects both men and women of all ages, women are more vulnerable to this illness, particularly during their childbearing years. Despite a much more sophisticated understanding of depression over the last few decades and the development of highly effective treatments for this illness, far too many women with depression do not receive the attention and treatment they need and deserve. Depression frequently goes undiagnosed, and it is estimated that only about a third of those with depression receive *adequate* treatment. The situation is even worse when depression emerges *during* pregnancy or the postpartum period, when even the most severe and disabling symptoms may be overlooked or erroneously considered to be a normal or expected consequence of having a child. Furthermore, an expectant or new mother, when she is not able to understand why she is feeling depressed at a time when she is expected to feel unambivalently happy, is frequently too ashamed to ask for help.

Understanding the Scope of the Problem

Let's start with the basics. Depression is one of the most common illnesses among Americans today. The National Institutes of Mental Health estimates that in any given year about 10 percent of the adult population in the United States—at least 18 million people—suffer from this disorder. Just to put this in perspective, about 17 million Americans suffer from asthma, 15 million from heart disease, and 10 million from diabetes. Although there has been a tendency to downplay depression or to consider this disorder as distinct from, and therefore less severe than, other types of medical illness, depression is a leading cause of disability throughout the world. According to a study conducted by the Harvard School of Public Health and the World Health Organization (WHO), depression-related disability is significant and exceeds that caused by other chronic medical conditions, including high blood pressure, diabetes, and arthritis. Furthermore, the WHO predicts that depression will become the second leading cause of premature death and disability worldwide by the year 2020.

Women are disproportionately affected by depression. In fact, depression is about twice as common in women as in men, with about 1 woman in 4 suffering from depression at some point during her lifetime. Depression may strike at any time, but women appear to be particularly vulnerable during their childbearing years. Women are at highest risk for depression during pregnancy and shortly after delivery. One recent study indicated that as many as 25 percent of women suffer from depression during either pregnancy or the postpartum period. The number of women affected by depression in this context is staggering. Each year in the United States, almost 4 million women give birth to a child, and at least a million of these women experience depression either during pregnancy or after childbirth. Add to that the significant number of women who develop depression in the context of infertility problems, and you have a major public health problem. Yet, in most of these women, the illness goes unrecognized and untreated.

A Neglected Problem

In her short story "The Yellow Wallpaper," written more than one hundred years ago in 1896, feminist writer Charlotte Perkins Gilman chronicled the experiences of a woman suffering from severe depression after the birth of her child: her inability to care for her infant and her deteriorating relationship with her husband, culminating in a profound and rather disturbing detachment from the world around her. One of the most striking aspects of the story is the narrator's struggle to make sense of what was happening to her as she tries to overcome her feelings of helplessness and hopelessness.

> John [her husband] is a physician, and *perhaps* — (I would not say it to a living soul, of course, but this is dead paper and a great relief to my mind) — *perhaps* that is one reason I do not get well faster.
>
> You see he does not believe I am sick!
>
> And what can one do?
>
> If a physician of high standing, and one's own husband, assures friends and relatives that there is really nothing the matter with one but temporary nervous depression — a slight hysterical tendency — what is one to do?

Gilman, like the narrator in her story, suffered from postpartum depression and was frustrated by her condition and the inability (or unwillingness) of others, including her physician husband, to recognize the severity of her problem. A century later, Susan Kushner Resnick, in her memoir *Sleepless Days*, wrote of her experiences with postpartum depression and described a similar struggle to understand and to recover from this illness. After months of sleepless nights and a steadily mounting sense of desperation, Resnick finally reached out to her physician for help. He diagnosed her with "housewife's anxiety" and suggested that she take a vacation. Despite a far more refined understanding of depression over the last hundred years, women who suffer from postpartum depression continue to be misunderstood and overlooked.

Even more invisible are the women who suffer from depression *during* pregnancy. Pregnancy has been heralded as a time of emotional well-being, and it has long been assumed that pregnant women simply do not get depressed. While pregnancy may bring joy and excitement, women are by no means immune to depression during pregnancy. Recent studies indicate that during pregnancy, about 20 percent of women experience significant levels of depression, suggesting that depression during pregnancy (also called antenatal depression) is just as common as postpartum depression. Particularly vulnerable are those women who have suffered from depression before becoming pregnant; they have about a 50 percent chance of becoming depressed during pregnancy. What is especially concerning is the lack of attention to this serious problem. Most women who suffer from depression during pregnancy go unrecognized, with one study revealing that 85 percent of them received no treatment whatsoever. Given that depression affects such a large number of women, depression during pregnancy is clearly a problem of immense proportions, an issue the public (and many health care professionals) have not yet addressed.

Also at high risk for depression are those women who are struggling to have children. For about 10 percent to 20 percent of women, pregnancy ends in miscarriage. Although the emotional impact of miscarriage is often minimized, many women suffer from depression after the loss of a pregnancy. In addition, it is estimated that about 9 million American women have experienced fertility problems, and as more women delay their plans to have children, this number is steadily rising. Obviously, discovering that one may be infertile is stressful and potentially devastating in and of itself; however, as a woman pursues infertility treatment and attempts to get pregnant, her emotional distress may be intensified and she is particularly vulnerable to depression. In fact, recent studies indicate that about one-quarter of women receiving infertility treatment may develop significant depression or anxiety. Particularly concerning is the long duration of depression under these circumstances, as treatment for most couples may drag on for several years.

Depression and the Family

What is most concerning is the unequivocally negative impact of maternal depression on the family. Because of the central role a mother occupies within the family, her depression sends ripples throughout the entire family and may have a significant impact on her children, her husband, and others close to her. One study after another has demonstrated that depression in the mother may lead to a constellation of problems in her child: sleep and feeding problems, developmental delays, and various behavioral problems, including aggression. There are also other risks to consider. The tragic deaths of five children at the hands of their mother, Andrea Yates, focused media attention on maternal depression and its potentially devastating effects on the family. While this case is unusual and certainly extreme, it has pushed us to understand the importance of emotional well-being in the mother. This tragic event has highlighted the importance of educating women and their families about depression and how it may affect the family.

How to Use This Book

A *Deeper Shade of Blue* will discuss depression as it occurs in childbearing women and will focus on the broad range of emotional problems women experience prior to conception, during pregnancy, and after delivery. Part One addresses the problem of depression in women, with the goal of understanding why women are so vulnerable to this disorder and recognizing the significant impact depression may have on the family. Part Two explores the immense psychological changes a woman must undergo as she becomes a mother and how these changes may make her more vulnerable to stress and depression during the reproductive years. There are specific sections on the emotional issues surrounding infertility and pregnancy loss. Part Three focuses on the issues many women face after delivery as they adjust to their new role and includes a detailed discussion of the many different types of emotional problems women may encounter, including postpartum depression.

Depression affects a woman's ability to function, to interact with others, and to derive pleasure from her life. Given a woman's central role in both her family and society, when a mother suffers from depression, everyone around her suffers as well. This is especially true for her children; thus, the final section of this book focuses on how to manage the symptoms of depression and how to minimize the negative effects of depression on the family. Depression is a highly treatable illness and the potentially devastating effects of depression can be prevented. Particularly when depression occurs *during* pregnancy, women often receive the message that there are no options for treatment. This is simply not true. You will learn strategies for improving your relationship with your partner and bolstering your support network, and you will find practical information on seeking professional treatment. Also included is a summary of the most up-to-date information on effective therapies for depression, with special emphasis on the use of medication during pregnancy and breastfeeding.

One of the most important goals of *A Deeper Shade of Blue* is to help you to learn how to recognize depression and to understand your risk for this illness. Too often, women who suffer from depression during pregnancy or after the birth of a child do not know where to turn for information or for help. They find that others, even health care professionals, may lack a good understanding of the problems they are experiencing. Furthermore, their efforts to seek help may be thwarted by the many myths surrounding this problem. They are told that what they are experiencing is normal. It is not serious. It will go away on its own. However, depression is never "normal" and should never, under any circumstances, be ignored. While this book should not be considered as a substitute for professional care, *A Deeper Shade of Blue* will provide the information you need so that you may obtain the care you need and deserve. And it may also help others understand what you are experiencing.

A *Deeper Shade of Blue* is not only for women suffering from depression; it is for those women who are planning to conceive or who are in the early stages of pregnancy and are concerned about their risk of developing depression. With the advent of newer and more effective antidepressants, a large population of childbearing women are now taking antidepressant medications on a regular basis. For these women, pregnancy is a more complicated issue, since the decision to become pregnant is mingled with questions regarding their risk for illness during pregnancy and the postpartum period and concerns regarding the types of treatment available. Many women have taken antidepressant medications for many years and have questions regarding the use of these drugs during pregnancy and while nursing. What is clear is the considerable anxiety these women must bear in making these decisions regarding their treatment and the paucity of resources for women who are seeking this type of information. A *Deeper Shade of Blue* will help to fill this gap and will provide accurate up-to-date data so that you, in collaboration with your own physician, can make the most informed decisions regarding your care during pregnancy and beyond.

Chapter 2

Hormones and Mood

Understanding What Causes Depression in Women

As long as we have known about depression, we have wondered about its causes. Although much attention has been focused on this area, many questions remain. Like other types of psychiatric illness, depression tends to run in families, and a vulnerability to depression is strongly influenced by genetic factors. But genes are not all that determines whether you will suffer from depression. Your early childhood experiences, your personality style, and life experiences all influence your susceptibility to this illness.

Particularly pressing is the question of why women are so much more vulnerable to this disorder than men. Many have attributed this disparity to the various stresses women face as a result of their gender and the demands women face as they occupy multiple—and often conflicting—roles within the family, in the community, and at work. Over the last decade, researchers have also focused on the role of reproductive hormones, particularly estrogen. While it seems that many different factors may cause depression in women, depression should never be considered a "normal" or expected consequence of being a woman.

What Is Depression?

What exactly is depression? In the simplest terms, depression is a mood disorder; people with depression feel sad or down or they are unable to feel pleasure. Depression is to some degree a more exaggerated form of emotions we normally feel; however, clinical depression is not merely having a bad day or feeling upset about a specific something. It is a more pervasive and persistent feeling of sadness that does not seem to lift, lasting for weeks or even months at a time. Depression affects how you think, how you act, and how you interact with others. When you are depressed, you may try to cheer yourself up and to pull yourself out of it; however, when it's a real depression, these efforts are usually only fleetingly successful.

Anyone may suffer from depression; however, it is an experience that is shaped by one's history, personality, religion, society, and culture. With so many different factors acting in concert, depression may present itself in a startling spectrum of forms. What perhaps is so confusing is that two people may suffer from the same disease and yet look so different. Here are some examples:

Susan is twenty-eight, single, and recently moved to New York to work as a management consultant. At first she was very excited about and enjoyed her new job, but she now finds it difficult to motivate herself. She feels bored. She has never missed a day of work and has received relatively good reviews, but her home life is a different story. She never has the energy to cook, her apartment is embarrassingly cluttered and dirty, and she is habitually late in paying her bills. She avoids the phone, and most of the time she prefers to stay at home, telling her friends that she is too busy or too exhausted to go out. She feels lonely but at the same time helpless to do anything to improve her situation.

Samantha is forty-six and the mother of two children. About five years after the birth of her second child, Samantha discovered her husband was having an affair. Although she wanted to try to repair the relationship, her husband was determined to leave. Samantha was devastated. She had always pointed to her relationship with her husband as one of the accomplishments in her life, and she was proud of the life they had built together. She felt like a failure. Over the past year, she has become progressively more depressed and despairing. Despite encouragement from friends and family, she cannot imagine that she will be able to go on with her life. She is not able to sleep and spends much of the night pacing around the house. During the day, she is too exhausted to do much. She sends her children off to school and spends the rest of the day in bed. She finds herself crying— sobbing, in fact—throughout the day. Recently, she even started to have thoughts about killing herself; she feels worthless and sometimes wonders if her family would be better off without her.

Jessica is twenty. She was originally from rural Pennsylvania but ran away from home at the age of fourteen in order to escape an abusive stepfather. She now lives in Los Angeles and since arriving two years ago, she has been homeless. She has a long history of alcohol problems, but occasionally she uses heroin. She has struggled with depression since she was eight or nine years old. She is able to enjoy herself only when she is high and finds herself using more and more heroin, particularly when she is at her lowest. She has tried to commit suicide by overdose on multiple occasions, and she has been psychiatrically hospitalized about a dozen times. She continues to feel that suicide may be her only way to escape her problems.

All three of these women suffer from depression, yet the manifestations of the illness and the factors that have contributed to it are so entirely different that it may be difficult to think of these three people as experiencing the same disease. Most people would agree that Samantha is depressed, whereas many would be more likely to describe Susan as going through a difficult transition. In contrast, Jessica has had problems with depression since her childhood, yet it has been overshadowed by her problems with alcohol and drugs.

Because it comes in so many different forms and appears to have so many different causes, depression is often difficult to diagnose and easily overlooked. There are no blood tests or diagnostic tests to confirm the diagnosis. The signs of depression are not visible on a CT scan or an MRI. So how do we know it's depression? To make the diagnosis, doctors must rely on identifying a constellation of characteristic symptoms.

What most people call "clinical depression" is what psychiatrists call **major depression.** No matter when or in whom depression occurs there are certain common features. At the core of this disorder is a disturbance of mood—a sadness, a sense of depression or despair, an inability to enjoy yourself. It interferes with your ability to function; it is more difficult to motivate yourself and to work productively. It diminishes your sense of confidence and can make you feel helpless or ineffective. It affects every aspect of your life.

Depression not only affects how you feel, but it also affects how you think. Even if you are normally a rational and levelheaded person, depression can distort and disfigure how you look at and interpret the world. If you are depressed, you may feel less attractive, less intelligent, less competent, and less likable. You may feel pessimistic about your ability to accomplish a task or project, or it may seem like everything is an uphill battle. You may feel like your situation will never get better. When depression colors your world, experiences and external events are often misinterpreted. You may feel overly sensitive and may feel that others are criticizing or attacking you.

Depression also affects how you respond to and interact with others. If you are depressed, it may become more difficult for you to be around other people, and you may find it exhausting to maintain a friendly, socially engaging façade. You may feel much less confident around others, even people who are very close to you. You may worry that, if you are honest about how you feel, you may bring others down or push them away. You may believe that you and your depression are a burden to others. When you feel this way, the easiest solution may be to isolate yourself.

It is fairly common to feel quite irritable or impatient with others when you are depressed, and for many women irritability is one of the earliest signs of depression. Everything gets under your skin: how other people drive, how slow the checkout line is, how your husband is always ten minutes late, how your mother always gives advice. Sometimes it may be difficult to contain your annoyance, and you may be more argumentative or openly critical of others. Most often it is a woman's relationship with her partner that is most affected by depression. However, if you have children, you may notice that you are less patient with them and snap more easily.

But depression is not only psychological; there are also physical changes that take place. You may feel extraordinarily tired, unable to generate the energy required to go about your usual activities. Or you may feel very restless or even agitated, finding it difficult to sit still. Most women complain of difficulty falling asleep or discover that they are waking too early in the morning and unable to return to sleep. Or you may find it hard to stay out of bed; you may notice yourself going to bed earlier than usual and resisting getting out of bed in the morning. Often depressed women experience an increase in appetite and a tendency to gain weight; however, if your depression is more severe, there is usually a loss of appetite, which can be particularly problematic if you are pregnant or nursing. You may also notice that it is more difficult to think clearly; this may be experienced as forgetfulness, feeling "foggy" or "scattered," or not being able to concentrate.

If the depression is very severe, you may feel hopeless and may even think that life is not worth living. If you feel that things will never improve or that you are a burden to other people, you may even think of killing yourself. Although some women do contemplate suicide, women more commonly imagine dying in an accident or having a life-threatening illness rather than actively thinking about killing themselves. However, suicidal thoughts should never be ignored. If you are having these thoughts, this is a serious problem you should discuss with your physician immediately.

Types of Depression

The Diagnostic and Statistical Manual of Mental Disorders, also known as the DSM-IV, contains detailed definitions of the vast spectrum of psychiatric disorders. It defines several different subtypes of depression. These sub-

SYMPTOMS OF DEPRESSION

Psychological Symptoms
Sadness
Tearfulness
Lack of interest in usual or pleasurable activities
Low motivation
Inability to start or complete tasks
Pessimism
Hopelessness
Feelings of helplessness
Lack of confidence
Feelings of incompetence
Difficulty making decisions
Irritability or intolerance of others
Feelings of tension or being on edge
Numbness, inability to feel intense feelings or intimacy
Feelings of guilt or shame
Sensitivity to rejection or criticism
Feelings of unworthiness
Thoughts of death or dying
Suicidal thoughts

Physical Symptoms
Fatigue or lack of energy
Restlessness or physical tension
Difficulty falling asleep or waking frequently or too early (insomnia)
Sleeping more than usual (hypersomnia)
Changes in appetite (either eating too much or too little)
Loss of libido
Difficulty concentrating or distractibility
Memory problems
Frequent physical complaints (headaches, back pain, stomach upset)

types share the same core symptoms of depression; however, there are some important variations. Although the name is somewhat misleading, **atypical depression** is the most common type of depression among women. In contrast to **melancholic depression,** where a person is profoundly depressed and loses pleasure in *all* aspects of life, those who suffer from atypical depression have a greater degree of mood reactivity. That is, they are able to feel pretty good when something good happens; however, they cannot consistently sustain this mood and find that their mood plummets when something bad happens. They also seem to be more sensitive to criticism or rejection. Those with atypical depression also have some other distinctive symptoms. Whereas those with a melancholic depression experience restlessness, agitation, insomnia, and loss of appetite, those with atypical depression most commonly describe an increased need for sleep, fatigue, and increased appetite or weight gain.

In the absence of treatment, the average episode of depression lasts between eight and ten months. For some an episode of depression may last for years at a time, and some research indicates that women tend to have longer episodes of depression than men. While most people have an episodic course of illness, where they have one or more discrete episodes of depression and then return to their normal level of functioning, up to 3 percent of people may have a more chronic problem with low-level depression, an illness that psychiatrists call **dysthymia** or **dysthymic disorder.**

The symptoms of dysthymic disorder persist for more than two years. In many cases, the symptoms may be hard to recognize, and it is often difficult to date the earliest beginnings of the illness; in fact, it is fairly common for a person with dysthymia to report that they have felt down or mildly depressed for most of their adult life. Those with dysthymic disorder also complain of other problems, including changes in appetite, sleep disruption, fatigue, poor concentration, low self-esteem, and feelings of hopelessness. Typically the symptoms of dysthymic disorder are less severe and do not impact one's ability to function to the same degree as the symptoms of major depression. However, those with dysthymia may also suffer from a superimposed episode of major depression. When the two problems occur simultaneously, it is called a "double depression." Although there is a tendency to think of dysthymia as a more benign version of major depression, it is not. Given its chronic nature, dysthymia may have a significant long-term impact on one's ability to function and to fully enjoy life.

Bipolar Disorder

In some patients, the downs are only one part of the problem. About 1 percent to 3 percent of the population have **bipolar disorder,** also known as "manic depression" or "manic-depressive illness." In contrast to garden-variety depression, or *unipolar* depression, where there are only periods of depressed mood, bipolar disorder is characterized by dramatic upswings in mood alternating with periods of depression. Those who have bipolar disorder have episodes of euphoric or elevated mood, which is called mania. During a manic episode, they may experience a constellation of symptoms, including increased energy and productivity, decreased need for sleep, an elevated sense of confidence, and increased sociability. Obviously there are certain advantages to this state of being, but for most it is difficult to ride in this perfect zone for a sustained period. People who are manic are often impulsive and lack good judgment regarding their behavior; they go on spending sprees, drive recklessly, act promiscuously, or quit their jobs and travel to unexpected places. And often they crash. They may be so disorganized or disoriented that they cannot function. They may become so irritable or agitated that they snap at others or, in the most extreme examples, they may become physically violent or self-destructive.

SYMPTOMS OF HYPOMANIA AND MANIA

Euphoric or elated mood
Rapidly shifting moods or more intense displays of emotions
Irritability or argumentativeness
Racing thoughts or "flight of ideas"
Increased energy, restlessness, or agitation
Increased productivity or hyperactivity
Talkativeness or rapid speech
Decreased need for sleep
Inflated sense of self-esteem or grandiosity
Disorganized behavior
Impulsive or reckless behavior (spending money, going on trips, quitting job, driving too fast)
Poor insight into own behavior
Increased use of alcohol or drugs

All patients with bipolar disorder have both manic and depressive episodes. In many women, however, the manic episodes often go unnoticed. This is because men, more so than women, tend to have more full-blown manias, and it is often difficult to ignore their symptoms. Women, on the other hand, are more likely to suffer from what is called *hypomania*, a milder, less dramatic form of mania. During a hypomanic episode, a woman may feel energized, elated, confident, and outgoing. She may be a bit more impulsive or careless. She may seem a little bit too happy or a little bit too excitable, but the symptoms are generally under control and usually do not cause too many problems. In addition, bipolar disorder may be more difficult to detect in women because they tend to ride at the depressive end of the bipolar spectrum; that is, they have more depressive symptoms and fewer hypomanic or manic episodes than men. And when women get manic, they more often have what is called a *mixed episode*, where they experience symptoms of depression *and* mania at the same time. In this situation a woman is depressed or down, but she may be more anxious, agitated, impulsive, or irritable than a woman with a simple major depression. In these women, it may be very difficult to recognize bipolar disorder, and it is no surprise that many women with bipolar disorder are mistakenly diagnosed with and treated for major depression.

Premenstrual Dysphoric Disorder

Women also differ from men in that they may suffer from depressive disorders specifically linked to reproductive functioning and driven, at least in part, by shifts in the hormonal environment. The best example of this phenomenon is PMS (premenstrual syndrome) or a more severe form of this problem, which is now called **premenstrual dysphoric disorder** or PMDD. Women with PMDD experience significant mood changes during the one to two weeks preceding their menstrual periods, and it is believed that these mood symptoms are triggered by the hormonal changes associated with the menstrual cycle. (Premenstrual mood changes will be discussed in greater detail later in this chapter.) Similar, but even more dramatic, hormonal changes take place during pregnancy and after delivery and again as a woman transitions to the menopause; these are all times at which women seem to be at greater risk for both depression and anxiety.

Searching for the Cause

Almost everybody who becomes depressed tries to find a reason for his or her malady. Often they can identify some source of stress in their life—an unstable situation at work, marital problems, the loss of a close friend—that may have caused or at least contributed to the depression. Sometimes, it is more difficult to find something wrong, and the appearance of depression is bewildering. This is especially true for the new or expectant mother. Having a child is supposed to be a joyful experience, and a woman is expected to be happy. When depression strikes then, it is particularly unsettling.

Often people try to construct an explanation for their depression, blaming somebody or something for how they feel. "If only my husband were more helpful, I wouldn't feel so distressed." "The baby has colic. Who wouldn't feel depressed in this situation?" It is natural to try to understand why one is depressed. After all, if you can grasp why the problem exists, then you might be able to do something about it or to avoid this problem in the future. But sometimes it is not so easy to find a satisfying explanation, and too often depression is interpreted as a sign of weakness: "Other people don't get depressed. There must be something wrong with me." But it's not so simple.

Depression is a complex disorder, and more often than not it is difficult to point to a single cause for its appearance. It is generally believed that depression may have many different causes and emerges within the context of a complicated interaction of genetic, biologic, psychological, and social factors. Even in one individual, many different factors may contribute to the onset of depression. While the role of external events in bringing on depression has long been studied, scientists now believe that certain people are more prone to depression than others due to their genetic endowment and/or early childhood experiences. A person may go through life without being aware of this vulnerability and without any signs of depression or other type of emotional problems. However, exposure to certain stressors, whether physical or psychological, may reveal this vulnerability to depression.

A Historical Perspective

While we tend to think of depression as a modern ailment, some of the earliest written and most accurate descriptions of this disorder can be found in the works of the early Greeks and in the Bible. The Book of Job provides some of the most evocative descriptions of grief and anguish.

So I am made to possess months of vanity, and wearisome nights are appointed to me.
When I lie down, I say, When shall I arise, and the night be gone? and I am full of tossings to and fro unto the dawning of the day.
My days are swifter than a weaver's shuttle, and are spent without hope.
O remember that my life is wind: mine eye shall no more see good.
When I say, My bed shall comfort me, my couch shall ease my complaints;
Then thou scarest me with dreams, and terrifiest me through visions:
So that my soul chooseth strangling, and death rather than my life.
I loathe it; I would not live alway: let me alone; for my days are vanity.
—Book of Job 7, King James version

While Job's suffering was not in Biblical times conceptualized as an illness, the symptoms of which Job complained—the sleepless nights, the loss of joy, feelings of hopelessness, and a wish to die—are identical to those used by clinicians today to diagnose depression. These words speak to the notion that depression is not a concoction of our modern society but a human condition.

Job, like many who have suffered from depression, questioned why he was suffering, what he had done to deserve such pain and anguish. For thousands of years, physicians, scientists, and philosophers have sought the answer. In ancient Greece, the physician Hippocrates believed that one's health derived from a perfect balance of the four bodily humors (blood, phlegm, yellow bile, and black bile) and that illness occurred when there was imbalance of the humors. He hypothesized that depression (which he called melancholy) occurred when there was an excess of black bile (or *melan chole*). Within this conceptual framework, the treatment of illness was focused on correcting this imbalance.

In the Middle Ages, depression was viewed within the religious context of the Christian church. The devil was blamed as the cause of all types of illness, and depression was believed to be an outward manifestation of moral weakness or sinfulness. Mental disorders, particularly when severe, were often caught up in the realm of demonic possession and witchcraft. The *Malleus Maleficarum* (hammer of witches), the authority on witchcraft and the handbook for the Inquisitors, stated that when doctors could find no cause for a disease or when the disease did not respond to traditional treatment (usually bloodletting or purging), it was the work of the devil. During this time women, in particular, were viewed with suspicion, and thousands of women, many of them mentally ill, were imprisoned or burned at the stake.

It wasn't until the late 1500s that a more benevolent attitude toward the mentally ill took hold, and philosophers and writers began to probe the workings of the human mind. Mental illness was not the purview of physicians but rather a rich source of material for creative thinkers. William Shakespeare provided some of the most accurate and poignant accounts of depression and other types of mental illness. Hamlet most likely suffered from depression, Lady Macbeth from obsessive-compulsive disorder, and King Lear from Alzheimer's dementia. It could easily be argued that Shakespeare, more so than any physicians of his time, helped to lead the field of psychiatry out of the dark ages. His works addressed a wide array of psychological issues and humanized, rather than demonized, the face of psychiatric illness. It was not until 1621, however, with the publication by Sir Robert Burton of the *Anatomy of Melancholy*, that a more analytical and scientific approach was employed in the study of mental illness. Burton provided a lengthy and well-researched text that endeavored to understand the causes and effects of depression and set the stage for more modern conceptualizations of this illness.

A More Modern View of Depression

In the early years of the twentieth century, Sigmund Freud revolutionized the field of psychiatry and promoted the concept that one's behavior is influenced by unconscious psychological processes. According to Freud, psychiatric illness is the product of unresolved childhood conflicts. In his landmark treatise *Mourning and Melancholia*, Freud conceptualized depression as an exaggerated grief response, a delayed reaction to the loss (either real or symbolic) of an important person (or object) early in life. Melanie Klein, like Freud and many of the psychoanalysts who followed in his footsteps, placed special emphasis on the early relationship with one's mother. Klein hypothesized that depression occurred when one did not have a positive and nurturing relationship with one's mother early on in life.

Other theorists have viewed depression within the broader context of social relationships both in and outside of the family. American psychiatrists Adolf Meyer and Harry Stack Sullivan proposed an interpersonal theory of depression. They suggested that those people who experience difficulty in establishing and maintaining successful interpersonal connections are more vulnerable to depression. Developing a supportive social network seems to offer some protection; depression occurs when one experiences disruptions of or conflicts within these important relationships. In support of this theory is the finding that marriage, especially when it is described as satisfying and a source of emotional support, appears to decrease the risk of depression. On the other hand, when a marriage falters or fails, the loss of this important source of emotional intimacy and social connection may be a potent trigger for depression.

The cognitive theory of depression emphasizes the importance of how one perceives oneself and the external world and how these core beliefs may influence vulnerability to depression or other psychological problems. The father of cognitive theory, Aaron Beck, theorized that depression occurs when one has certain distorted patterns of thinking (or cognitions) and behaviors. Specifically, those with depression have a negative concept of themselves and view themselves as deficient, helpless, incompetent, and unlovable. They tend to view the world as very demanding and likely to present obstacles. They do not expect to gain pleasure or gratification from their endeavors, and they readily anticipate their own failure. It is not difficult to imagine how these negative thoughts may help to perpetuate a depressive state of mind and more negative thoughts.

Interesting as they are, many of these early theories have fallen by the wayside in favor of a more biological conceptualization. While it may be appealing to reduce the problem of depression to a simple chemical imbalance, it is important to understand how depression fits within the context of your life. Have there been any losses or childhood experiences that have left you more vulnerable to depression? Are there any current issues that may be contributing to the problem? Questions like these not only help you make sense of your depression, but also this process of understanding these psychological issues lies at the core of talk therapy. For many people, addressing these sorts of questions may help to alleviate the symptoms of depression and may relieve suffering.

Depression Is a Biologically Driven Illness

In the 1950s and 1960s, there was a move within the field of psychiatry to identify and categorize different types of depression. Depression was initially divided into two categories: *neurotic* and *endogenous*. Neurotic depression was thought to be driven by external events, a psychological response to stressful life events. In contrast, endogenous depression came from within or was caused by some type of biological process or genetic factors. As our understanding of depression advances, these distinctions blur. Current research indicates that, regardless of the specific factors that cause or trigger depression, there are specific biochemical changes that occur within the brain that are characteristic of depression. No matter what type of depression is observed clinically, these biochemical changes are present and believed responsible for the feelings of sadness and despair that define this disorder.

Despite extensive research, our understanding of exactly what causes depression remains incomplete. Over the last fifty years, researchers have studied the biochemical or structural abnormalities in the brain that may be responsible for causing depression. Researchers have observed a remarkable array of abnormalities within the brains of depressed patients. While an exhaustive discussion of these findings is beyond the scope of this book, clearly, depression is associated with specific changes in brain function. These changes are not evident on a standard physical examination, and it may be difficult to detect these alterations using standard laboratory tests or imaging techniques; however, there are distinct changes detectable in the brains of each and every person who suffers from depression.

Scientists now postulate that depression is the result of a chemical imbalance, a disruption of neurotransmitters in the brain. Neurotransmitters are the chemicals that carry signals between brain cells (or neurons). Every thought, every action, and every reflex is governed by thousands of neurons communicating with one another via these neurotransmitters. We know that those with depression produce lower levels of certain monoamine neurotransmitters, including norepinephrine, serotonin, and dopamine. It is interesting to note that all conventional antidepressants used today seem to "correct" this imbalance by increasing levels of these monoamine neurotransmitters within the brain. For example, the widely used selective serotonin reuptake inhibitors, or SSRIs, including Prozac, Zoloft, and Paxil, increase levels of serotonin. The older tricyclic antidepressants increase levels of norepinephrine, epinephrine, and to a lesser degree, serotonin, while bupropion (Wellbutrin) has a more potent effect on dopamine systems.

The monoamine hypothesis, which has prevailed over the last forty years, is probably only one part of a larger puzzle. Recent research has focused on the body's response to stress and how that response is altered in patients with depression. In mediating the effects of stress on the brain, the hypothalamic-pituitary-adrenal (or HPA) axis appears to be the driving force. This is a primitive survival response to stress or danger that prepares the body for "fight or flight." In humans with depression, however, the HPA system is working in overdrive. In response to even relatively mild stressors, the HPA axis goes wild and generates abnormally high levels of stress hormones. Researchers hypothesize that this pathological response to stress causes depression. And if this theory holds true, it helps to explain the importance of stressful life events in making a person more vulnerable to depression and serves as a link between the earlier theories regarding adversity and loss experienced in early childhood and the more recent conceptualizations of depression as a biological illness.

Why Are Certain People More Susceptible to Depression?

Depression tends to run in families. If you have a first-degree relative (mother, father, or sibling) with depression, your chances of having depression are about two to four times higher than a person with no family history of depression. If you have several affected family members, your chances are even higher. Within a typical family, all members are exposed to essentially the same living conditions and experience many of the same stressors. They also share, at least to some degree, the same genes. Is it the environment within the family that determines risk for depression? Or is it the genetic heritage that determines whether or not a given individual will suffer from depression?

Since the last decade research has sought the precise genes that may be responsible for causing depression. Unlike Down syndrome, for example, where an abnormality on a single chromosome is responsible for the disorder, depression is probably transmitted by multiple genes located on different chromosomes. This, coupled with the fact that depression may take so many different forms, has complicated the search for the depression genes. Recent attention has focused on the genes governing the production and function of certain neurotransmitters in the brain, including serotonin and norepinephrine; however, no studies have yet identified a consistent linkage between any specific gene or chromosomal region and this disorder.

While genes play an important role, it seems that vulnerability to depression cannot be attributed entirely to one's genetic endowment. Sigmund Freud first popularized the notion that early childhood experiences may influence one's susceptibility to emotional problems later in life. For example, he suggested that a child who is estranged from his mother or father is more likely to develop depression than a child raised in a nurturing family with emotionally available and loving parents. Although modern psychiatry has moved away, to some degree, from the teachings of Freud, considerable evidence suggests that early childhood events are of critical importance in determining vulnerability to depression.

We are only beginning to fully appreciate the long-term impact of early stressful life experiences on the human brain, but we do know that stress experienced at an early age can significantly and permanently affect how the brain functions. Researchers hypothesize that early exposure to stressful life events, experienced while the brain is still developing, appears to induce an oversensitivity to stress that persists into adulthood. Later, when these individuals are exposed to stress, the HPA axis, which dictates how we react to stress, is *too* responsive: the body is sent into a flight-or-fight response with little provocation and produces higher than normal levels of stress-related hormones. When the brain is exposed to high levels of these stress hormones, certain changes may occur, and it is believed that individuals who have this pathological response to stress may be more vulnerable to depression.

This research indicates that the seeds of depression are sown early in life, even before the baby is born. At the time of birth, one possesses certain genes that play an important part in determining predisposition to depression later in life. Superimposed upon that genetic inheritance are the earliest experiences of childhood. By adulthood, one's vulnerability to depression is almost predetermined, a by-product of genes and early experiences. The missing ingredient is a trigger, some event that uncovers this vulnerability and allows depression to manifest.

What Triggers Depression?

When a person talks about her own depression, it is common, almost universal, to refer to the external events—health problems, marital tension, stress at work—that may have triggered an episode. Researchers, too, have focused on stressful life events and how they may either cause or contribute to depression. It is clear that stress, particularly when chronic, has damaging effects on both the body and the brain. Certain individuals appear to be exquisitely sensitive and may develop depression, anxiety, or other emotional problems in response.

What kinds of life events can trigger depression? One of the most powerful triggers is loss. Grief is a natural response to a loss of a loved one; however, it seems that in vulnerable individuals, grief may be prolonged and may lead to a significant depression. Furthermore, loss need not be restricted to the death of an important person; a sense of loss may arise in many different situations. Leaving one's childhood home, changing jobs, experiencing the breakup of an important relationship—these are all losses that may cause depression or other emotional problems.

Myriad other stressors may trigger depression. Probably one of the most potent stressors is being a victim of physical or sexual abuse, particularly when the abuse is chronic. Other life stressors include separation and divorce, financial difficulties, and unemployment. Medical illness appears to be another important trigger of depression. But there are also a few surprises on the list, including marriage and the birth of a child. In general, transitions, even when they are believed to be positive in nature, may create significant stress.

How one responds to stress or stressful life events depends on multiple factors. As we discussed earlier, stressful early childhood experiences may cause physiologic changes that make certain individuals particularly sensitive to stressful experiences. Temperament and personality, which are to a great extent determined by genetic factors, are also important in determining how one responds. For example, people who are naturally easygoing and relatively flexible may deal with stress better than those who are rigid or prone to anxiety. Those who are more assertive are better able to find solutions to a problem and often seem to fare better in stressful situations than those who are more passive or prone to feelings of helplessness.

But sometimes there isn't an easily identifiable trigger. If you survey adolescents and young adults with depression, they typically relate the onset of depression to a stressful life experience. However, if you survey older adults with depression, this connection between stressful life events and depression becomes less obvious. What researchers now believe is that in a given individual, the first few episodes of depression are often brought on by some type of stressful life event, but after time, especially in those who have had multiple episodes of depression, there is no specific trigger. Those who have suffered from depression often comment: "I don't know what happened. I don't really have a good reason to be depressed." It seems that, over time, depression acquires a life of its own.

Depression-Prone Personalities

We have all met people who seem to be teetering on the edge of depression. No matter what, they always seem to see the world from a negative vantage point. It is unclear whether this type of personality develops in response to chronic or recurrent depression or depression is more common among people with a negative outlook. Experts have proposed the existence of *depressive personality disorder*, a personality that is dominated by persistently negative patterns of thinking. Those with depressive personality disorder are overly serious, humorless, and seemingly unable to enjoy themselves. They tend to be very critical and judgmental of others, but seem to reserve the harshest criticism for themselves and are prone to feelings of guilt and remorse. They are fervent pessimists and, convinced that things will never go well, tend to dwell on negative, unhappy thoughts. It is not difficult to imagine how this persistently gloomy outlook on life may lead to depression, and some experts argue that this type of personality is actually a precursor to clinical depression.

However, other attributes of personality may render one more susceptible to depression. For example, a person who is a perfectionist is more self-critical and is likely to repeatedly fall short of her own expectations, contributing to feelings of incompetence, a sense of failure, and ultimately depression. Another personality trait that appears to increase one's vulnerability to depression is being dependent on others. A dependent or needy person ends up feeling ineffectual, with little control over her own life. Over time, this pattern of thinking hinders a person's ability to take charge of difficult situations, leading to feelings of helplessness and, eventually, depression.

Why Are Women So Vulnerable?

It is interesting to note that before adolescence, rates of depression are about the same among girls and boys. Things begin to shift between the ages of eleven and thirteen. Over these years, there is a dramatic rise in the prevalence of depression in girls, and by the age of fifteen, females are twice as likely as males to suffer from depression. What happens to create this gender gap during adolescence is a topic of intense debate and research. There is no doubt that adolescence is a time characterized by dramatic psychological and physical changes for women, and it is easy to imagine that this tumultuous transition may render adolescent girls more vulnerable to depression. However, a woman's risk for depression persists beyond puberty and she remains at higher risk for depressive illness than a man throughout her entire adult life.

At no other point are women *more* vulnerable to depression than during their childbearing years. How can we explain this susceptibility to depression? From a psychological standpoint, this is a time when she is faced with many life-changing and potentially stressful transforming events; during this span of years a woman pursues her education, career, marriage, childbearing, and child rearing. These changes provide the emotional context within which depression may take hold. However, in addition to being an emotionally charged time, the childbearing years are also characterized by dramatic hormonal shifts related to reproductive functioning. Every month a woman completes a menstrual cycle and is exposed to rising and then falling levels of reproductive hormones. During pregnancy and after delivery, a woman experiences even more dramatic shifts in this reproductive hormonal environment. Many specialists in the field of women's mental health have postulated that it is this combination of psychological stressors and hormonal events that make women so vulnerable to depression during the childbearing years.

How Hormones Affect the Brain

We can all agree that women are different from men. At a physiological level this difference is determined by the steroid hormones estrogen and testosterone. Prior to puberty, these hormones are produced by the body but circulate at very low levels. With the onset of puberty, there is a dramatic rise in their levels. In men, testosterone is the dominant hormone, produced in the testicles. In females, the ovaries produce several different types of estrogen (estriol, estrone, and estradiol) and progesterone. These hormones are essential for sexual development and reproduction. Estrogen and testosterone also trigger the appearance of secondary sexual characteristics, such as breast development in women and facial hair in men, and are also responsible for the many more subtle physical and physiological differences between men and women.

Not only do these sex steroid hormones affect the body, they have important effects on the brain. Receptors for estrogen, progesterone, and testosterone are found in many different regions throughout the brain. One region that appears to be relatively rich in these sex steroid receptors is the limbic region, an evolutionarily ancient region of the brain that governs our emotions and moods. The effects of estrogen are complex; however, it appears that estrogen interacts with both serotonin and norepinephrine neurotransmitter systems in the limbic region. In fact, many people think of estrogen as a natural antidepressant because it increases levels of both of these neurotransmitters, which is exactly what conventional antidepressants do. The effects of progesterone are mixed. On one hand, progesterone may counteract the positive effects of estrogen. On the other, progesterone is metabolized by the body to form allopregnanolone, a barbiturate-like compound that seems to have calming and anxiety-relieving effects. The actions of testosterone are less well understood, but it is believed that testosterone may also have a mood-elevating effect, although too much of this hormone may lead to irritability or hostility. In both men and women, testosterone is important for sexual drive.

Not only is a woman exposed to different types of hormones and different levels of these hormones than a man, throughout her reproductive years she experiences constant hormonal fluctuations. During the menstrual cycle, there is a typical pattern of hormonal shifts linked to ovulation. In the first two weeks of the cycle, called the follicular phase, the egg follicles within the ovary grow and produce a steady rise of both estrogen and progesterone levels. Somewhere around day 14 of the cycle, ovulation occurs, and, if conception does not take place, the follicle starts to wither, causing a fall in estrogen and progesterone levels during the last two weeks of the cycle, called the luteal phase. Without the nourishing effects of estrogen, the uterine lining, or endometrium, can no longer support its growth and begins to disintegrate and slough off, resulting in a menstrual bleed. This cycle takes place every month, year after year, for about thirty to forty years.

As a result of these fluctuating hormone levels, many women experience both physical symptoms and mood changes. In general, women tend to feel better during the first half of the cycle, the follicular phase, when levels of estrogen and progesterone are on the rise. After ovulation occurs, during the last one or two weeks of the cycle, when levels of these hormones are falling, most women note some minor physical symptoms, including fatigue, bloating, breast tenderness, headaches, muscle aches, and carbohydrate cravings. When women experience symptoms that are more severe and occur nearly every month, they may suffer from what clinicians call **premenstrual syndrome (PMS)** or premenstrual tension.

When a woman has, in addition to these physical symptoms, significant mood symptoms or changes in her behavior, she may be suffering from a more severe type of mood disturbance called **premenstrual dysphoric disorder (PMDD)**. The hallmark symptom of PMDD is irritability, but women also commonly complain of mood swings or feeling depressed or easily overwhelmed. Others may have more prominent anxiety symptoms and describe feeling tense or edgy. Obviously not all women experience these symptoms, and it appears that only about 3 percent to 5 percent of menstruating women have full-blown PMDD. In contrast to women with premenstrual symptoms or PMS who are able to function quite well despite these symptoms, women with PMDD note that their symptoms cause problems both at work and at home.

There is significant overlap between the symptoms of PMDD and those of clinical depression. In fact, there has been some debate as to whether PMDD is a distinct illness or merely the premenstrual unmasking of a mood disorder. It is clear that many women suffer from depression throughout their cycle and notice worsening of their symptoms during the last one or two weeks. However, it should also be noted that women with PMDD experience mood changes *only* during the premenstrual phase of their cycle. Experts believe that these hormonal shifts may act as a trigger for depression in some women and that women who have premenstrual mood changes may also be more vulnerable to depression at other times when exposed to significant hormonal fluctuations, such as after childbirth or during the transition to menopause.

While it is clear that certain women may be more vulnerable to these hormonal shifts, it is not clear whether hormonal factors increase vulnerability to depression in *all* women. Some researchers hypothesize that these monthly hormonal changes act as a type of recurrent stressor, and with these repetitive insults, the underlying architecture of a woman's brain is somehow altered so that it is more susceptible to depression. While this is an interesting speculation, it has yet to be proven.

The Interplay of Psychology and Society

While it may be appealing to blame everything on hormones, this would be an oversimplification. British researchers George Brown and Tirril Harris have demonstrated that the link between stress and depression is much stronger in women than in men and that most episodes of depression in women occur subsequent to some sort of adverse life event. While losing an important person or relationship is an important trigger for depression, the effects are intensified if the loss leads to feelings of humiliation or entrapment. Furthermore, women are not only vulnerable to the losses in their own lives, the intricate and far-reaching social networks that women build make them susceptible to the traumatic events occurring in other peoples' lives as well.

In most societies, women are exposed to higher levels of stress and adversity than men, and many have cited this fact as an explanation for the higher prevalence of depression among women. Women are more often than men the victims of physical and sexual abuse, and this type of severe trauma is a risk factor for depression, as well as other psychological problems. Women are more likely than men to live in poverty. With poverty comes a constellation of problems that may further increase a woman's vulnerability to depression, including teen pregnancy, single parenthood, inadequate social supports, and violence.

Women must also contend with other less extreme sources of stress that may contribute to their increased vulnerability to depression. Women receive less education than their male counterparts and have access to fewer and less lucrative careers. When compared to college-educated women, those with only a high school education have a fourfold higher risk for depression. And for those women who lack paid employment, the risk for depression is twice as high, regardless of their level of education.

More so than men, women usually play multiple roles both within and outside of the home, further increasing their stress. While a satisfying career may help to decrease the risk of depression and protect a woman from stressful events that occur within the family, women who experience financial pressures to work and feel that they have been forced to work outside of the home while being the primary provider of child care are more likely to report higher levels of stress and depression. This is particularly true for women caring for young children at home. The effects of chronic strain may be further intensified when women do not feel adequately compensated or appreciated for the work they do both in and outside of the home.

Several researchers have presented evidence suggesting that it is actually the act of parenting itself—being the primary caregiver in the family—that makes women so vulnerable to depression. If a woman's ability to fulfill her role as a mother is compromised in some manner or if she feels that she is not able to perform this role competently, she is at risk for depression. For a woman, events that threaten her core relationships—with her partner or with her children—are the most potent triggers of depression. Thus, it seems that when a woman accepts the traditional female role as a mother and primary caregiver, she becomes more emotionally vulnerable within the context of the family. Evidence for this hypothesis is the finding that women are at highest risk for depression during their childbearing years, a time during which differences in gender roles are the most pronounced; the gender gap in risk for depression is less pronounced in college-aged and older adults. Further supporting this theory are several studies that have examined risk for depression in less traditional families. In the families where the responsibility of child care and other domestic activities is shared more evenly, men and women have about the same vulnerability to depression.

Other theories suggest that the problems start much earlier in a woman's life and focus on how women are socialized, arguing that girls are taught to behave differently than boys and that this early difference in gender roles makes women more vulnerable to depression. Parents and our culture at large tend to have different expectations for female and male children, fostering the belief that girls should be more nurturing and more attentive to their social connections and position. In contrast, boys are expected to be more independent and focused on their own accomplishments. For women, this stereotypical gender socialization leads to a lower sense of self-esteem and mastery and a greater concern regarding others' opinions. It is theorized that girls encouraged to behave in this manner are more passive, less confident, and more dependent on others, traits that may ultimately make them more vulnerable to depression.

In addition, girls grow up with different attitudes and expectations regarding emotional expression. From an early age, boys are encouraged to keep their feelings in check, whereas girls are more often encouraged to express their feelings of anxiety and sadness. Parents are also more likely to talk about their own worries or feelings of sadness in front of their daughters than their sons. This degree of emotional awareness may be of benefit to girls, and typically women grow up with a better grasp of their own emotions and a greater facility in expressing their feelings than men. However, psychologist Susan Nolen-Hoeksema at Yale University points out that there may be some disadvantages when girls are socialized in this manner. Parents may be tolerating and reinforcing feelings of anxiety and sadness rather than teaching their daughters how to overcome difficult situations or how to develop other, more positive coping strategies. In drawing girls' attention to these negative feelings, parents may also create a sense of despair, painting the world as a place where unhappiness abounds and one is helpless to change the situation.

A recent study has taken a closer look at the link between gender roles and depression. Sociologists Anne Barrett and Helene Raskin White demonstrated that children and adolescents who show more stereotypically masculine traits (such as assertiveness, aggression, and self-reliance) as opposed to feminine traits (such as being gentle, affectionate, and emotionally expressive) were less susceptible to depression in adulthood. Interestingly, this result held up in both males and females, suggesting that there may be certain traits (ones that are more commonly associated with stereotypically male gender roles) that may help protect both men and women from depression. This is consistent with other research indicating that some traits, such as independence and assertiveness, which are labeled in this study as more masculine traits, are associated with better psychological adjustment. But Bartlett and Raskin White take the data one step further and go on to hypothesize that being more masculine confers a more desirable and privileged social status, another factor that may protect men from depression.

Depression Is *Not* a Normal or Expected Consequence of Being a Woman

Many different factors increase your risk for depression: genes, stressful situations in your life, hormonal fluctuations, the roles and societal expectations for women. While a better understanding of what causes your depression may shed light on your situation, it should not breed complacency. Just because there is a fairly good reason for your depression does not mean that you should learn to live with it. Depression may be very common, but that does not make it "normal." Depression is a disease that demands treatment.

Chapter 3

The Ripple Effect

How Depression Affects the Family

Depression does not occur in a vacuum. It can have a devastating effect on the people around a woman, affecting her partner, her children, other family members, and her friends. Even if she is aware of her depression and how it affects her, it may be difficult to shelter others from its detrimental effects. Whether a woman's depression is relatively mild or very severe, whether she has had one episode or many, depression leaves a mark on the people around her.

A mother is clearly one of the most important persons in a child's life. The relationship between a mother and her child during the first years of life lay the foundations for the child's social, emotional, and intellectual development. At its worst, depression may interfere with a mother's ability to attach to and care for her infant, and this early disruption in attachment may result in a broad spectrum of problems as the child grows older. But even when it is relatively mild, depression may cause subtle shifts in the interactions between mother and child, and a mother's depression may negatively affect her child's development and well-being.

If you are a mother who has suffered from depression, this is likely a very difficult message to hear. You care deeply for your child, and it is unbearable to think that your depression may have in some way harmed your child. Certainly young children are extremely vulnerable to events during the early years of their life; however, it must be emphasized that children are also remarkably resilient. Acknowledging your depression and the problems that may stem from a child's exposure to this illness opens up an opportunity to intervene. Depression is a treatable and in some cases preventable illness. It is of utmost importance to recognize this problem and to intervene as soon as possible in order to protect the family from its ill effects.

Bonding and Attachment

Let's review the fundamentals of the mother-child relationship. Everybody talks about bonding, but what exactly is it? Bonding is a term coined by the animal behaviorists that refers to the capacity of a young animal to identify and to form a close connection with its mother. Austrian researcher and Nobel laureate Konrad Lorenz was one of the first to study this phenomenon in his experiments with baby geese. Lorenz discovered that babies are born with the capacity and instinct to attach to their caregiver. This drive is so fierce that young animals often bond with the first figure that appears before them during the first hours of life, even if it is not their mother.

Not surprisingly, human babies exhibit similar, albeit slightly more complicated, bonding behaviors. Believe it or not, even before the baby is born, an important bond has already started forming between baby and mother. A fetus has the capacity to hear sounds at about 25 weeks of gestation, and soon thereafter, the unborn baby is able to recognize and show a preference for his mother's voice, his heartbeat quickening whenever he hears her speaking. As the baby is bathed in amniotic fluid, he also becomes familiar with how his mother smells. Soon after birth, a baby is able to detect and to turn toward his mother's smell and prefers the scent of her breast milk over all others'. After birth, the bond between mother and child intensifies. Although a baby initially accepts indiscriminately whoever holds or comforts him, within a few days, a newborn develops a distinct preference for his primary caregiver, usually his mother. In her presence, the baby becomes more alert and sucks more vigorously every time her voice is heard. Her touch provides a calming influence.

At the same time, the mother also engages in her own bonding behaviors. How a mother interacts with her baby is certainly influenced by social and cultural norms. However, much of the bonding process is biologically driven, operating largely outside of a mother's consciousness. There are probably many physiologic and hormonal changes that contribute to the bonding process, but research shows that oxytocin, a hormone produced by the pituitary gland at the time of delivery and after birth, may play a central role. Oxytocin is essential for inducing labor (hence its name from the Greek for "swift birth"), but oxytocin levels remain elevated after delivery. Experiments have demonstrated that a sheep deprived of oxytocin will reject her own lambs, whereas one injected with oxytocin can be coaxed to care for a lamb even if it is not her own. While oxytocin is likely to play a somewhat different role in more advanced mammals, like humans, it is believed to promote early maternal behaviors. In humans oxytocin seems to have a calming effect, and some suggest that it is responsible for the contented and loving feelings mothers experience as they hold and nurse their infants. Oxytocin is also found at high levels in the breast milk, and it is possible that this hormone may enhance bonding behaviors in the infant as well. Obviously, oxytocin is not the whole story, but it is one aspect of the bonding process where a new mother becomes caring, loving, and protective of her own child.

And the early bonding process is just the beginning. "Attachment" most commonly refers to the close social or emotional bond a young child forms with a primary caregiver. The attachment object, usually the mother, serves as a secure base. She is reliably available to protect the infant and provide food, warmth, and love. Not only is attachment mandatory for survival, this relationship between caregiver and child is an important template for all other social interactions, and within the context of secure attachment a child's development can take place.

John Bowlby, a British physician and psychoanalyst, began to study the process by which infants "attach" to their mothers during the 1950s. He noted that when a mother cares for her infant, she attends to the baby's basic physical needs—feeding, diapering, and bathing her baby—but in the process she also engages the baby socially. He saw that basic caregiving activities were combined with social interactions: touching, holding, hugging, rocking, talking, and singing. Bowlby recognized that the interactions between a mother and her infant are driven by a natural tendency in both mother and child to engage socially. The mother communicates with her child, both verbally and through gestures and facial expressions, interpreting her child's signals and mirroring them with her own responses. When the infant withdraws, the mother gently works to again engage him and to restore the intimacy of their interaction. When the infant cries or is in distress, the mother is able to understand and to respond quickly to his needs. These small yet important interactions contribute to an ongoing dialogue between mother and child that helps to foster the child's emotional and cognitive development.

According to Bowlby, a secure attachment develops over the first one to two years of a child's life, as a by-product of consistent and attentive caregiving. Although many mothers expect bonding and attachment to occur in the moments immediately following delivery, attachment is a gradual learning process whereby the baby "teaches" the mother to understand and respond to his nonverbal signals. With the mother serving as the baby's guide, the baby learns to interact with and negotiate the environment. A young baby confronted with an unfamiliar situation will be clearly distressed and cling to his mother. However, over time, the mother helps her child to develop a sense of security and he begins to explore the world independently, knowing that his mother is there if he needs her.

Although many people may help to care for a human newborn, the relationship between mother and child is of prime importance during the first years of life. In most families, it is the mother who is the primary caregiver and the source of most of her child's social interactions. Mary Ainsworth, a psychologist who worked with John Bowlby, helped to identify the characteristics in the mother that foster the development of secure attachment between infant and mother. These factors include emotional availability and responsiveness, an accepting attitude, and sensitivity to the infant's signals and needs. These attributes help the growing child to successfully and confidently explore the world, a process that will help him become self-reliant.

How securely an infant is attached to the primary caregiver may be measured by observing how he behaves during and after a period of brief separation from his mother. Mary Ainsworth observed that most infants and toddlers, when separated from their mothers, stage a protest. They became upset and sometimes angry. They stop playing and begin to look for their mother. When their mother returns, they go to her, cling to her, and are comforted by her presence. But not all of the infants behaved in this manner. Some of the children were almost impossible to console, even after their mother returned; other infants seemed not even to notice that their mother had reappeared. Ainsworth suggested that these patterns of behavior were indicative of insecure attachment to the primary caregiver. She described two different patterns of insecure attachment. Children with an "ambivalent" attachment seem to be more anxious and cling to their mother; they are very distressed by her absence, yet they do not seem to really trust her when she returns and are difficult to console. Children with "avoidant" attachment do not protest after their mother leaves, and when she returns, they seem to ignore or avoid her. Subsequent to Ainsworth's work, a third pattern of attachment was identified and labeled as "disorganized." After the mother returns, these "disorganized" children seem confused and chaotic, alternately rushing to or avoiding their mother.

Depression May Affect How Mothers Interact with Their Children

In 1972, pediatrician Dr. T. Berry Brazelton and developmental psychologist Dr. Edward Tronick began to carefully observe the everyday interactions between mothers and their infants using a novel technique. They filmed the face-to-face interactions of mothers with their infants and then analyzed these films frame by frame in order to capture the most subtle changes in behaviors in the mothers and their babies. From this innovative research, we have gained a much better understanding of the communication that occurs between mother and infant. These studies clearly showed that even the youngest babies, while lacking the full capacity of spoken language, exhibit complicated and well-organized patterns of communication. Shortly after birth, not only do they have a full range of emotions but, using gaze, facial expressions, vocalizations, and gestures, young infants can effectively relay information regarding their emotional state to their caregivers. When the infant looks intently at the mother and coos, the message is "I like what you are doing." When the baby looks away, physically withdraws, or cries and whimpers, the message is "I do not like what is happening now."

Prior to Brazelton's and Tronick's work, researchers believed that the ideal mother-infant relationship moved in perfect synchrony, with the mother precisely in tune to her infant, understanding and responding to every one of her child's gestures or vocalizations. Tronick and Brazelton discovered that a mother and her child do not always work together in perfect harmony. Rather, there is a complicated pattern of interactions. What emerged from these studies was the notion that the mother and infant form a closely knit dyad where both the mother and her child regulate their own behavior in response to the other's behaviors. There are frequent mistakes and missteps in communication—about one every three to five seconds—but what seems to matter in this process is the mother's willingness and ability to recognize these communication errors and to make the appropriate adjustments. Confirming Mary Ainsworth's earlier hypotheses regarding attachment, Tronick and his colleagues found that the most successful interactions were characterized by attentiveness, sensitivity, and responsiveness in the mother. While a mother may not instinctively understand all of her child's cues and signals, she does have the capacity to learn and this is the cornerstone of secure attachment.

It is easy to imagine how depression may affect these basic interactions between a mother and her infant and disrupt the process of attachment. Depression clearly has an effect on how one interacts with and responds to others. When suffering from depression, a mother may be more withdrawn and less responsive to the people around her. Or she may be more angry and irritable when interacting with others. Given the emotional intimacy of the mother-child dyad in the first year of life, a young infant may be particularly vulnerable to fluctuations in the mother's behavior. In fact, researchers have discovered that an infant can perceive even relatively subtle changes in how the mother behaves and these may have a profound effect on the child's behavior.

Decades of research on the interactions between depressed mothers and their infants have demonstrated that depression clearly affects how a mother responds to and behaves with her child. Dr. Tronick and his coworkers have studied videotapes of hundreds of depressed women with their young babies. They have discerned several different patterns of behavior in depressed mothers as they engage with their infants. Most often, depressed mothers were more withdrawn and less responsive to their infants' signals. Their facial expressions and displays of emotion were more muted or flat, and their voices more monotone. They remained disengaged and did little to support their child's activities or exploration of the environment. Other depressed mothers displayed a more intrusive style of engaging with their infants. These mothers tended to use an angry tone of voice, and they more often poked at their infants or handled them roughly. In general, these mothers were more emotional and looked overly distressed in response to their child's cries. When playing with their children, they were involved but tended to interfere with, rather than support, their child's activities.

How the infants behaved depended on what type of behavior their depressed mothers exhibited. In response to the withdrawn and disengaged mothers, infants were clearly distressed and fussed and cried frequently and forcefully to attract their mothers' attention. When their efforts to maintain connectedness with their mothers failed and their needs were not satisfied, they became increasingly withdrawn and passive. They were less playful and less likely to be interested in novel stimuli or to engage with other people. They began, after a time, to look just like their mothers: withdrawn, unresponsive, and depressed. What is particularly alarming is that this becomes a persistent pattern of responding to others. Even when encountering a friendly and engaging stranger, the infant was less engaged and more likely to show negative emotions. It seems that after repeated failures to effectively engage their mothers, these infants had adopted a coping strategy: they simply disengaged, and they learned to use this strategy automatically, even before knowing if it was warranted or not. They learned to view their mothers, as well as others in their environment, as unreliable and unresponsive and they experienced being ineffective and helpless.

When the mother's behaviors were more intrusive, the infants initially expressed anger or frustration. They tended to pull away from and to look away from their mother; at other times, they attempted to screen her out. On occasion, they would even push the mother away. While the infants of the withdrawn mothers experienced helplessness in relation to their mothers' behaviors, the children of the intrusive mothers fared a bit better. Their behaviors were sometimes successful in preventing their mothers' intrusiveness, and the babies' efforts were rewarded in that the mother was able to modify her behavior according to her child's wishes. Although these infants tended to display, with less provocation, anger or hostility toward others and exhibited more frustration when engaging in activities, they were able to maintain social interactions with others instead of withdrawing.

How a mother interacts with her child may affect the process of attachment, and the young children of depressed mothers are more likely to show signs of insecure attachment than those children raised by nondepressed mothers. Many young children who initially show signs of insecure attachment ultimately develop more secure forms of attachment as they grow older. However, many children never grow out of the problem, and insecure attachment, when it persists, may be a harbinger of other problems. Children who are insecurely attached may have difficulties making and sustaining friendships and other types of relationships. They often have problems showing affection; either they are overly or inappropriately affectionate or they remain distant and detached. They may have problems regulating their own emotions and tolerating stressful situations. They often suffer from low self-esteem and tend to view the world with pessimism and negativity. As a result of these interpersonal difficulties they may be more prone to academic difficulties and certain behavioral problems, including aggression.

Most studies thus far have addressed the interactions between mothers and their babies; however, there is evidence that depression also disrupts a mother's interaction with older children. In observations of mothers relating to their older children, it was noted that depressed mothers were more likely than nondepressed mothers to be critical of their children and to describe their children in negative terms. What is particularly concerning is that these negative opinions were not concealed from their children, and children were often openly criticized, more so than the children of nondepressed mothers. When these children were interviewed, it appeared they had adopted their depressed mother's view of themselves. They were more likely than the children of nondepressed mothers to suffer from low self-esteem and a sense of helplessness. This is a concern because these negative attitudes may make these children more vulnerable to depression later on.

Maternal Depression May Affect a Child's Intellectual Development

While a baby's body grows rapidly during the early months of life, it is her brain that undergoes the most tremendous transformation. At birth, a child's brain is only one-quarter of its adult size, and within the first six months of life, it doubles in size. Not only does the brain grow in size, there is also a dramatic increase in the complexity of its organization. During this stage of development brain cells, or neurons, will form more than 1,000 trillion synapses; these connections allow neurons to communicate with one another, forming networks that are responsible for all the infant's perceptions, vocalizations, and behaviors. The most dramatic phase of development occurs within the first several years after birth, but recent studies suggest that the brain continues to develop and mature during the first two decades of life.

Exactly how this developmental process takes place lies at the heart of the nature-nurture debate. Many developmental psychologists now believe that this process of development is essentially preprogrammed, unfolding according to the instructions encoded within the inherited genetic material. It is now generally accepted that one's IQ is determined at an early age and remains relatively constant throughout life, and there seems to be little that can be done to affect IQ. Within this theoretical framework, only the most extreme disruptions of the external environment can derail this naturally unfolding process, and what would be considered as normal development occurs in the vast majority of cases.

On the opposing side of this debate are those who believe that, while this process may be largely predetermined, we cannot ignore the impact of external events on intellectual development. During the earliest years of life, as the brain is developing so rapidly, it is possible to create an environment that stimulates and enhances cognitive development. There may also be environmental factors that delay or interrupt this process. Severe stress or deprivation can impede physical and intellectual development. We now know that less extreme changes in a child's external environment may have a significant impact on the child's cognitive development.

Drs. Lynne Murray and Peter Cooper, researchers at Cambridge University in Great Britain, followed a group of first-time mothers with postpartum depression and compared them to a similar group of women who remained well after delivery. When they tested the women's children at eighteen months of age, they discovered that, on several tests of cognitive functioning, the children of depressed mothers did not perform as well as the children of nondepressed mothers. Since this report, several other studies have also observed similar cognitive delays in children who were exposed to maternal depression in their first few months. Furthermore, these studies have demonstrated that even relatively mild depression in the mother, especially if it lasts over a long period of time, may affect a child's development.

How long these deficits in intellectual functioning persist is an important but unresolved question. When Murray and Cooper retested the children at five years of age, they did not observe any differences between the two groups. This study is reassuring in that it demonstrates that the children of depressed mothers, despite early setbacks, were able to catch up in terms of intellectual development. Other studies, however, have demonstrated less positive outcomes. Perhaps the most unsettling study is one recently published by Dr. Dale Hay from Cardiff University in Wales, suggesting that the effects of depression experienced during the first few months of a child's life may be evident many years later. Dr. Hay followed a group of women with postpartum depression and then assessed their children at eleven years of age. The children of mothers who were depressed at three months postpartum had significantly lower IQs than the children of nondepressed mothers. They were also more likely to have problems with attention and to have special educational needs. This lingering effect may be explained, in part, by the fact that quite a few of the women who were depressed after delivery continued to have episodes of depression throughout the child's life. Clearly, the children whose mothers had either chronic or recurrent depression demonstrated the most significant cognitive problems at a later age; however, even if the mother had only one episode of depression during the postpartum period and was well for the remainder of her child's life, there was an appreciable effect on the child's intelligence and cognitive abilities.

While studies suggest that maternal depression can affect a child's cognitive development, exactly how this happens is unclear. One theory holds that the mother is largely responsible for the child's learning environment and surmises that depression may affect a mother's capacity to perform this essential role of teacher or facilitator. Under normal circumstances, the mother keeps her child alert and engaged in activities that stimulate brain development. She is able to assess her child's aptitudes and to appreciate his level of frustration, adjusting her activities and behaviors accordingly. She praises her child for successful completion of a task and encourages him or her to engage in new activities. When a mother is depressed, she may be more disengaged and less motivated to engage in these important activities. Or within the context of these activities, she may not be adequately sensitive or appropriately responsive, making the learning experience more difficult for her child. As depression may have the capacity to interfere with this learning process, it may also have the potential to disrupt or delay cognitive development in the child.

An important developmental task in the first year of development is mastering the ability to sustain attention. One of the major roles a mother plays is to help her child to focus his or her attention on objects and events. This exercise takes place over and over again: "Oh, look at that dog. He's so white and fluffy," "Look, it's raining outside." If a mother is depressed and withdrawn, less responsive, or less communicative, these exchanges cannot take place. Without the mother's presence and involvement, a young child may have difficulty maintaining his attention. Unfortunately, it is suspected that these early deficits in attention may persist and may later interfere with other developmental tasks and make learning more difficult. This belief is supported by some studies that have examined the older children of mothers who suffered from postpartum depression. At school age, these children demonstrate more attention problems and are more likely to have academic problems in school. They are also more likely to be diagnosed with attention deficit-hyperactivity disorder.

While there is ample evidence to support the assertion that postpartum depression negatively affects a child's development, it is apparent that not all children with depressed mothers are affected to the same extent. There may be factors that protect children from the negative effects of depression. For example, several studies indicate that when mothers have achieved higher levels of education prior to pregnancy, their children do better on cognitive testing, despite being exposed to maternal depression. Many researchers believe that depression does not act on its own in disrupting or delaying a child's development. There are many other factors—such as marital disharmony and parenting problems—that may derail this process of development, and postpartum depression may interact with or accentuate the effects of these other factors.

Children at Risk for Behavioral Problems

Behavioral problems occur frequently and, in most cases, are part of a normal childhood. Even with the most well-informed and consistent parenting, children are bound to have one problem or another. The types of problems one encounters depend on the age of the child. Infants typically exhibit sleeping and feeding problems. Preschool children frequently have temper tantrums, whereas school-age children may present with more complex problems, like inattentiveness, hyperactivity, or oppositional behavior. Obviously, there is a wide range of problems, but most are relatively benign and do not merit any type of professional treatment or intervention. However, some children do have more serious or disruptive behavioral problems.

Certain behavioral problems may be more common in children whose mothers are depressed. In all infants, sleep problems are common, affecting up to 50 percent of infants under one year of age. Depressed mothers are even more likely to report significant sleep problems in their infants, most commonly difficulty initiating sleep and frequent nighttime awakenings. There may be several reasons for this finding. First, depressed mothers frequently have difficulty sleeping and consequently may be more aware of their infant's awakenings during the night than nondepressed mothers who sleep well. There is also some suggestion that the infants of depressed mothers may be more difficult to soothe, and so may have more difficulties falling asleep and may wake more frequently. While these explanations are compelling, some pediatricians see the problem from a different angle and have suggested that problematic sleeping patterns in the infant may actually *cause* depression in new mothers. It seems that depressed mood is a very common problem among women who experience prolonged disruption of their sleep by their infants, and there is evidence that behavioral interventions that improve infant sleeping patterns may actually lead to a significant improvement in the mother's mood.

A different spectrum of behavioral problems has been observed in older children. In the toddlers of depressed mothers, there have been more reports of temper tantrums, as well as complaints of disruptive or aggressive behavior. In addition, the toddlers of depressed mothers are more likely than the children of nondepressed mothers to show signs of insecure attachment, and it is believed that insecure attachment, whether or not the mother is depressed, may be a predictor of behavioral problems. It must be noted, however, that not all studies have demonstrated significant behavioral problems in the younger children of depressed mothers, and it appears that other factors may be important in determining risk for behavioral problems. The children who seemed to have the most problems were those from households where children were exposed to marital conflict, inadequate social supports, or other types of adversity. These factors, as well as depression, may contribute to creating a family environment that does not support positive patterns of parenting.

What is especially concerning is that several studies have indicated that many of these behavioral problems may persist over time. Some studies have reported that the children of depressed mothers are more likely to exhibit hyperactivity and distractibility in the classroom, and to suffer from attention deficit disorder. These children are also more likely to engage in oppositional behaviors or aggression. In these older children, behavioral problems were more prominent in children whose mothers were depressed at the time of the evaluation or who had been depressed more recently; however, it appears that children exposed to maternal depression during their infancy exhibit similar problems. Looking at a group of eleven-year-old children, Dr. Dale Hay found that those whose mothers had suffered from postpartum depression at three months after delivery were more likely to have problems with violent behaviors, such as bullying, fighting, or using weapons, than the children of nondepressed mothers. In general, studies indicate that while girls may engage in aggressive behaviors, boys are more likely than girls to exhibit behavioral problems. Furthermore, the negative effects of maternal depression are the most pronounced in economically disadvantaged households.

Why are the children of depressed mothers more likely to have behavioral problems? And how can we explain the finding that depression occurring so early in a child's life may translate into problems many years later? Although not all depressed mothers experience parenting problems, experts believe that depression, particularly if it is chronic or recurrent, may contribute to a toxic family environment. For example, when a depressed parent is angry, irritable, or hostile and is verbally or physically abusive to other family members, a child may adopt these aggressive behaviors and use them to resolve conflicts. But having a depressed parent who is more withdrawn or emotionally unavailable is not good either; these children may suffer from inadequate supervision, and disruptive behaviors may be the only way to get attention. In addition, depressed parents often have problems setting limits. They may lack the strength and stamina required to parent consistently—giving in to the child's demands, allowing rules to go unenforced, and inadvertently rewarding bad behavior. Or depressed parents may be too controlling or punitive, and this may push a child to be more disruptive or oppositional. Even when depression is not an ongoing problem and the family environment appears to be relatively healthy, some children may be more vulnerable to behavioral problems.

Children at Risk for Depression

Probably one of the most concerning, yet overlooked, aspects of maternal depression is that it may be transmitted to one's children. Several large-scale studies unequivocally indicate that the children of depressed parents are much more likely to suffer from depression than children raised by nondepressed parents. While many factors determine a child's vulnerability to depression, parental depression is one of the strongest.

Since the 1980s, Dr. Myrna Weissman, a psychologist now working at Columbia University in New York, has followed a large group of families from the New Haven, Connecticut, area. She found that when compared to the children of nondepressed parents, the offspring of depressed parents were three times as likely to suffer from depression. But depression was not the only disorder that affected the children of depressed parents. In this group of children, aged sixteen to thirty-four, it was startling to find that 78 percent had some type of psychiatric problem, and many had more than one diagnosis. Anxiety disorders, particularly phobias, separation anxiety, and panic disorder were three times as common in the offspring of depressed parents. These children were also about five times more likely than the children of nondepressed parents to develop a substance abuse problem.

What is startling about this study's finding is that depression tends to occur very early in the offspring of depressed mothers. The average age of onset for depression is somewhere in the mid-twenties; however, depression most commonly emerges in the children of depressed mothers between the ages of fifteen and twenty, with girls being at higher risk than boys. Anxiety disorders emerged even earlier, most commonly between the ages of five and ten.

Another striking finding from the New Haven study is that the children of depressed parents were not only vulnerable to psychiatric illness, they were in poorer physical health. These children were seen more often by a physician, were at greater risk for injuries and accidents, and were hospitalized more frequently. They were more likely to suffer from a wide range of medical problems, including headaches, respiratory problems, head injury, and seizures. Exactly how parental depression may cause or contribute to health problems in these children is not entirely clear. Dr. Weissman suggests that certain problems, such as head injuries and other accidents, may be the result of inattentive or negligent caretaking by a depressed parent. Children of depressed mothers are less likely to receive routine well-baby care, including vaccinations. Depressed parents are also less likely to consistently use child safety devices, such as car seats or safety restraints on a changing table, which may make these children more vulnerable to injury and accidents. It has also been hypothesized that depression itself, which is present in about half of the offspring of depressed parents, may cause certain physiologic changes that increase vulnerability to certain medical problems.

One of the challenges in understanding how maternal depression may affect children has been figuring out what part of this effect is genetic and what part is environmental. As we discussed in chapter 2, one's vulnerability to depression is determined, in part, by the genes one inherits from one's parents. But vulnerability to depression is also influenced by one's early childhood experiences. Exactly how these genetic and environmental factors interact is not fully understood; however, it is clear that the children of depressed mothers are at high risk for depression. Not only do these children inherit from their mother a genetic vulnerability to depression, but living with a parent who is depressed may be a stressful life event, and being exposed to this type of stress at an early age may render a child more susceptible to depression later. In addition, by watching and interacting with a depressed parent, a child may adopt a more depressed style of interacting with others. He may become more withdrawn and emotionally unavailable. This child, like his depressed parent, is more likely to make negative appraisals of himself and the world around him. And as we discussed in chapter 2, these sorts of negative patterns of thinking, especially when combined with other factors, may make a child more vulnerable to depression.

Sorting this all out is complicated by the fact that depression is a highly variable illness. Do all types of depression carry the same risk? Or is there some threshold that must be crossed before the negative effects of depression become apparent in the child? Dr. Constance Hammen, a psychologist at the University of California at Los Angeles, has attempted to answer this very important question. Her research group interviewed 816 women and their children at various points during the first five years after birth and then again when the children were fifteen years old. She demonstrated that by the age of fifteen, the children of depressed mothers were about twice as likely to suffer from depression or anxiety than the children of nondepressed mothers. The children exposed to moderate or severe maternal depression fared the worst. Even if their mother had been depressed for only one to two months, they were at higher risk for depression. If the children were exposed to milder forms of depression, the duration had to be longer than twelve months to have an effect.

Children Are at Risk Even Before They Are Born

Most research in this area focuses on how depression affects a child after birth, but many experts believe that a mother's depression can also influence her unborn child. Infants born to depressed mothers *look* depressed; they are more irritable, less physically active, and less expressive than children born to mothers who are not depressed. They are more difficult to soothe and show more signs of being stressed than babies born to nondepressed mothers. Like their depressed mothers, these infants are also more likely to have disrupted sleep patterns and decreased appetite.

So how does this happen? We know certain physiologic changes take place in a woman who is depressed, and it has been hypothesized that an unborn child exposed to these changes may experience long-lasting negative effects. At the time of birth, infants born to depressed mothers appear to have a dysregulation of their stress response system and elevated levels of certain stress hormones, including cortisol and norepinephrine. Like depressed adults, they also have lower serotonin and lower dopamine levels. In addition, their brain activity (as measured using an electroencephalogram, or EEG) is similar to what is seen in adult patients with depression. What concerns experts the most is that the hyperreactivity of the body's stress response system may persist into childhood and young adulthood. In older children, elevated levels of stress hormones may interfere with memory and attention and may impede learning. These children may also not be able to tolerate stress well, and when exposed to stressful life events, may be more prone to develop anxiety or depression.

Some Children Are More Vulnerable Than Others

While it is clear that maternal depression may have a negative impact on a child's development and well-being, not all children do poorly and some appear to be rather resilient. This is because some factors appear to protect the child from the mother's depression. One important variable is the timing of the mother's depression. Several studies have reported that infants appear to fare relatively well when the mother has had a brief episode of depression lasting only a couple of months. In contrast, infants do not do as well when the mother has had a more chronic course of depression. About one-third of women with postpartum depression remain depressed one year after delivery, and most women who have one episode of depression will have others. When a child is exposed to her mother's chronic or recurrent depression, the effects are magnified and the child is more likely to experience long-term difficulties at school and at home.

A child's age and developmental stage also determine how he or she will respond to changes in the mother's mood or behavior. When the mother is the primary caregiver and figure of attachment, maternal depression may have a more pronounced effect. On the other hand, an older child may be more independent and self-reliant and may have access to a broader range of caregivers, including the father, other family members, day care workers, and teachers. Gender may also play some role here. Several studies have demonstrated that preadolescent boys, more so than girls, are more affected by a mother's depression and are more likely to exhibit developmental delays and behavioral problems. Things seem to shift, however, as children enter into adolescence. Then, girls are more vulnerable and more likely to show signs of depression and interpersonal difficulties when cared for by a depressed mother.

In many families, depression is not the only factor to consider. Inadequate social support, lack of education, chronic medical problems, and poverty all may compromise the health and well-being of infants and children. They may magnify the negative effects of maternal depression; some researchers believe that these factors may be even more powerful than the depression itself and have been associated with developmental delays, behavioral problems, and psychiatric illness in children. Marital discord and divorce are more common in families where a parent has a psychiatric illness, and this factor is particularly important in determining how a child will fare when a mother is depressed. There is no doubt that living in a house where there is parental conflict is extremely stressful. This stress takes a toll on a child's well-being, but there are other problems that may occur. Children may mimic their parents' interactions and adopt some of their parents' patterns of behavior, which may lead to behavioral problems and interpersonal difficulties both in and outside of the home. But even when there is not overt conflict, parenting may be inconsistent or unpredictable, and parents may not be fully available to deal with their children's needs. Given that marital conflict may be a strong predictor of problems in the child, interventions that address conflicts between the partners and improve the quality of the marital relationship may be particularly beneficial for children. Another situation where a child is at high risk is when he or she has a depressed mother *and* a depressed father. Although depression tends to be less common in men than in women, women with depression tend to marry men with depression or other psychiatric problems. While having a supportive and nondepressed partner can help to buffer the effects of a mother's depression, a child exposed to depression in *both* parents is particularly at risk.

What Makes a Child More Resilient?

While most children feel, at least to some degree, the negative effects of their mother's depression, some children seem to do better than others. This may be because they are not forced to contend with certain factors (such as marital discord) that intensify the effects of a mother's depression. However, there may be certain factors that help to protect a child and make him more resilient. A child's temperament or personality may influence this vulnerability. A child who is easygoing and relatively confident will be more impervious to a mother's negative behaviors. Children who have good interpersonal skills and are able to maintain satisfying relationships with friends, other family members, and teachers also appear to fare much better. A child who is intelligent and insightful can better understand a parent's illness and recognize that she is not to blame for the illness or how a parent behaves.

When there is a supportive and emotionally available partner in a family with a depressed mother, both the mother and her children fare better. The father can serve as a positive role model, helping the child to regulate his own emotional responses and to cope with stressful situations. He can also help to maintain an environment where there is consistent and effective parenting. Several studies indicate that even when there is marital conflict, children are better adjusted if they have a parent who has the capacity to be supportive, appreciative, and emotionally engaged. Creating an environment where good communication is encouraged can also help a child to share feelings about his situation at home and can promote a better understanding of his parent's illness.

How to Minimize the Impact of Depression

If you suffer from depression, you will undoubtedly worry about how your depression may affect your child. However, it is important to keep in mind that children are remarkably resilient and there are many ways to minimize the impact of your depression on the family and help your child to grow up healthily and happily.

Get Treatment

If you are depressed, the first item on the agenda is to treat your depression. Although sometimes depression goes away on its own, not getting effective treatment may cause unnecessary problems for your family. Chapters 12 and 13 outline the many effective strategies available: talk therapy, behavioral techniques, support groups, or medication, or a combination of two or more approaches. If you are pregnant or breast-feeding, your options in terms of medication are more limited, but under no circumstances should your depression be ignored.

For most women, depression tends to be a recurrent or chronic condition, and the vast majority of women experience multiple episodes. That is why it is so important to focus not only on how depression is treated but on how to *prevent* it. Protecting yourself from future episodes of depression may entail long-term or "maintenance" treatment, either psychotherapy or medication. But there are other things that you can do to minimize your vulnerability to depression. If you are aware that there are certain triggers for your depression, you may be able to eliminate or avoid them. Learning how to better manage stressful situations and how to bolster your support network may also help to make you more resilient. It is also important to learn how you and your family can recognize the earliest signs of depression; the earlier the depression is picked up and treated, the better you and your family will do.

Rely on Other Caregivers

When you are depressed, you may pull away from other people. However, this is when you need the help and support of others. One of the important roles that these people may play is to help you take care of your children. You may be reluctant to rely on others in this fashion; however, bringing other supportive and loving people into your child's life can help your child when you are not feeling your best. Friends, family members, child caregivers, teachers, and coaches may also help to buffer the effects of your depression. With their support, you can create a stable and loving environment for your child.

Improve How You Interact with Your Child

New research suggests that interventions that focus on improving the interactions between mother and child not only improve the quality of this relationship but may also have positive effects on the mother's mood and may alleviate her symptoms of depression. Dr. Tiffany Field and her colleagues at the Touch Research Institute at the University of Miami School of Medicine have developed a number of innovative approaches that help new mothers and their children. These techniques have been helpful not only for depressed mothers but in other cases where mothers are experiencing parenting problems.

One of the techniques Dr. Field promotes is infant massage, a common child-care practice in other parts of the world, including Africa and Asia. Although infant massage is not used commonly in the United States, there appear to be many benefits for the child; compared with infants who were rocked, massaged infants cried less, were easier to soothe, showed fewer signs of being stressed, gained more weight, and slept better. While awake, the massaged babies were more alert and more vocal and active in their play with their mothers. The researchers also noted improvement in how the mothers interacted with their babies. Depressed mothers who used the massage therapy for their infants were more engaged and showed more positive interactions with their infants. Exactly how infant massage works is not known, but Dr. Field believes that one of its most important elements is touch. Her research indicates that simply by touching her child more often, a depressed mother can help her child to engage with her and to respond more positively.

Dr. Field's group also explored the use of coaching to develop more positive parenting techniques. This is sometimes called interaction coaching. It seems to work best when it is specifically tailored to the mother's style of interaction. For mothers who are more withdrawn and less emotionally responsive, the coach teaches the mother how to keep her child's attention and how to be more sensitive and responsive to her child's cues. She is taught how to play with her child; these games can help the mother to actively engage with her child and help the infant to learn how to sustain his attention. Mothers who tend to be more intrusive or overstimulating are taught to step back and slow down, allowing the child to be more independent. Not only can these interventions lead to more positive parenting styles, they seem to reduce levels of maternal depression.

While it may be difficult for you to find an expert in the area of interaction coaching, there are some resources that provide many of the same benefits. Every new mother can benefit from a supportive and knowledgeable person advising her on how to solve certain problems and providing reassurance. Traditionally, this has been provided by the extended family, a mother, an aunt, or an older sister. Many women do not have these resources or feel uncomfortable asking others for help; in other cases, a woman's family may not be able to provide the support and reassurance she needs. In this situation, it may be helpful to seek professional support, the services of child psychologists, psychiatrists, and other mental health professionals.

There are a growing number of programs and organizations that offer support to the mother as well as the child. These organizations, like the Parents as Teachers programs, are dedicated to providing education and support to parents and families. They typically rely upon parent educators to work with parents, providing them with practical information on their developing child and parenting support. They also help parents to access other family-oriented resources in their community. Research indicates that children who participate in these types of programs, when evaluated at age three, are significantly more advanced in language, problem solving, and other cognitive abilities and social development. Their parents are more confident in their parenting skills and are more involved in their child's school activities.

For mothers with infants and younger children, there are also home-visiting programs. Initially, these programs—such as Healthy Start and Healthy Families America—were designed for women at high risk: those who are single, under the age of eighteen, or living in poverty; however, this type of intervention may help *all* women. These programs, such as the Visiting Moms program organized by Jewish, Family, and Children's Services in Boston, rely on volunteers—usually experienced mothers—to visit and help with new mothers in their homes.

Educate Your Child About Depression

Nobody likes to talk about depression, and parents are often reluctant to share information regarding their mental health with their children. Although younger children may not have the intellectual capacity to grapple with the concept, children of all ages can tell that there is something amiss. Children often blame themselves for their parent's depression; they worry that they have done something to cause their parent's grief, and they feel guilty if they cannot make them better. They fear that things will get worse, and they do their best to hold their family together. Thus, the silence that often surrounds depression can make the situation even worse.

For decades Dr. William Beardslee and his colleagues at Children's Hospital in Boston have studied how families cope when there is a depressed parent. He argues very strongly that when a mother is depressed, her children, even if they are young, must be made aware of the situation. He advocates the use of a mental health clinician to help educate both the depressed parent *and* family members about depression, and encourages family meetings where the whole family gets together on a regular basis to talk about the depression and how it affects the family. Dr. Gregory Clarke from the Kaiser Permanente Center for Health Research has designed a similar educational program for the adolescent children of depressed parents where the children learn about depression and how to cope with it. The children who have participated in these programs have a much better and more sympathetic understanding of depression and are less likely to blame themselves for the problem. The adolescents who participated in Dr. Clarke's study also appeared to be at lower risk for developing depression later on.

When talking to your children about your depression, it is important to remember that children of *all* ages often imagine the worst. They may fear that their family will fall apart, or they may worry that you are very sick and may die or may be taken away. Your children need to know how you feel, but they also must be reassured that you are getting help for your problems and that you will eventually feel better. And they need to know that *they* did not do anything to make you feel this way, nor should they worry about trying to make you feel better. Most important, you have to emphasize that you love them and will do everything you can to take care of them.

The Last Word

Mothers so easily succumb to feelings of guilt and inadequacy, and many women, when confronted with the issues discussed in this chapter, may feel like they have failed their families. But this is not the message you should leave with. Many women who suffer from depression do raise happy and healthy children. Although depression has the potential to cause significant problems, it is a highly treatable illness. Depression should never be ignored, tolerated, or lived with. Depression is a signal to you that something must be done; there are many ways to intervene and to protect your children from the negative effects of this illness.

Part Two

Pregnancy

Chapter 4

Modern Technology Meets Mother Nature

Getting Pregnant

In the United States, about 1 out of every 5 or 6 couples experiences infertility. Discovering that you may have a problem with your fertility is both distressing and emotionally devastating; it is not surprising that most women describe infertility as one of the most stressful life events they have ever experienced. Most couples do not anticipate problems conceiving the child they desire, so infertility comes as a tremendous shock, a stumbling block that threatens their future plans and aspirations. Modern technology has given women much greater control over their reproductive lives. While there are many techniques and treatments to help couples have the children they desire, having a baby in this manner is not so simple. Infertility treatment is an enormous financial burden for most couples and takes a tremendous toll on their emotional and physical lives.

It appears that women who experience problems with infertility are more vulnerable to depression than their male partners. As a woman journeys through the dizzying world of infertility treatment, her life is quickly consumed and she is subjected to repeated cycles of hope and disappointment. In addition to the emotional distress, a woman is exposed to various hormonal treatments that may have a significant impact on her mood, sometimes causing depression or severe anxiety. Among women who undergo infertility treatment, about 25 percent to 30 percent suffer from clinical depression. This chapter will focus on the many emotional challenges of infertility and its treatment. It will provide strategies for relieving that stress and will help you and your partner recognize the signs of depression and anxiety that may occur in this setting. With accurate information you can recognize and manage the emotional problems that may arise under these difficult circumstances.

Understanding the Scope of the Problem

Experts define infertility as the inability to become pregnant after one year of regular unprotected sexual intercourse or the inability to carry a baby to term. According to data collected by the National Center for Health Statistics in 1995, it is estimated that in the United States about 6.1 million women of reproductive age suffer from fertility problems. Although there are both male and female causes of infertility, one of the most significant factors affecting fertility is a woman's age. Fertility begins to wane as a woman reaches her late twenties; by the time a woman approaches the age of forty, the chance of having a fertility problem is about 30 percent. Men also begin to experience a decline in their fertility as they grow older, although this appears to be a much more gradual process. With couples now waiting much longer to start their families, infertility—or what some experts prefer to call reduced fertility—has become a relatively common problem.

Infertility may be transient or permanent and is the result of a variety of medical conditions. Although there is a tendency to think of infertility as a woman's problem, it is due to a female factor about 35 percent of the time and to a male factor about 35 percent of the time. In 20 percent of cases, infertility is the product of combined male and female factors. In the remaining cases, it is not possible to determine the precise cause. Over the last twenty years, infertility treatment has evolved tremendously and continues to move forward rapidly, offering a wide and steadily growing array of treatments. While some treatment options are relatively benign, others are physically and emotionally demanding and, for many people, prohibitively expensive. Furthermore, success rates vary widely. A thorough discussion of these procedures is beyond the scope of this book. In the Recommended Reading section, you will find listed several books that provide more detailed information on infertility and its treatment.

Does Stress or Depression Cause Infertility?

Since it is not always possible to identify a precise cause for infertility, many experts have questioned whether infertility may be caused by stress or depression. It is well established that women who experience higher levels of stress in their daily lives are more likely to have irregular menstrual cycles, and women experiencing extreme stress may stop menstruating altogether. When the menstrual cycle is disrupted, ovulation does not occur regularly and it becomes more difficult to conceive. And there is some evidence to suggest that even the stress we experience on a daily basis may affect fertility. In a large study from Denmark, researchers found an approximately 25 percent reduction in pregnancy rates among women who described higher levels of stress during their attempts to conceive.

Although many have postulated a link between stress and infertility, the extent to which depression affects fertility is not clear. In one study, infertility problems were about twice as common among women with depression than women who had no history of depression. Exactly how depression may cause this reduction in fertility is not well understood. It is possible that depression itself is not the issue, but rather that depression is associated with a number of behaviors that reduce a couple's chance of conceiving. People suffering from depression often complain of a lack of sex drive, and many antidepressants taken to treat depression may affect sexual function. We also know that people who are depressed are also more likely to smoke or to use alcohol and recreational drugs, all of which may negatively affect fertility and lead to premature menopause. Furthermore, recent studies indicate that consuming even moderate levels of alcohol (one to five drinks per week) may significantly reduce a woman's chance of conception.

Dr. David Rubinow and his colleagues at the National Institutes of Mental Health go one step further. They believe that depression itself *is* the problem and that depression may actually cause infertility in some women. Rubinow hypothesizes that depression exerts its negative effects on fertility by activating the body's stress response system. When this occurs, stress hormones, such as cortisol, are produced and these block the production of various hormones, including gonadotropin-releasing hormone (GnRH) and luteinizing hormone (LH), the hormones that trigger ovulation and allow conception. When the production of these hormones is disrupted, ovulation may not occur on a regular basis, resulting in impaired fertility.

While there is at least one study that documents the negative effects of depression in women attempting to conceive naturally, the literature also includes several studies that suggest women who are undergoing infertility treatment are less likely to be successful if they are depressed. In a study of 330 women undergoing in vitro fertilization (IVF), success rates were markedly lower (less than half) in women who were depressed at the outset of treatment as compared to women who were not depressed. A similar study involving forty women undergoing IVF also demonstrated lower success rates in depressed women. Anxiety also appears to have negative effects. In one study, women who experienced higher levels of anxiety prior to artificial insemination required more cycles to get pregnant, and there were higher rates of miscarriage among women with higher levels of anxiety.

Depression is a relatively frequent complication of infertility and its treatment. With evidence that depression may diminish the effectiveness of infertility treatment, it simply cannot be ignored. Furthermore, it may make the stress of infertility treatment unbearable, causing some women to lose hope and to drop out of treatment prematurely. Recognizing this, many infertility clinics offer counseling or more structured programs to help couples to manage the stress of treatment and to reduce the risk of depression. Not only do these interventions help to decrease the stress associated with infertility, there is some evidence that they may actually improve the chances of getting pregnant.

Infertility Takes Its Toll

Although most women have entertained the possibility that they may have problems getting pregnant, infertility still comes as a shock. While many infertile couples ultimately become pregnant, with treatment or on their own, infertility feels to many like a terminal illness. Not surprisingly, discovering that you may have a problem with infertility unleashes many intense feelings and affects every aspect of your life.

Several years after getting married, Alice and Jack decided to start a family. They stopped using contraception, but after a year Alice was not yet pregnant. When her gynecologist suggested that Alice and Jack meet with an infertility specialist, Alice was stunned; she was totally healthy and only thirty-two; she felt like there was something horribly wrong with her and was too uncomfortable to talk about it with her friends. Jack and her family were supportive, but Alice was distraught. What if she and Jack could never have a child?

Alice was diagnosed with mild endometriosis and underwent surgery to correct the problem. In addition, Jack had a low sperm count. They again started to try to get pregnant on their own. For several months, Alice got her period and was gripped with feelings of disappointment. She felt herself focusing more and more on getting pregnant and found herself retreating from her friends and not interested in many of the things she used to enjoy. Despite her many successes in other areas of her life, she felt like a complete failure. She sensed her husband's disappointment and began to worry that he would leave her.

After six months, Alice and Jack again met with the infertility specialist and were presented with a list of possible treatments. Alice's doctor felt optimistic about their situation. Initially Alice felt hopeful, but it was difficult for her to press onward without knowing exactly how things would work out. She so much wanted to have a child but she did not know if she could bear any more disappointments. The thought of going through infertility treatment was so overwhelming; she wanted to take a break but worried that she couldn't waste any time. Sometimes she felt like giving up.

Recent studies indicate that 60 percent to 90 percent of those diagnosed with infertility experience significant psychological distress. Although both women and men suffer considerably, it appears that women almost always report higher levels of distress than do men. Infertility affects every aspect of a woman's life: self-identity and self-esteem, physical well-being, relationship with a partner, relationships with friends and family, career. While sadness is likely to be at the top of the list of the many intense, sometimes overpowering emotions, it is not the only uncomfortable feeling that you may grapple with. As you try to make sense of your situation, anger and frustration are bound to come to the surface. Although you may be given a medical explanation for what is happening, there is certainly no good reason for you to have to suffer this way. It is simply unfair. Why are you being denied the opportunity to have a child? And why is it that so many others around you seem to have no problem having children? Unfortunately, this line of thinking often drifts into self-blame and feelings of guilt. Although it is irrational, you may believe at some level that you are to blame for your infertility or that you have done something to deserve it. And as you look at other women who are pregnant or who have children, you may find yourself struggling to hold back feelings of envy. It may also be very difficult for you to relate to women who do not seem to value their ability to have children—for example, a woman who has had several abortions or one who abuses or neglects her children.

Although you may want to talk to other people about your situation, you may find that it is difficult for others, including your partner, to appreciate the intensity of your feelings. You may also feel that others minimize the impact of infertility; however, the truth is that the distress you may feel in this situation may be extreme. In fact, one study indicated that infertile women experience levels of distress similar to those reported by women recently diagnosed with cancer.

The distress a couple feels may be exacerbated by the cost of infertility treatment. In most states, insurance companies do not cover the cost of infertility treatment or they limit the number and types of treatments available. Further, the emotional and physical demands of infertility treatment are often so great that many women find it necessary to quit their jobs, reduce their time at work, or delay promotions.

The distress that you experience may wax and wane over time. It is often most intense soon after you learn that there is an infertility problem and during the early stages of treatment. Feelings of sadness, loss, and frustration are at their most intense after a treatment cycle fails. Although you may start to feel less upset over time, you may find that intense feelings resurface every time important decisions regarding treatment must be made, particularly the decision to pursue a different type of treatment or to take a break. Over time, many women adjust to this situation and do relatively well, seemingly buoyed by their hopefulness that over time they may conceive. However, when a couple makes repeated attempts to become pregnant, they pass through one cycle after another of hope and disappointment. Confronted year after year with the inability to have a child, many couples feel increasingly hopeless or despairing.

To make matters worse, this grief is often experienced in isolation. Not wishing to burden others with their problems or too ashamed to talk about their situation, couples often withdraw from family and friends. Having to deal with friends or family members who are pregnant or having children can be extraordinarily painful. Sometimes it is even difficult or too painful to discuss this issue with one's partner, and many women end up feeling that they must contend with their feelings of sadness or anger on their own. Many women find themselves leading two separate and equally consuming lives. They have their daily activities: their work, their friends, their usual responsibilities. Then they have their more private and painful world of infertility.

Infertility Is Experienced As a Loss

In the broadest sense, infertility is experienced as a loss or, more accurately, a series of many different losses. Having a child carries many different and complex meanings, and these meanings color how each woman experiences and responds to the crisis of infertility. Having a child is seen as a mix of deeply gratifying and life-transforming opportunities: the opportunity to join with your partner, to carry your family line into the future, to be a parent, to explore a new dimension of your life, to make a unique and enduring contribution. When confronted with infertility, couples feel that these dreams and opportunities may be lost.

Women today occupy many different roles outside of the home. These diverse opportunities add richness to their lives and can bring much satisfaction and happiness. Yet, most women still consider motherhood the most important and gratifying of their roles. Even a woman who plans to have children later in life probably considers the potential to become a mother at the core of her identity. When this is threatened, her sense of self and self-esteem are in jeopardy. Infertility is seen as an obstacle to having a fulfilling life. An infertile woman may feel that she is a disappointment to her partner and to her family, that she has let them down. She may also feel incompetent, unable to do what women are "supposed to" do. And, regrettably, these feelings of inadequacy and failure can permeate other domains of her life.

When confronting infertility, many couples feel that they have lost control over an important aspect of their lives. Most of us function with the notion that all we have to do is decide *when* to have a child. The harsh reality is that no matter how much you want a child or how hard you work to achieve this goal, what ultimately happens is largely out of your control. As you embark upon infertility treatment, this loss of control becomes even more apparent. Your reproductive life is transformed from spontaneous and natural to a series of procedures orchestrated, scheduled, and monitored by a team of medical professionals. Everything seems to change; work schedules are rearranged, vacations are postponed, social engagements are canceled. In this new reality, all decisions must consider the demands infertility treatment places on your time, energy, finances, and emotional resources.

You and your partner will likely go through some sort of grieving process where you confront and come to terms with the many losses you have suffered as a result of your infertility. As you pass through the various stages of this grieving process, you will encounter the same types of strong emotions we experience after the death of a loved one. Grief ebbs and flows; it is set into motion as you come to grips with your infertility, and although treatment may bring hope of having a child, feelings of loss and sadness may reemerge and intensify with each attempt to conceive.

Denial. Although you have not been able to conceive, it may be difficult for you to accept that there is a problem. Many couples blame their childlessness on other things—such as stress or a hectic lifestyle—and it may take a long time to entertain the possibility that there is a fertility problem. Without acknowledging that there is a problem, you may delay or avoid seeking further evaluation or treatment.

Partially because the chances of conceiving naturally decrease over time, it is very important to realistically evaluate your situation sooner rather than later. Sometimes it is not so easy to tell if you are in denial. (If you are reading this chapter, you probably aren't.) Yet it is also important to remember that denial is not always an appropriate response to a difficult situation. Although most of us use this very effective defense mechanism to protect ourselves from experiencing painful feelings, denial can prevent you from getting help in a timely manner. Here are some signs to help you determine if you are avoiding the problem:

- You avoid talking to others about having children or the fact that you are having problems doing so.
- You become defensive when others bring up the topic or if anybody suggests that there may be a problem.
- You are doing things just to keep busy, to avoid thinking.
- You are using alcohol or recreational drugs to make yourself feel better.
- You find yourself feeling more anxious or depressed but are unsure why.

Anger. You may feel angry at your body for failing you. You may feel angry at yourself or your partner for having waited so long to have children. And you may feel especially angry at those women and couples who seem to have no problem getting pregnant. However, sometimes it may feel like there is no clear target for your rage, and you may end up directing it toward innocent bystanders. Often your partner is a convenient target. You may also be angered by women who do not seem to value their ability to have children. Another common target for your anger may be your doctors; you may be angry that they did not make you aware of the problem earlier or that they did not act more aggressively. You may blame them when a particular treatment fails.

Guilt and self-blame. Women often feel responsible for a couple's inability to conceive, even if that's not really the case. It may be difficult to rationally appraise your situation, and in the back of your mind, you may believe that infertility is a punishment for some real or imagined transgression. If you have previously terminated a pregnancy, you may find it especially difficult. You may start to doubt yourself, believing for some reason that you do not deserve to have children.

Withdrawal and isolation. Although infertility looms large in their lives, most women do not openly discuss it with family members, friends, or coworkers. Infertility is often viewed as socially or personally unacceptable. Because it is so often perceived as a failure or a shortcoming, you may feel too ashamed or embarrassed to talk about it. Or it may just be too painful to bring up this topic with others, especially if you feel that they may not be able to understand your situation or may make well-intentioned but inappropriate comments.

Even when your friends or family try to be supportive, you may not feel that they can appreciate the intensity of your distress. It may be extraordinarily difficult to be in situations where there are other women who are pregnant or who have children, and you may end up avoiding many social situations, further limiting your opportunities to connect with others and increasing your sense of isolation. Even within the relationship with your partner, you may experience a sense of isolation when you feel that he does not appreciate your situation or has his own competing needs.

Grief. At some point after a fertility problem is made apparent, you will feel a profound sadness related to your inability to have children as you had planned. Although there may be alternatives to having children naturally, you may sense that you are being forced to abandon your most important dreams for the future.

The grieving process is complicated. With infertility, the nature of the loss is ambiguous. You are not grieving for a specific someone you have lost—you are grieving for the dreams you have lost. Grieving is also complicated by the fact that with infertility, in most cases, it is never entirely clear how things will work out. One day you may be ready to accept the fact that you can never have children, and another day you may feel hopeful that you will have children. It is a loss you experience over and over again.

Acceptance. Over time, you will be able to come to some degree of acceptance. But what exactly is acceptance? It does not mean that you will ever completely stop wanting to have children. Nor does it mean that you will feel unaffected by your situation. It does mean that at some point you will come to some resolution of your more intense feelings. While it is likely that from time to time you will feel considerable sadness, this acceptance allows you to move forward and to derive pleasure from other aspects of your life.

Infertility Is Experienced As a Physical Illness

To many women, infertility feels like a physical deficit or flaw. The inability to have a child, to do what women are naturally supposed to do, represents a failure, palpable evidence that one's body is not healthy or is somehow defective. Furthermore, in our society, infertility becomes a prolonged and sometimes chronic medical condition. When you choose to pursue infertility treatment, you, a previously healthy woman, become a *patient*. As you attempt to have a baby, you are subjected to invasive tests and procedures. It is not surprising that, in many respects, as you are exposed to the rigors of infertility treatment, you may confront many of the same issues faced by those who suffer from a chronic medical illness.

You may be preoccupied with your physical health and well-being. As an infertility patient, your physical being is closely scrutinized and monitored by your medical team. You are specifically told what to eat, what activities to pursue, and what things to avoid. No wonder you may become extremely focused on or even obsessed with maintaining your health. You may also find that you are overly attentive to and disturbed by any sign of illness or any medical problem that may compromise your fertility.

Your sense of your body image may change. Infertility does change how you think about your body. Although previously you probably thought of yourself as being relatively healthy, infertility transforms your body into something that is imperfect. If you are not able to have a baby, you may feel less attractive, less feminine, or less sexual. Not being able to have a child may be an indication that you are getting older, and you may find yourself focusing on and being more distressed by any signs of aging.

You may feel more vulnerable or helpless. Being a patient makes it difficult to think of yourself as healthy and strong. You have doctors, nurses, and other medical professionals *taking care* of you and telling you exactly what to do. You may end up feeling that your body, and your ability to have a child, are under someone else's control, and this may make you feel helpless.

You may feel less confident or inadequate. When you cannot attain a goal that is highly valued and important to you, when your body is not able to do what it is supposed to do, you may lose confidence in yourself and your other abilities. You may feel unable to handle certain tasks and to accomplish other important goals. Even though you may engage in many other pursuits that are rewarding and highly regarded by others, you may feel that you have fallen short of what is expected of you.

You may have a sense of a foreshortened future. Although, in most cases, a woman with infertility is just as healthy and likely to live a long life as a woman who is fertile, infertility may change how you look at your future. Whereas there is a sense that having a child will allow you to enter a new phase of your life and will present you with many new opportunities, infertility may make it feel more like your life is coming to an end. You may feel that a large portion of your life has been taken away from you.

Making Decisions Regarding Treatment

Fifty years ago, if you were infertile, all you could do was cross your fingers and hope for good fortune. Today you have many different and promising ways to conceive. However, the decision to pursue treatment must take into account that infertility treatment can be a grueling process, one that may last for many years and is likely to take a significant toll on you and your partner's lives. It is important to remember that infertility treatment is only one of several options. Many couples decide to adopt. Some couples decide to use a surrogate or gestational carrier. Others decide to live without children. It is important to consider all of these options before you leap into treatment.

Infertility represents a crisis. To survive it, you must be able to face this crisis with your partner and you must work as a team. You will be making many important decisions that both of you must feel comfortable with. Although couples often feel that time is of the essence and that they need to push ahead quickly, it is important to take the time to make sure that you and your partner have the same goals in mind. First of all, learn what options are available to you. How successful are these procedures likely to be? What if they do not work out? What about other alternatives? What are your feelings about adoption? It is crucial that you be able to talk openly about these decisions before you embark upon treatment. Talking can allow the two of you to understand each other, and it can also help diffuse the intensity of your feelings. Knowing how both of you feel about other options or having some sense of when you would both feel comfortable switching to "Plan B" can alleviate some of the stress. If you have problems discussing these decisions with your partner now before you start treatment, it is unlikely that things will get any easier as time goes on.

Contrary to popular belief, not everyone who has infertility pursues treatment. In fact, only about a quarter of infertile women receive treatment and less than 2 percent undergo any sort of high-tech procedure. Some women are not good candidates for treatment because they have a problem that cannot be corrected or the chances of a successful and healthy pregnancy are very low. For other women, artificial reproductive techniques are simply not an option. Some women have very strong personal and/or religious beliefs regarding the importance and sanctity of a naturally conceived pregnancy. Many couples simply cannot afford these expensive interventions. Ultimately you may not want to live without children, but circumstances may force this choice. And it is understandable how in that sort of situation you may experience intense feelings of envy or anger directed toward those who have more options.

Some women and their partners make the decision to live without children. Typically, this is not an alternative that a couple comes to early in the process. Some couples make this decision after infertility treatments have failed; for others, living without children feels like the best option. Unfortunately, many women who make the decision to live without children end up feeling alone and misunderstood. If everyone around you has children or is actively trying to conceive, it may be difficult for you to explain why you are not. Many will not understand the decision you have made. While there are many sources of support for couples who suffer from infertility, most often support is offered within the context of treatment. Although a few organizations have sprung up to address the emotional needs of those who decide to live without children, much less is available in this circumstance.

How Fertility Drugs May Affect Your Mood

If you have made the decision to pursue treatment, you will find that infertility treatment encompasses a broad spectrum of diagnostic and medical or surgical procedures and a steadily growing list of medications. In many situations, medications will be used to enhance fertility. The vast majority of the medications used to treat infertility are taken by the woman to regulate her hormonal environment so that a successful pregnancy may take place. As we discussed in chapter 2, the hormones essential for pregnancy—estrogen and progesterone—have potent effects on the brain. Not surprisingly, many of the infertility drugs used to regulate these hormones may have mood-altering effects, too.

Exactly how often full-blown psychiatric symptoms occur as a result of exposure to these drugs is not entirely clear. While there is a tendency to focus on the more serious and potentially life-threatening side effects of these drugs, less attention has been directed toward the impact of these medications on mood. The situation is further complicated by the fact that it may be particularly difficult to recognize the emergence of psychiatric symptoms, given that so many women with infertility describe significant problems with depression and anxiety before they initiate treatment. While most infertility specialists agree that the overall incidence of significant psychiatric symptoms in patients treated with fertility-enhancing drugs is relatively low, women with an underlying vulnerability to depression may be at higher risk for medication-induced mood changes. Also women who are more sensitive to hormonal fluctuations (e.g., women with a history of premenstrual mood symptoms or those who have experienced mood changes while taking other hormonal preparations, including oral contraceptives) may experience similar mood changes when exposed to infertility drugs. If you feel that you are at risk for depression or anxiety or are already experiencing these symptoms, discuss your concerns with your infertility specialist. There are many different options available for treatment, and it may be possible to select a regimen that is less likely to cause significant mood changes.

One of the simplest and most popular treatments for women with infertility is the drug clomiphene citrate, also known as Clomid. Clomiphene citrate interacts with estrogen receptors, blocking the effects of natural forms of estrogen. As estrogen appears to have positive effects on emotional well-being, it makes sense that the clomiphene citrate may cause some mood changes. Depression, irritability, insomnia, and anxiety have been reported in women taking this medication. Typically, the duration of exposure to Clomid is relatively brief, only five days per cycle, yet some women may experience persistent and significant symptoms lasting long after the treatment stops. Data from the manufacturer suggests that in the general population, these symptoms are relatively uncommon, affecting less than 5 percent of women. The effect of the medication may be magnified, however, when the medication is used at higher doses or when it is taken repeatedly, cycle after cycle.

Progesterone is also used extensively and is administered for up to six weeks during early pregnancy to protect the uterine lining and promote the development of the placenta. Unfortunately, progesterone may undermine the positive effects of estrogen and may thus lead to significant depressive symptoms. This is especially a problem since progesterone is usually used for a relatively long period during the early stages of pregnancy. Although typically used orally, there are vaginal progesterone suppositories that may be less likely to cause mood changes because lower dosages are used.

The GnRH agonists, including leuprolide acetate (Lupron) and nafarelin acetate (Synarel), are important in regulating the hormonal environment during infertility treatment. These medications interact with the hypothalamus to shut off the hormonal signals that induce ovulation. What the body experiences is a drug-induced menopause and, unfortunately, all the negative effects of estrogen deficiency. Although this phase of infertility treatment is often brief, it can bring a host of symptoms, including mood swings, depression, and anxiety. There have also been reports of mania induced by GnRH agonists in patients with a history of bipolar disorder. The GnRH agonists may also cause other symptoms associated with estrogen deficiency, including memory problems and loss of libido.

Oral contraceptives may also be used to regulate the menstrual cycle. While most women find that oral contraceptives have no impact on their mood or actually increase their sense of well-being, some women experience significant mood changes within a few days of starting this regimen. Steroid hormones, including prednisolone and dexamethasone, are sometimes used in these procedures. For most, this is not a problem as the doses are relatively low and the treatment brief. However, some women, especially those with bipolar disorder, may be exquisitely sensitive to the steroid hormones and may experience anxiety, irritability, or mood swings.

Although reports of mood changes and anxiety have been reported in conjunction with the use of infertility drugs, the incidence of these side effects is probably relatively low. If you have had a bad reaction to hormonal preparations or steroid hormones, like prednisone, in the past, you should discuss this with your physician. Also, if you have had a history of depression or anxiety, you may be more vulnerable to the effects of these medications. Discuss this with your physician.

Fertility and the Mind-Body Connection

Over the last few decades there has been a growing interest in the interplay between the mind and the body. Not only does having a serious medical illness affect your sense of well-being, there is clear evidence that stress and depression may increase your risk for or may worsen the course of many different illnesses, including heart disease, high blood pressure, and cancer. Psychologist Alice Domar, founder of the Mind-Body Program for Infertility in Boston, is a pioneer in the field and has developed highly effective programs to help women and their partners cope with the stress of infertility.

Domar's programs use many different techniques: yoga, meditation, deep breathing, progressive muscle relaxation, and guided imagery. (These techniques are described in detail in Alice Domar's book *Conquering Infertility*.) Other stress reduction skills are also emphasized: helping women to take better care of themselves, to increase their supports, to improve communication skills, and to eliminate negative patterns of thinking. The results are quite impressive. Domar's research indicates that not only do these techniques help to alleviate stress and depression, they may actually *increase* a woman's likelihood of conception. In one study, among women with infertility who attended Domar's mind-body program, 55 percent conceived within one year. In contrast, among the women who received no intervention, only 20 percent were pregnant after one year. Furthermore, the women who used mind-body techniques were also much more likely to conceive naturally, with no medical intervention. The message seems clear: reducing levels of stress and depression may make it easier for you to get pregnant.

Managing the Stress of Infertility and Its Treatment

If you are planning to undergo infertility treatment, it is important to acknowledge and accept that this will be a challenging time for you and your partner. While pursuing your usual activities may help distract you, this approach may backfire, leaving you feeling overloaded and completely depleted. As you embark upon this project, it is important to recognize that you and your partner are going to need more time and emotional space, and it is unrealistic to assume that life can go on as usual. Here are some strategies that will help to reduce the stress you are likely to experience.

Educate Yourself

Confronting infertility, it is easy to feel bewildered and lost. Many couples feel that they are bombarded with highly technical information and long lists of options. They end up feeling overwhelmed, confused, and uncertain about which direction to go. In addition, the many myths and misconceptions surrounding infertility and its treatment may generate significant anxiety and, at the worst, they may lead some infertile couples to make decisions that are not in their best interest. Becoming an educated consumer is one of the best ways to feel like you are taking control of the situation.

- Find a reputable infertility specialist, one that you feel comfortable with. He or she should be able to understand your concerns and take the time to address them.
- Attend consultations with your partner.
- Always ask questions.

- Write down information for later reference.
- Contact RESOLVE, a nonprofit organization that provides educational materials and can help you connect with health professionals and support groups in your community.
- Familiarize yourself with your options for treatment and their rates of success. There are several good books on the reading list at the end of this book that may be useful sources of information for you.
- Beware of the Internet. While it offers an endless bounty of information, you must take into careful consideration the source and the quality of the information you receive online. At the end of the book, you will find a list of helpful and reputable Web sites.

Formulate a Plan

Many couples feel a great deal of pressure to plunge right in, but taking the time to educate yourself and to formulate a sensible plan may save you pain and disappointment down the line. Before starting evaluation or treatment, it is important that you and your partner sit down and discuss your goals and your expectations. Do you both want the same thing? How far are you willing to go? Some couples find that once they get started, it is almost impossible to stop. The decision to stop treatment is always a difficult one, but it is easier if you start thinking about it at the beginning.

- Discuss with your partner and your infertility team what options you are planning to pursue.
- In advance, determine when it is time to stop treatment. What are your financial, emotional, and physical limits?
- From the outset, discuss your feelings regarding adoption. This is not a good choice for everybody, but it is important to think about how you feel about this option.
- On a periodic basis, reevaluate your plan and make sure that both of you are still comfortable with it. Revise the plan as needed. Your goals may change as certain options are eliminated or others appear.

Try to Eliminate Other Sources of Stress

Try to make an accurate assessment of *all* the sources of stress in your life and focus on those things that you have some control over. What can you change? Come up with a list of possible solutions for each problem. Keep in mind that even positive changes, like buying a new house or getting promoted, may cause stress. Although this list is far from complete, consider the following potential sources of stress.

Relationship	Disagreements related to infertility treatment
	Poor communication
	Sexual difficulties
Family	Caring for family members (elderly parents, children)
	Domestic responsibilities
	Social obligations
	Pressure to have children
Work	Inflexible or long work hours
	Unrealistic demands
	Conflict with coworkers
	Inadequate pay
	Lack of job security
	Job dissatisfaction
Financial	Cost of infertility treatment
	Impact of missed time at work

Though your list may be long, remember: it's not your job to solve *all* the problems. Give your attention to the problems that seem the easiest to solve or to those that seem to cause the greatest stress in your life.

- Be realistic about what you can actually accomplish with your time. This is not a time to stretch yourself in too many different directions.
- Try to reduce your responsibilities.
- Try not to take on new projects or responsibilities.
- If possible, delegate stressful or unpleasant tasks to others.

Learn to Communicate More Effectively

Although you may not want to share this problem with everybody, you do need to find at least a few people to whom you can talk openly and honestly. First and foremost on this list is your partner. Although infertility is a problem you share, you cannot assume that your partner feels exactly the same way that you do. Having a child may have very different meanings for you than for your partner. Because you bring to this crisis different experiences and different expectations, how each of you responds to and copes with infertility may be very different. Only by working to understand these feelings can the two of you learn to support each other.

It is also important to learn to talk to and to share at least some of your concerns with your friends and family. All too often infertility becomes a secret, a source of shame and embarrassment. While you may ultimately decide not to share this issue with some friends or family members, there should be *some* people to whom you feel comfortable talking. Emotional support from others is tremendously helpful and by sharing the pain you are feeling, you may also enrich and strengthen your relationships with certain friends or family members. By sharing, you give them the opportunity to be more sensitive to your needs, and they can avoid making excessive demands of you in this difficult time. However, as you bring up the topic of your infertility, you want to remain in control of it and of when you want to talk about it.

From time to time you are sure to hear: "I know exactly how you feel." In reality, *nobody* knows exactly how you feel. Many, even those that are the closest to you, may not know exactly how to help you. Sometimes you may want their helpful words of advice or their capacity to be optimistic. At other times, you may not want them to try to solve your problems, but you may just need them to listen, to hear your sadness or anger. Try to be patient; even the most empathetic of your friends or family will get it wrong from time to time, and it is important that you communicate to them what is helpful to you. You should feel comfortable telling them what it is okay to talk about and when. Conversely, you must be able to tell them when they have said something that has hurt your feelings or has made you angry. If you feel too uncomfortable to be around certain people, try, as hard as it may be, to let them know why you need a little bit of distance.

Adopt a Healthy Style of Living
Adopting a healthy lifestyle can help to diminish your stress levels and may make you feel healthier and stronger. It may also improve your chances of conception.

- Eating a healthful diet helps you maintain a steady, healthy body weight. If you have questions, discuss your nutritional needs with your doctor or with a nutritionist.
- Take care of your physical self. Many infertility programs encourage you to curtail your physical activity, but moderate activity shouldn't be a problem. Walking may be one good way to get some exercise. Yoga is

also a good option because it strengthens your body and helps you to relax. Whatever you choose, you should always discuss your activity program with your doctor.

- Avoid alcohol and recreational drugs. These may exacerbate feelings of depression and anxiety and may also have a negative impact on fertility.
- Stick to a consistent sleep schedule. (Healthy sleep habits will be discussed in chapter 11.)

Learn to Live in the Present

Living in the here and now is not always easy. It is even harder when you are struggling with infertility. You may have regrets about the past and worries about the future. Try to hold on to the things that give you pleasure, whether it is reading the Sunday paper in bed or walking your dog on a sunny day. Instead of focusing on the negative aspects of your life, try to focus on the things around you that bring you joy.

Set Aside Time to Enjoy Yourself

If you are undergoing infertility treatment, it may seem that there is little time for anything else. Infertility becomes a full-time career, and couples often find themselves with little time to enjoy themselves or to tend to other aspects of their lives. But being able to relax and enjoy yourself is vital; it helps to renew your emotional resources and will help to keep things in perspective.

- Set aside some time each day where you can relax.
- Set aside time each week to do something special.
- Plan a vacation. You need to take a break from infertility and the other stresses of daily living from time to time.

Bolster Your Support Network

When you are dealing with infertility, it is easy to feel that you are the only one with this problem and you may convince yourself that your situation is hopeless. This is simply not true, and it is important to take advantage of the available resources. Finding somebody who has had problems with infertility, with whom you can share your experiences and concerns, can be life-transforming.

- Make time to spend time with your friends or family.
- Give yourself permission to avoid those people who are insensitive to

your situation and instead spend time with those who are sensitive and sympathetic.

- Contact RESOLVE (www.resolve.org). There are more than fifty local chapters in the United States offering support groups and other services to couples with infertility.
- Consider professional sources of support. It may be helpful to meet with a counselor or therapist to discuss issues related to infertility. RESOLVE or your infertility clinic can help you find a professional with expertise in this area.

Avoid Situations That Are Too Painful

Couples undergoing infertility treatment may find it particularly painful to participate in or to attend activities related to having or raising children, such as baby showers, christenings, and children's birthday parties. Often these events are pleasurable, but sometimes they may be too painful to endure. In most situations, avoidance is not the best solution to a problem and a less-than-ideal coping strategy. But it does work, and may, on occasion, be necessary.

Protecting Your Relationship with Your Partner

Infertility, like any long-term problem, may take a tremendous toll on your relationship with your partner. For most people, infertility is the first crisis they will face as a couple. Old issues with communication may become more evident as the couple attempts to make difficult decisions and new problems may arise. While the integrity of the relationship may be jeopardized, it should also be recognized that with this crisis comes opportunity, the chance to make important and positive changes in the relationship. Many couples actually feel that their experience with infertility brought them closer and strengthened their relationship. Although almost all of your attention is likely to be focused on the pursuit of pregnancy, every effort must be made to nurture your relationship with your partner.

Further complicating matters is the fact that men and women often respond differently to the crisis of infertility. Many women complain that their male partners do not seem to be affected, that the situation just doesn't appear to upset them. This is simply not true. Men are clearly concerned about and committed to having children, and men *do* experience distress. However, men and woman have different communication styles. While women tend to be more outwardly expressive of their emotions, men are more likely to keep their distressing feelings to themselves. Even when a man spends a tremendous time thinking about a problem, he may not share his thoughts openly. While women want to talk about their sadness, men tend to be more action-oriented and are eager to solve the problem. Men often feel the need to be the "strong one" and thus feel that there is no room for them to express their sadness or frustration, fearing that their display of emotion may add to their partner's pain. To a woman, this silence may be perceived as an inability to understand her feelings or, at worst, a lack of interest or concern.

In this situation the differences between men and women run even deeper. Although you and your partner both want to have a child, what it actually means to have a child may be different for each of you. For some men, fatherhood, while very important and meaningful, does not appear to be as crucial to their sense of identity and self-esteem. Most women, on the other hand, do feel that being a mother is an important aspect of their identity. For many women, missing out on the experience of having their own child affects how they feel about themselves and may hinder their ability to feel confident and competent in other aspects of their lives.

And of course, women, more so than men, bear the burden of infertility treatment even when infertility is determined to be due to a male factor. It is the woman who usually undergoes the vital diagnostic tests, most of the hormonal treatments and procedures, and it is the woman who ultimately carries the pregnancy. No matter how supportive and available her partner may be, this inherent inequality in shouldering the burden of childbearing may make a woman feel overburdened and resentful while her partner may feel shut out from the experience.

If your partner is unable or reluctant to talk about the problem, you may feel as if he is not concerned about you or is not able to acknowledge the intense emotions you are experiencing. You may end up feeling distanced from your partner at a time when you need him the most. Infertility may also make you feel much less secure about your relationship. You may feel that your partner is disappointed in you. You may even worry that your partner will leave you to find a woman who can give him a child. Obviously, this type of thinking can undermine even the strongest of relationships. At a time when you need to be honest about your feelings, you may find yourself holding back, worried that if you burden your partner too much, he may end up leaving.

Many women who struggle with infertility also find themselves struggling with depression. If you are feeling depressed, you may find yourself avoiding your partner at a time when you need each other the most. And your emotional state may have an impact on how your partner interacts with you. If you are sad or irritable, your partner may find it difficult to spend time with you. If you are feeling persistently pessimistic or hopeless, it may be difficult for him to talk to you about the issues surrounding your infertility and to make plans for the future.

The strain of infertility is often felt most intensely in the bedroom. Many couples experience some level of dissatisfaction with their sex lives. Feelings of resentment or anger toward your partner may make it difficult to be close physically. The feelings of inadequacy that often accompany infertility may make a woman feel less attractive or desirable, and many women feel less interested in sexual intimacy with their partner. For men, fertility is inextricably connected with their sexuality and potency, and their inability to have a child may leave them feeling inadequate or less "masculine." Some men have problems with impotence. When lovemaking becomes "baby making," sex is not simply something to be enjoyed or a way to be close to one's partner. Women may find themselves avoiding sex because the experience brings with it feelings of disappointment and sadness, rather than pleasure. Undergoing infertility treatment may add to these problems, as a couple's intimate activities are being closely scrutinized and scheduled. When sex must be performed according to these strict guidelines, both partners may feel anxiety or pressure. Needless to say, this is not going to make lovemaking an enjoyable event. Sexual intimacy is an important form of communication, and without it the couple faces another loss.

It is, however, possible to protect your relationship during this difficult time; there is even opportunity to strengthen and enrich it.

Avoid placing blame. Even if only one person is infertile, it is important to keep in mind that infertility is a shared problem and no one's fault. Blaming your partner for the problem is not going to help you feel better about your situation, and finger-pointing is likely to lead to resentment that may undermine the relationship. Conversely, feeling that you are at fault is not going to help your situation either.

Learn to compartmentalize. Many infertile couples complain that there is one partner (usually the woman) who is more focused, or even obsessed with, infertility. The other partner seems better able to compartmentalize the problem and to go on with life, keeping the infertility problem in the background. While good communication is important, it can be taken to an extreme. A never-ending discussion of infertility is not going to help either of you or improve your chances of conceiving.

Compartmentalization is not necessarily a synonym for avoiding painful issues; it is a technique that you may use to gain control over a difficult situation and maintain perspective on other aspects of your life. Some couples use the twenty-minute rule, where the couple agrees that they will talk about infertility-related issues for no more than twenty minutes each day. The time of this discussion is predetermined so that it cannot disrupt work or an enjoyable activity. Each member of the couple is given time to talk, without interruption, while the other listens.

Set aside couple's time. No matter how crowded and hectic your life gets, it is absolutely essential to set aside time for your partner. Even the most compatible relationship needs time to be tended. At least twice a week, choose an activity that you both enjoy doing; it can be as simple as taking a walk together or watching a television show. This time you set aside should be considered an infertility-free zone where the two of you simply enjoy your time together. Spending this time with your partner helps to strengthen your bonds and keeps you focused on the positive aspects of your relationship.

Join an infertility support group. Even the most supportive and sensitive partner may not be able to understand exactly what it feels like to be a woman struggling with infertility. In a support group, you will find a place to openly share your feelings. If you feel that your feelings have been validated and are understood by others, it will help to take some of the pressure off of your relationship.

Look for warning signals. Although it may be your instinct to look the other way, it is important not to ignore the signs that there may be problems between you and your partner. It is also important to recognize that the difficulties you are encountering may not simply disappear after you have a child. There may be more significant issues that could cause problems down the line and affect your ability to parent effectively. If you are having any of the following problems, try discussing them with your partner.

- If you are angry or frustrated by your partner's inability to understand your feelings.
- If you are feeling hostile or resentful toward your partner.

- If you are having more arguments or are more focused on the negative aspects of your relationship.
- If you find yourself turning more often to others for support.
- If you are spending less time with your partner.
- If you think you would be better off with someone else.

If you are not able to discuss these issues with your partner, or you are unable to resolve these issues, it may be helpful to meet as a couple with a counselor. View this as an opportunity to improve communication and to better learn how to support each other.

The Decision to Stop Treatment

Infertility treatment must stop at some point. The best reason is that you may become pregnant. But if you do not conceive after multiple rounds of treatment, it may be difficult to figure out when is the right time to stop. Some couples feel that it is almost impossible to abandon treatment; they are unwilling to give up and the beginning of each new cycle brings new hope. For many, stopping treatment feels like admitting defeat. It is for this reason that it may be helpful to decide early on—even before starting treatment—what type of treatment you would like to pursue and how far you will go. It is also important to revisit this decision from time to time along the way. Your experiences during your treatment may be different than what you expected. Often there is intense pressure to keep going ahead, and you may quickly pursue one cycle after another. This approach works for some people, but may end up making you miserable if you feel that you are on a treadmill and cannot get off. Sometimes a doctor will suggest that you take a break, but more often than not couples feel propelled forward by their own wishes.

If you are not sure when to stop, it may be helpful to take a break for a few months and allow your life to settle back into its normal shape. This is a good time to again explore the meaning and importance of having a child. How has pursuing infertility treatment affected your life? What have you had to give up? With these things in mind, do you still want to continue treatment? This is also a time to start thinking about other options. Here is a list of signs that it may be beneficial for you and your partner to take a break from treatment.

- If you feel that you are just going through the motions of treatment and have lost sight of your original goals.

- If you and your partner are experiencing more tension or are drifting apart.
- If it is difficult for you to relate to anybody other than your partner or your infertility team, or you are avoiding your friends and family.
- If you have given up activities that you used to enjoy.
- If infertility is interfering with your ability to work and to derive pleasure from your work.
- If you are in debt and can no longer afford treatment.
- If the fertility drugs are causing significant physical or psychological side effects.
- If you are showing signs of depression or significant anxiety.

Pregnancy After Infertility

The good news is that many couples become pregnant with or without treatment. The bad news is that while pregnancy is an event viewed with much happiness and considerable relief, the experience of pregnancy may not be entirely positive and may be colored, at least to some degree, by your previous experiences with infertility. Many women with infertility problems continue to experience significant emotional distress during pregnancy. Most of all, they worry about losing the baby. A fair number of women with infertility have had repeated miscarriages, and it can be particularly difficult for them to feel confident that the pregnancy will succeed. While this fear is the most intense during the early stages of pregnancy, this is a concern that may be difficult to give up, even as the pregnancy progresses, and it may not fully disappear until after delivery when a woman is able to hold her baby in her arms.

More so than women who conceive naturally, women who become pregnant after infertility treatment tend to be more focused on their bodies and are more likely to worry about any unusual physical symptoms that may occur during pregnancy. They worry that something may be wrong with the baby. Their anxiety may be intensified by the fact that many women who have become pregnant through artificial reproductive technology (ART) may be considered to be a high-risk pregnancy, based either on their age or other complications associated with their infertility treatment. The experience of having a high-risk pregnancy is undoubtedly distressing, and for women who have experienced infertility, this may generate feelings of sadness or anger over the inability to have a "normal" pregnancy. The risk for preterm labor is also higher in women with a history of infertility, particularly if they are carrying multiples. Bed rest, especially when it is prolonged, is disruptive and emotionally draining; it intensifies a woman's feelings of vulnerability and reinforces the notion that the pregnancy is more fragile and less likely to succeed.

Even after you become pregnant, being an "ordinary" pregnant woman may not be so easy. Visiting your obstetrician monthly will probably seem odd, as compared to what you experienced during infertility treatment. Without your infertility treatment team, you may feel as if you have lost a large chunk of your support system. Remembering how difficult it was for you to spend time with your pregnant friends when you were *not* pregnant, it may feel awkward to share your excitement with your nonpregnant friends who are continuing their infertility treatment. On the other hand, after finally getting pregnant, you may feel that you do not deserve to complain about anything and it may also be difficult to express any less-than-excited or ambivalent feelings about your pregnancy.

Are You Depressed?
Even though you may work very hard to manage the stress of infertility, it is possible that you may become depressed. This is no fault of your own. If you are experiencing problems having a child, you should remember that this is one of the most stressful experiences for a woman. Even the strongest and most resilient may experience depression when forced to endure such significant demands on their emotional and physical resources.

Unfortunately, the problem of depression among infertile couples has been, up until very recently, ignored. Several recent research studies indicate that women who suffer from infertility are vulnerable to significant depression or anxiety: among women who undergo infertility treatment, it is estimated that about 25 percent to 30 percent suffer from clinical depression. That's about a twofold to threefold increase in risk for depression among women of childbearing age. While any woman may become depressed, research indicates that certain women appear to be more likely to experience significant emotional problems. Women who are younger seem to find the experience to be more stressful, especially if no cause for the infertility can be identified. In addition, if you practice a religion that places an emphasis on childbearing, it also may make it more difficult to accept your situation, and if your religion prohibits the use of infertility treatments, this may make the situation worse. Not surprisingly, the women who have experienced infertility for a longer time or have undergone more years of treatment seem to be the most vulnerable. Rates of depression are very high in women who have received three or more years of treatment.

But perhaps the most vulnerable in this situation are those women who have a history of depression. The stress associated with infertility and its treatment can be a potent trigger for depression, and many women who have been treated with an antidepressant discontinue this treatment while receiving infertility treatment, further increasing their vulnerability to depression. As we discussed earlier, this group of women may also be more likely to experience the mood-altering effects of infertility drugs.

Many women with infertility who develop depression view this as a natural response to being infertile rather than a separate problem that must be addressed. They are often overburdened with the intensity of the process, and many women are understandably reluctant to seek treatment for their depression and to add yet another doctor to their list. Although counseling is usually available to women undergoing infertility treatment, most do not take advantage of this option.

The symptoms of depression in this situation are identical to those discussed in chapter 2. You may feel sad or down a great deal of the time, or you may find that you have lost interest in your usual activities. You may notice changes in your appetite, have problems sleeping, or complain of feeling tired all the time. Although depression can be quite severe, sometimes it may be very difficult to figure out if you are depressed. Are the feelings of loss you contend with normal or are they a sign of depression? What about those feelings of hopelessness you have after a cycle fails? Is that depression? In the midst of infertility treatment, all of your regular routines are disrupted and there may simply not be time for you to pursue the activities you usually enjoy. It may be difficult for you to be around other people as you go through this ordeal. But does that mean you are depressed? The answer is not always obvious. You are experiencing a constellation of feelings that you most likely have never dealt with before, and it may take a while to figure out if this is a normal response to a difficult situation or something more serious.

The warning signs below may not mean you are depressed, but they do signal a significant amount of distress. It may be helpful to meet with a mental health professional.

- If you find it difficult to control your emotions and spend a lot of time crying.
- If you are having problems functioning at work or at home.
- If you find that your relationship with your partner is deteriorating.
- If you are feeling very irritable and have more difficulty getting along with others.

- If you are feeling persistently hopeless.
- If you are thinking about death or about killing yourself.

If you are experiencing any of these problems, you should ask your obstetrician for referral to a specialist experienced in working with women who suffer from infertility. Infertility clinics often have social workers or psychologists available to meet with patients who are receiving treatment. Another resource you may consider is RESOLVE; this organization maintains lists of mental health professionals who work with women and couples who have infertility problems. In chapter 12, you will find more information on how to find a professional who is appropriate for you.

You don't have to be profoundly depressed to ask for help. Often women are reluctant to share their feelings with others because they are afraid the intensity of their emotions may overwhelm or overburden them. Psychotherapy or counseling gives you a place to discuss your sadness and the other difficult feelings you may have with somebody who can be understanding and supportive. Therapy may also help you figure out better ways to relate to others in this situation and find other ways to support yourself.

When a depression is very severe or does not respond to psychotherapy, you may consider using an antidepressant. However, women who are actively pursuing infertility treatment are understandably reluctant to take any medications, including medications to treat their depression. They are afraid to jeopardize their chances of becoming pregnant or are fearful of the effects that a medication may have on their baby or on the viability of the pregnancy. While there is no data on the impact of these antidepressant medications on fertility in women, it is reassuring to note that women who take these drugs do often become pregnant while taking them. Although many antidepressants may have a negative effect on sexual functioning in women, causing lowered libido and difficulties attaining an orgasm, there are no reports in the literature to suggest that antidepressants reduce fertility.

A full course of treatment may last six months or longer, so many women feel that they have to choose between treating their depression or pursuing infertility treatment. Some women decide to suspend their infertility treatment while completing a course of antidepressant therapy. However, you should know that it is possible to take certain antidepressants during pregnancy. In chapter 13, you will find information regarding the safety of medications commonly used during pregnancy. Although you may ultimately decide not to use medication, it is important to know what your options are. You should not simply assume that nothing can be done about the way you feel.

The Importance of Protecting Your Emotional Well-Being

Infertility is an event that challenges your sense of yourself and your visions for the future. It puts a strain on even the strongest relationships. Remember that depression, although a common problem in this setting, is not normal and may further accentuate the strain of infertility and its treatment. However, the stress of infertility *is* manageable. Using the techniques outlined in this chapter, you and your partner can learn to cope with infertility and its treatment.

Chapter 5

Unexpected Tragedies
Coping with Pregnancy Loss
and Other Complications

Although most women have some worries about their pregnancy, in most cases there is the expectation that pregnancy will proceed without significant problems. Women are aware that there may be some physical discomfort or other minor difficulties along the way, but most women expect that they will have a healthy baby. Unfortunately, this is not always the case; some women encounter significant complications during their pregnancy. While many of these problems are relatively benign, others may threaten the pregnancy or place the unborn child and/or the mother at risk. Any complication—benign or life-threatening—may dramatically affect how you experience your pregnancy.

About 15 percent to 20 percent of pregnancies are not carried to term. Most pregnancies are "miscarried," or lost, early during the first trimester, while a smaller number of losses occur later during pregnancy. Other losses may occur while the baby is very young, within a few weeks of delivery. While the experience of losing a pregnancy is relatively common, the emotional repercussions of this event are frequently overlooked or neglected. Whether the loss occurs early or late, whether this is the first pregnancy or one of many, the loss of a pregnancy is described by most women as an event that causes significant emotional distress. Most women are eventually able to negotiate the loss and to move forward; however, many others may find it difficult to disentangle themselves from this painful event. And for some, the loss of a pregnancy may lead to a more profound and persistent state of depression. The first step in dealing with such a painful loss is learning to tolerate and express your intense and sometimes overwhelming emotions. Most women are eventually able to move beyond the loss and are able to lead happy and fulfilling lives. Relying on your inner resources and the support of others, you will find how you can best cope with the various problems that you may encounter during pregnancy and minimize the effects of these events on you, your family, and your plans to have a baby.

Prenatal Testing: Good News or Bad News

Over the last several decades, our ability to detect medical problems in the unborn child has improved considerably. Long before the baby is born, we are now able to know much about her health and well-being. A fetal heartbeat can be detected as early as six weeks. Later on, an ultrasound may be used to get a closer look at the developing fetus. Most women view the ultrasound as one of the highlights of their pregnancy—their first glimpse of their baby. While this is an event that most women look forward to, it may also bring with it some uncertainty. Will everything be okay? What if there is a problem with the baby? Most of the time, the ultrasound is normal. Having this piece or information can be tremendously reassuring and can help to relieve many of the anxieties you may have had early on in the pregnancy. After crossing this hurdle, you are likely to feel more confident that things will work out and that your baby will be healthy.

But what happens if some of these screening tests are abnormal? Ultrasounds are very sensitive and can detect a wide range of congenital malformations (birth defects). Down syndrome, as well as many other types of genetically inherited diseases, may be picked up with amniocentesis or chorionic villus sampling (CVS). If the tests indicate a problem that is very severe or compromises the chances of your baby surviving, you and your partner may have to make the difficult decision of whether or not to proceed with the pregnancy. Although you may ultimately decide that it is the best decision for your family, terminating a pregnancy under these circumstances is a traumatic experience. However, making the decision to proceed with the pregnancy may be just as painful, as you must come to the realization that you may give birth to a child who may die shortly after birth or may suffer from illness or disability the rest of her life. The decision may be even more difficult when the results of a particular test are uncertain. For example, these tests often provide little information on the severity of a particular illness, and you may find yourself struggling to guess how the illness will affect your child.

Carrie was thirty-eight. Her obstetrician recommended that she have an amniocentesis, and she knew she was at higher risk for having a child with Down syndrome but she was not prepared to discover that her child had another type of chromosomal abnormality called Turner syndrome.

Although Carrie and her husband initially thought they would terminate the pregnancy if there was a problem, it did not feel right to have an abortion knowing that their child could possibly lead a happy, satisfying life. They were told that their baby was likely to be short in stature and to be infertile, but they were also given a long list of other less common problems their child might have: heart malformations, obesity, high blood pressure, orthopedic problems, an increased risk of certain types of cancer. Carrie and her husband made the decision to continue the pregnancy, but initially Carrie felt very sad. It was hard to imagine that this child would have such a hard life and might not be able to do the things that other children get to do. Over time, however, she started to feel more optimistic about her situation. She and her husband learned more about Turner syndrome, and began to work out ways they could help their child reach her full potential. By the time Carrie delivered, she was excited about having a child.

Unfortunately, prenatal testing is not a perfect science, and sometimes these tests generate information that is ambiguous or difficult to interpret. For example, ultrasounds are very sensitive and can detect structural abnormalities that have no impact on the baby's health, such as a deposit of calcium in the baby's heart or an unusual collection of fluid in the baby's kidney. Although these may be associated with a serious problem in some cases, they are often inconsequential findings. Amniocentesis is used to detect problems like Down syndrome, but sometimes it reveals rare genetic abnormalities that we know much less about. Parents are thus left with the knowledge that their baby is not "perfect" but do not know the significance of this imperfection.

Although an abnormal test finding does not always signify a life-threatening or chronic problem, it is difficult to come to terms with the fact that there may be something wrong with your baby. You may find it difficult to emotionally invest in your pregnancy, and you may feel detached or disconnected. You may also find yourself dealing with intense feelings of sadness and loss. Whether the problem is relatively benign or more severe, it is experienced as a significant loss. You had hoped to have a healthy baby, and that wish was not granted. While this type of information is difficult to come to grips with, it does give you an opportunity to prepare yourself and your family, so that you can give your new child what she needs. Even under these difficult circumstances, it is possible to be happy and excited about the birth of your child.

Coping with Other Complications
Although many pregnancies are relatively problem-free, a fair number of women experience serious medical or obstetric complications. Although

modern medicine can do much to limit the occurrence of serious and potentially life-threatening problems during pregnancy, many complications simply cannot be prevented. During the first trimester, a significant number of women develop severe nausea and vomiting and about 1 percent of women suffer from a more intractable pattern of vomiting called *hyperemesis gravidarum*. Gestational diabetes and high blood pressure are relatively common problems encountered during the latter half of the pregnancy. Near the time of delivery, women are at risk for preterm labor and delivery, as well as other serious complications, such as preeclampsia and eclampsia, conditions characterized by high blood pressure and other potentially life-threatening problems for the mother and her baby.

Fortunately, most of the problems women encounter during pregnancy, like gestational diabetes, come on gradually and do not, with appropriate treatment, present an imminent threat to the pregnancy or the woman's life. Nonetheless, experiencing these medical complications is stressful. If you are having any type of medical problem, it is likely that you will find yourself worrying more about your pregnancy and the well-being of your unborn child. It may be difficult to be optimistic and you may even blame yourself for what is happening. For example, women who develop gestational diabetes may feel very guilty, convinced that they have not been responsible with their diets. Some women who experience premature labor believe that they brought it on by being either too physically active or too emotionally reactive, even though in the vast majority of cases these factors do not play any role.

There are also medical emergencies, such as preeclampsia or premature labor. When these occur, there is little time to analyze the situation and to react to it. After the fact, you may end up feeling a sense of emotional overload, as you come to grips with what did happen or what could have happened. You may remain cautious or apprehensive for a period of time, fearful that you may encounter more problems. Or you may end up feeling numb or somehow disconnected from the people around you. It is likely to take some time to fully recover, and many women find that these painful memories are easily triggered, even long after the event has occurred.

Whether the problems you experience are relatively benign or very serious, they can transform what is supposed to be a wonderful experience into something that is much more complex. Rather than being able to focus on the pregnancy and to fully invest in it, you must devote a certain amount of your mental energy to these other issues. You may feel that you have been deprived of the pregnancy you had imagined and expected, and in confronting this reality, you may experience feelings of sadness, anxiety, frustration, and possibly anger.

Bed Rest

Many women at some point during their pregnancy are put on either partial or total bed rest. It is often recommended when women show signs of premature labor, but there are also a broad range of medical conditions that might prompt your doctor to recommend bed rest. These include high blood pressure, preeclampsia, bleeding, and cervical problems (such as an incompetent cervix). If you are carrying multiples or are at risk for premature labor, your doctor is likely to recommend bed rest during the last weeks of your pregnancy. Bed rest might also be recommended if you have had previous pregnancies that ended in a premature birth or fetal loss.

While some women seem to tolerate or even enjoy bed rest, it may cause significant stress for others. If you are aware early on in the pregnancy that you may need to go on bed rest at some point, you will have at least some time to prepare yourself and to put things in order before you go on bed rest. In the majority of cases, however, you are forced to go on bed rest immediately and without warning. Being unexpectedly pulled out of your everyday activities can cause a tremendous amount of stress and chaos. While trying to take care of yourself, you undoubtedly will also have to spend much of your time trying to reorganize your life. If you already have children at home, it may be particularly difficult to give yourself time to rest, and they may be unable to understand your limitations. You may also feel very guilty that you are not able to spend more time with them. When it feels that there are still many things to accomplish before having your baby, you may feel like you are unprepared for the birth of your child.

The range of activities you will be allowed to pursue depends on why bed rest is recommended. Some women are on very strict bed rest and may only get up to use the bathroom, while others may enjoy a broader range of activities. But even when there is a rather liberal definition of bed rest, it can take a toll on a mother's emotional well-being. If you are stuck at home, it is almost impossible to maintain a social life or pursue the activities that you normally enjoy. Without these diversions, you may end up feeling isolated and bored. When you are alone and without enough to engage your mind, you may also find yourself worrying excessively. Being cut off from social activities and the usual routines can lead to depression and feelings of hopelessness.

Twin and Multiple Pregnancies

Thanks to artificial reproductive technologies, multiple pregnancies are becoming increasingly common. Although for most couples with infertility, having more than one child is a welcome thought, having twins or multiples is never easy. Multiple pregnancies are by definition high risk, and a multiple pregnancy is often associated with various problems, including premature labor and delivery, low birth weight, various complications at delivery, and medical problems in the newborns. Having a high-risk pregnancy is potentially very stressful, and, under these circumstances, the fear of losing the pregnancy may be quite intense.

One of the difficult decisions many couples confront in this situation concerns fetal reduction, the targeted removal of one or more of the fetuses during the first trimester of the pregnancy. Given the risks associated with carrying multiples, fetal reduction is often recommended for women carrying three or more children. While this is a common, highly successful technique, it causes much emotional distress. While you may be able to rationally accept that fetal reduction may lead to a significantly better outcome for your pregnancy and for your children, this procedure may seem to run counter to your goal of having a child and it may be a violation of your personal or religious beliefs. Making this decision can be excruciating, and many couples feel that they are placed in an untenable situation where they are being asked to sacrifice one of their babies to ensure the safety of the others. Most women undergoing this procedure view fetal reduction as a traumatic event and experience feelings of sadness, loss, and guilt. While this type of grief may be particularly intense during the pregnancy, it seems to resolve more completely after the birth of the remaining child or children. The good news is that most women do well in the long run, and few have any long-lasting effects.

Premature Delivery

About 6 percent to 8 percent of women deliver prematurely (before week 37 of gestation). Low-birth-weight infants are more common in women who have undergone infertility treatment, especially if they are carrying twins or multiples. Other causes of premature delivery include cervical and uterine abnormalities, infection, and other medical problems, including high blood pressure and diabetes. While modern medicine often performs miracles and has significantly improved outcomes in low-birth-weight and premature infants, babies born under these circumstances have more medical problems and require specialized care. If you give birth to a child prematurely, you are likely to feel considerable and sometimes overwhelming anxiety. You may wonder if your baby will survive. Is the baby putting on enough weight? Will he have any lasting effects? You may be deluged with information and be forced to make difficult decisions regarding your child's medical care. Many parents describe feeling numb, especially during the early days and weeks of their child's life. It is only much later that the reality of their situation starts to sink in.

Like many mothers who give birth prematurely, you may feel guilty, convinced that you did something that caused this unfortunate outcome. You may also feel frustrated that you were not able do anything to prevent this. It is difficult to feel so helpless; there is nothing you wouldn't do to help your child, yet there is very little that seems under your control. When faced with a baby who appears so small and so fragile, it may be very hard for you to feel competent and confident in your new role as a mother. You may also feel a sense of grief. You had hoped that you would have a healthy baby; there is nothing more painful than to see your child suffer.

Making the Decision to Terminate a Pregnancy

The decision to terminate a pregnancy is never easy, and some women who have an abortion continue to have intense feelings about their decision long afterward. It can be even more distressing when it leads to disagreement or conflict between you and your partner, or if you have strong religious or personal beliefs regarding abortion. Abortion is a tremendously controversial topic, and women may feel uncomfortable discussing it with others. Abortion can generate feelings of sadness, self-doubt, shame, and guilt, but with time these feelings usually subside.

Taylor was forty when she became pregnant for the second time. She and her husband had been trying to get pregnant for the past year and they were delighted to discover that Taylor was pregnant. Although Taylor had felt well during her pregnancy, the ultrasound revealed that the baby had several serious birth defects. Even with surgery, the doctor said, the baby's chances of survival were not good. Taylor and her husband made the difficult decision to terminate the pregnancy. They felt that they did not have the emotional or financial resources to care for a child with a significant disability. Taylor had wanted a child so badly, and she felt as if somebody close to her had died. She felt horrible telling their son that he would not have the little brother he had been asking for. Her feelings of loss were further intensified by the fact that they knew, given Taylor's age, that they would probably never have another child. Although many friends and family members knew Taylor was pregnant, Taylor and her husband did not feel that they could talk openly with them because they were worried about the reactions others might have regarding their decision to have an abortion.

Most women who terminate a pregnancy do so because the pregnancy is unwanted or unplanned. Other women terminate a pregnancy because the baby has a serious medical problem or because the pregnancy threatens the mother's health. For many women, terminating a pregnancy that is desired and planned for is a devastating event. Many of these terminations take place later in the pregnancy, usually in the second trimester. At this stage, there is often a stronger attachment between the parents and their unborn child; thus, the sense of loss is often more intense. Late-term abortions, where labor is induced and the fetus is delivered, seem to be particularly traumatic. One study indicated that as many as 95 percent of mothers and fathers experience significant psychological difficulties, including depression, irritability, loss of self-esteem, and marital problems, in the months following a second-trimester abortion. The good news is that, for most, this intense grief resolves over time.

Miscarriage

A miscarriage, or what doctors call a spontaneous abortion, is a relatively common event. Approximately 15 percent to 20 percent of all documented pregnancies end in miscarriage, and the risk of losing a pregnancy is probably even higher. Some experts believe that as many as half of all pregnancies are lost, with most of these miscarriages occurring before the mother is even aware that she is pregnant. Miscarriages usually occur unexpectedly, without any real warning signs. With a miscarriage, a woman may experience bleeding, with or without some cramping. However, many women have no symptoms whatsoever; at a regular visit with their obstetrician, it is determined that there is no detectible heartbeat or that the fetus has failed to develop properly.

Miscarriages occur most often during the first trimester, before the twelfth week of pregnancy. Although the risk of losing a pregnancy declines significantly as the pregnancy enters into the second trimester, pregnancy losses do occur during the later stages of pregnancy. When a pregnancy is lost after the twentieth week or when the baby shows no signs of life at the time of delivery, doctors call this a stillbirth. This type of loss occurs much less frequently than miscarriage but is by no means rare. In fact, in the United States there is about 1 stillbirth for every 115 live births.

There are many different reasons for a woman to miscarry. The single most common cause for a miscarriage is a chromosomal abnormality in the fetus. In the majority of cases, the parents' chromosomes are normal, but at some point in the fertilization process, there is either a duplication or elimination of certain essential chromosomes. These abnormalities in the genetic material make it impossible for the fetus to mature normally. Miscarriages may also occur when there are hormonal, anatomical, or immune abnormalities. Women with certain illnesses—for example, diabetes, lupus, and high blood pressure—have a higher risk for miscarriage. Women who are either very young or older (over forty) are more likely to have miscarriages. Also women who conceive using assisted reproductive techniques are at higher risk for miscarriage.

In general, if you have had only one miscarriage, an extensive workup will not be performed. Doctors assume that this is an unfortunate but not unusual outcome of pregnancy and odds are that you will have a normal pregnancy the next time around. If you are healthy and have had only one miscarriage, your chances of having a healthy pregnancy are the same as those of a woman who has never miscarried. However, if you have had two or more miscarriages, it will usually be recommended that you undergo a more thorough evaluation to determine the cause. About 1 in 100 women have recurrent miscarriages, or what is called fetal loss syndrome, a topic that will be discussed in greater detail later in the chapter.

The Emotional Aftermath of Miscarriage

Many people fail to recognize that just because miscarriage is common it is not without significant emotional consequences. Whether the loss occurs early or late, whether this is the first pregnancy or one of many, a miscarriage can be devastating. After a miscarriage, it is normal to feel sad. Yet many women are surprised to find how deeply a miscarriage affects them. Even when the pregnancy has lasted for only a few weeks, this is more than enough time to become emotionally invested in the pregnancy. Your connection to your child is felt deeply and may be as strong as your connections to other people in your life. No matter when or why it occurs, miscarriage is a significant loss. Not only have you lost the child that you have hoped for and dreamed about, your dream of becoming a mother has also been threatened.

After getting married, Debbie and her husband Chris waited several years to have a baby and were excited to find out that Debbie was pregnant. Debbie felt great but around the eighth week, she started to have some bleeding. Although her obstetrician tried to reassure her that bleeding was not always a sign of a problem, it became heavier and a few days later, they were not able to find a heartbeat on the ultrasound. Debbie was crushed. She had so looked forward to having a baby and had so many fantasies about what it would be like to take care of her child. Now it was difficult to imagine that she would ever be a mother. Her feelings of guilt and responsibility for the miscarriage were overwhelming. Over and over again, she enumerated all the things she had done wrong during the first weeks of her pregnancy. She had continued to jog and work out. Maybe she put in too many hours at work. On a few days, she was so busy she skipped lunch. She sometimes forgot to take her prenatal vitamins. And why had she and her husband waited so long to have a baby? Often she felt furious; she just could not understand why this had happened to them.

Why me? You are certain to ask this question; everybody does. It is natural to try to understand why bad things happen. It's how we learn to accept our experiences, and it also helps us to feel more in control of our lives. Many women who have had a miscarriage spend a great deal of time trying to figure out exactly why the miscarriage occurred. Although you may be given a medical explanation for what might have taken place, you may not be satisfied and may search for other ways to explain the loss. Unfortunately, this process of questioning easily drifts into self-blame and feelings of guilt. Did the miscarriage occur because you were under too much stress? Did you not sleep enough? Was it because you had sex a few days before the miscarriage? It is very unlikely that you did anything to contribute to the loss of your pregnancy.

Many women believe, at some level, that they are being punished for something that they have done. You may wonder if you lost the pregnancy because at first you had some ambivalent feelings about being pregnant or you did not want the baby enough. Or you may believe that the miscarriage is some type of message; maybe you should not or do not deserve to be a mother. Are you being punished because you had terminated another pregnancy several years ago? Although these sorts of questions may be quite irrational, you may still find yourself replaying over and over the events of your miscarriage as you try to find an explanation.

After a miscarriage, you may also have a different sense of yourself. While pregnant, you may have envisioned yourself as being full of potential, having the awe-inspiring power to carry and bring forth a child. After losing a pregnancy, you may be left with the feeling that something is wrong with you—that you are unhealthy or deficient in some way, unable to do what other women can do. These feelings may creep into other aspects of your life, making you feel less confident in yourself at work and at home, with your partner and with your friends.

Multiple Miscarriages

For the approximately 1 percent of women who have recurrent miscarriage (defined as three or more miscarriages), there is most often an identifiable cause—anatomical, hormonal, immune, or environmental. In many cases treatment may help to correct the problem. It is estimated that 60 percent to 70 percent of women who have recurrent miscarriages will go on to have a healthy pregnancy.

Women who suffer recurrent miscarriages have the same kind of emotional responses to these repeated losses as women experiencing only one miscarriage. However, these painful feelings are often more intense. As a woman tries over and over to become a mother, her self-esteem suffers tremendously, and it is easy to lapse into feelings of hopelessness and despair. Pregnancy becomes something yearned for, yet many women who have had multiple miscarriages actually start to dread getting pregnant, as they are so fearful of suffering another loss. Like those who suffer from infertility, women who have experienced multiple miscarriages may reach a point beyond which they cannot go. There is a limit to the number of losses that one can endure, and after experiencing one miscarriage after another, it may be necessary to take a break or to pursue alternatives.

As recurrent miscarriage is more of a chronic condition, the grieving process may be more prolonged and more difficult to resolve. Given the intensity of psychological distress that may persist over a long period, women who have recurrent miscarriages are particularly vulnerable to depression. Several recent studies indicate that about a third of women with recurrent miscarriage experience clinically significant depression. Even among women who already have children, the levels of distress and anxiety are intense and can interfere significantly with a woman's ability to function.

The Process of Grieving for Your Loss

After you have lost a pregnancy, there is no "right" way to respond. Everybody reacts differently, and how you respond will be colored by your own personal experiences and will depend in part on the other losses you may have suffered. It is important to remember that after you have lost a pregnancy, recovering is a gradual process, one that involves many different steps: accepting and mourning the loss, learning not to blame yourself, seeking support from others, regaining your sense of health and well-being, and allowing yourself to be hopeful about the next pregnancy. For some this process may occur relatively quickly; for others the process may take longer.

Grief is not just feeling sad. It is a complicated, sometimes prolonged process by which you learn to cope with a loss and ultimately to move beyond it. Usually the term refers to the complex and painful feelings that come to the surface after the death of a loved one, but grief occurs after any type of loss. Although losing a pregnancy is not exactly like losing a loved one, many of your feelings may be similar and perhaps as intense. The process of grieving requires time, patience, and the support of others. Although some people think of grieving as being an excessively morbid or self-indulgent exercise, you can reassure yourself that it is a natural response to a loss. It is important not to resist or try to suppress your feelings, though when you allow yourself to experience these strong emotions, it may be quite frightening. You may feel that your emotions are totally out of control. You may wonder if things will ever get better. Although the pain may be very intense and all-consuming in the beginning, it becomes easier to bear as time goes on.

It is normal to feel numb at first. Yesterday, you were on your way to having a baby and today you are not. At first, you may be unable to comprehend what has happened, and it may take some time to adjust to the new reality. Over time you will become more aware of your sadness and a sense of loss. In fact, you may go through a period where you find yourself totally preoccupied with your loss, and it may be difficult to focus on other things. During this time of intense grieving, you may notice some changes in your sleep patterns, either difficulty falling asleep or waking up in the middle of the night. You may have dreams or nightmares about your pregnancy and the events leading up to and including the loss. You may lose your appetite. You may feel fatigued, with little energy to carry out your usual activities. It may be more difficult to concentrate on other things. You may find yourself withdrawing from other people. All this is normal. When you are in this stage of grieving, it is hard to imagine that you will ever feel better, that you will ever be able to get on with your life.

You may also experience feelings of emptiness. The pregnancy was part of you, and losing that part of you may make you feel incomplete. Although being a mother is only one aspect of your identity, it may be difficult to find pleasure or satisfaction in your other pursuits. When compared to being a mother, they may seem unfulfilling or meaningless. And it is hard to imagine that, without a child, you will ever feel happy again.

You may also find yourself feeling quite angry, and it is often difficult to figure out what to do with your anger and where to direct it. Your body? Your circumstances? Your doctor? Losing a pregnancy simply isn't fair! It is perfectly understandable and appropriate that in this situation you feel anger or even rage. With no clear target for your anger, it may end up seeping into other aspects of your life. You may find yourself having outbursts of anger, often with no clear reason or seemingly out of proportion to the event at hand. And even though you know it is irrational, you may find yourself feeling envious of and angry at those women around you who are pregnant or have children. Anger is one of the most difficult emotions to deal with. Many women are uncomfortable expressing their anger; they are ashamed or frightened by these intense feelings, and they feel out of control. But remember that communicating these strong feelings is an important part of the grieving process.

While your partner is affected by the miscarriage, he may experience a less intense grief reaction. A mother feels a profound sense of loss whether a miscarriage occurs early or late. For the father, a pregnancy usually feels less tangible, especially in its earliest stages. The intensity of a father's response to this loss is determined by how far the pregnancy has progressed and how attached he is to the pregnancy; a father is more deeply affected by a miscarriage if he has had the opportunity to hear the baby's heartbeat or if he has seen the baby on a sonogram. Nonetheless, fathers tend to talk less about miscarriages than mothers and tend to keep their feelings to themselves. They are usually able to return to their normal routines more quickly. If your partner's response is less intense than your own, you may feel that he does not understand what you are experiencing or you may feel that he is insensitive or uncaring. Your relationship may become strained; however, many couples find that such a crisis may help to bring them closer together.

With time, you will move toward acceptance of the loss and will be able to settle back into your life. It is unlikely that you will completely obliterate these painful feelings, but you will eventually be able to give them their allotted space in your emotional life. You will be able to think about the loss without having it overwhelm you, and you will be able to imagine a future for yourself and your family. For most women, the manifestations of grief tend to wane over time. The symptoms of grief after a miscarriage typically last about six months to a year and do not usually affect your ability to function for a prolonged period of time; however, some women may have a grief reaction that is more intense or more prolonged. When the grieving process seems unbearably intense or seems to persist for a longer period of time, this may be a sign of what is called "pathological" or unresolved grief, or this may be an indication that depression has complicated the picture.

Why It May Be Difficult to Grieve After a Miscarriage

Most miscarriages occur without warning. While many women, in the back of their minds, are aware that there is some risk of a miscarriage, they do not have the chance (or the inclination) to prepare emotionally for this loss. In most cases, there is usually no advance warning. A miscarriage is usually not a gradual thing, it just happens: one day you are pregnant, and the next day you're not. When such a significant loss occurs so suddenly, you are caught off guard, and it may take much longer than you expect to adjust.

The loss is somewhat ambiguous. With a miscarriage, there is no tangible object to grieve for. There is no "baby"; you have never met the child that you have lost. In this sense, mourning is much more complicated. Your loss lacks clear boundaries, and it may be quite difficult to fully comprehend the extent of it.

Most women mourn for their miscarriages alone. In most situations, miscarriages occur early, before you may have had the chance to tell others that you are pregnant. On the surface, this decision to keep this painful experience to yourself may seem protective. You do not have to discuss your painful loss with a lot of people; however, this may deprive you of emotional support and impede the grieving process. In general, it is difficult to grieve alone. Losses bring up feelings of loneliness and isolation; grieving done alone may intensify these painful feelings. While much of your grieving may take place privately, it is helpful, at least some of the time, to share your pain with others.

Others may not be able to understand your loss. It may also be difficult to mourn because those around you may not consider miscarriage a "real" loss. On one level, it may be encouraging to hear from your doctor that a miscarriage is a common event, but your doctor's words may make your loss seem less important, or even trivial. You might find yourself asking, "If so many women have miscarriages, does it really make sense to feel so sad about it?" Women often comment that their friends and family members seem to minimize the emotional impact of their situation. Even your part-ner may not be able to understand exactly how you feel. You may want a place to express your sadness, yet what you hear from your friends and fam-ily is "Don't worry, you can always try again." Or some people may appreci-ate the sadness you feel but still not be able to help you talk about it. They may be worried about how you will respond and are unsure that they would be able to comfort you.

Pregnancy After Miscarriage

You will get your first period four to eight weeks after you have a miscar-riage. At this point while you may be physically ready to try again, you may not be ready emotionally. Especially when a woman is in her thirties or for-ties and is concerned about the steady ticking of her biological clock, she may feel a pressure to try again as soon as possible. However, many women need more time to recover. How long you should wait is not well defined. You should allow yourself time to grieve, which typically takes anywhere from a couple of months to a year. Not doing so can cause problems later on. If you are still grieving when you are pregnant, it may be difficult to fully invest in the pregnancy. You may feel somewhat detached from your preg-nancy and it may be difficult to feel excited about having a child. When a pregnancy follows soon after a miscarriage, women may find themselves thinking about the new baby as a "replacement" for the one lost. While this may be a natural response, it does not allow the new child to develop his or her own individual identity in your mind.

Even when you think you have recovered from a miscarriage, there may be a situation or an event—the due date of the baby you lost, the anniversary of the miscarriage—that stirs up strong emotions. This is normal. Although the painful feelings that you experience after a miscarriage will never be completely erased, there will come a time when it feels right to try again. At this point, you will feel that you are ready to love another child and that you are strong enough to accept any disappointments you may encounter.

Although pregnancy is the desired outcome, it may generate unexpected distress. Once you have had a miscarriage, you may view your new preg-nancy as being more tentative or more fragile, and you may be more anx-ious or apprehensive this time around. You try to protect yourself from getting too excited about the pregnancy until you pass a certain point, the end of the first trimester or the time at which you had the miscarriage dur-ing your last pregnancy. As you cross this line, you may find some relief, but it may be difficult to fully let down your guard and to trust that everything will work out.

Many women find it helpful to share their concerns, especially with other women who have had a similar experience, and there may be support groups in your community for women who have suffered from a pregnancy loss. However, if you feel that your anxiety is interfering with your ability to enjoy your pregnancy or other aspects of your life, it may be helpful to meet with a professional to discuss your concerns.

Ectopic Pregnancy

An ectopic pregnancy occurs when the fertilized egg is implanted outside of the uterus, usually in the fallopian tube but occasionally in the abdomen, ovaries, or cervix. As the pregnancy grows there can be pain, bleeding, and, in the worst case, rupture of the fallopian tube, making this a life-threatening condition. An ectopic pregnancy may occur when there is blockage of or damage to the fallopian tube, as may occur when women have had endometriosis, pelvic inflammatory disease, or prior abdominal surgery. Infertility treatment can also increase the risk of ectopic pregnancy. Since 1970, the risk of ectopic pregnancy has been increasing, and it is now estimated that about 1 percent to 2 percent of all pregnancies are ectopic.

Having an ectopic pregnancy is a frightening and emotionally wrenching experience. Once discovered, an ectopic pregnancy must be terminated; the fetus cannot develop to term outside the uterus. The longer such a pregnancy progresses, the greater the risk to the mother. After an ectopic pregnancy, you will take some time to recover, physically and emotionally. Doctors usually recommend that you wait three to six months before trying to conceive again. If you have undergone surgery, even if it was laparoscopic surgery (which is less invasive than a major operation), you must understand that your body has just suffered a tremendous insult and it will take you several months to return to your usual self. Many women experience abdominal discomfort for a prolonged period, and this may also make it difficult to return to your usual activities. You may also experience symptoms that are the result of the hormonal shifts that take place after a pregnancy is lost, including night sweats, hot flushes, sleep disturbance, and fatigue.

Although for most women the physical recovery proceeds without complication, your emotional recovery is likely to take much longer. Because an ectopic pregnancy is, in most cases, a medical emergency, you will not have had a chance to prepare for this event, which can make the emotional recovery more difficult. To further complicate matters, the medical aspects of an ectopic pregnancy often overshadow its emotional consequences. During the first few weeks after an ectopic pregnancy, you will have to tend to your physical well-being. In the weeks following this event, you may feel numb or confused by what has happened, but after the reality of your experience begins to set in, you may find yourself grappling with more intense and painful emotions. This is a significant loss. Others may tell you that you should feel lucky, that you have survived a potentially life-threatening situation. You survived, but you have lost your pregnancy. And this loss is likely to bring up many painful feelings for you. You will likely go through a period of grieving for your pregnancy, experiencing many of the intense emotions we discussed earlier in this chapter. Your recovery is contingent upon allowing yourself the time to go through this grieving.

As you come to grips with your experience, you may wonder if you will ever be a mother. You may have sustained some damage to your fallopian tubes or ovaries, and you may worry that this may make getting pregnant harder. You may worry that you will have another ectopic pregnancy. If you have had one ectopic pregnancy, your chance of having another is about 20 percent. If the pregnancy was life-threatening or was followed by any medical complications, you may not be able to embark upon another pregnancy without significant anxiety. After such an experience, many women wonder if they should *ever* try to conceive again; some women ultimately decide that it is not worth the risk.

Stillbirth and Neonatal Death

While most pregnancies are lost early on, a small but significant number of pregnancies are lost during the third trimester. *Stillbirth* refers to a pregnancy that is lost after 20 weeks of gestation or when the baby dies near or at the time of delivery. The causes of stillbirth are different from those of early pregnancy loss. Often there is a problem with the placenta or the umbilical cord. Severe birth defects may cause stillbirth. In about 50 percent of cases, no specific cause can be identified. When the baby is born alive but dies within the first four weeks of life, this is called a *neonatal death*. Each year in the United States, about 1 in 19,000 babies dies within one month of delivery. About 25 percent of neonatal deaths occur when the baby is born with a severe birth defect. Babies born prematurely, especially those under 26 weeks of age, are also at higher risk for neonatal death. Other causes of neonatal death include abnormalities of the placenta or umbilical cord, complications during delivery, and infection.

Losing a child during the later stages of pregnancy or shortly after birth is a devastating experience. Childbirth is experienced as a tragic event. In most cases of stillbirth, there is no warning of a problem, and the loss of the pregnancy comes as a tremendous shock. With prenatal diagnostic techniques, including amniocentesis and ultrasound, it may be possible in some cases to detect a problem before the time of delivery, such as a severe birth defect that may increase the risk of a stillbirth or neonatal death. This may give parents a chance to prepare to some degree and may help to initiate the grieving process. But no matter how much time you have to prepare for this event, losing a baby in the first hours or days of his or her life is a heartbreaking experience.

This loss is similar to miscarriage, but with some important differences. You, your family, your friends, and your coworkers are all expecting that the baby will be born and you have made plans surrounding that date. You have started to prepare, or to make plans for, your baby's nursery. Perhaps you have chosen a name. Because the pregnancy has gone on for some time, your connection with your baby and your sense of yourself as a mother have had a chance to grow in complexity; this baby has become very much a real part of your life and you have formed a powerful bond with your child. When you lose a baby at this late stage, it feels like your life has been totally derailed.

The feelings you will experience after a stillbirth are similar to those that occur after any type of significant loss, and you will go through a process of grieving as described earlier in this chapter. Undoubtedly during the first days and weeks after your baby's death, you will be in shock. There is no way you could have ever prepared for such a catastrophe, and it will take some time to fully believe that you have lost your baby. It may be particularly hard to accept that the baby is not with you because you will physically feel as if you have just had a baby. And your body will be undergoing the physical changes that occur after delivery. In addition, you may find yourself on a maternity ward, where mothers around you are caring for their newborns.

Eventually intense feelings of sadness will come to the surface. After a stillbirth or a neonatal death, there will be a period of time when you are preoccupied with your baby's death, reliving over and over again the events surrounding the loss. It may be difficult to sleep. Some women describe having recurrent vivid dreams or nightmares about their baby. Even though there is no baby around, you may sometimes hear a baby crying. During this time, it may be difficult to feel close to other people and to feel pleasure in your usual activities. When you have suffered such a traumatic loss, everything else seems less important.

As you go through this grieving process, you will also find yourself asking why this happened and perhaps analyzing the events leading up to the birth. You may ask yourself whether you did anything to cause the loss. Were you too active during the last weeks of the pregnancy? Was it the flu you had? Was some problem missed during your last prenatal checkup?

Anne's pregnancy was difficult in the beginning; she had a lot of nausea and felt extremely fatigued, but she felt well for the remainder of her pregnancy. In week 39 she went in for her obstetric visit. The doctor could not find a heartbeat and informed Anne that her baby had died. The reason for the death was not obvious. Anne looked back over the last week and struggled to understand what had gone wrong. She had moved a bookshelf on Monday. She had forgotten her prenatal vitamin on Tuesday. She slept only for five hours last night. Then she realized that she could not clearly remember if the baby had moved over the last day. She felt devastated. Her baby had died, and she hadn't even noticed. What would have happened if she had come in earlier? Could the baby have been saved?

After an autopsy was performed on the baby, Anne was told that there was a blood clot in one of the major blood vessels of the umbilical cord, which cut off the blood supply to the baby. The doctor reassured her that it was a random event, and that she had done nothing to cause the problem. Still Anne blamed herself for not monitoring the baby's movements more closely. Perhaps the outcome would have been different if she had come to see the doctor earlier.

Many women, as they attempt to make sense of their loss, hold themselves responsible for the death. It is so easy to blame yourself for what happened, especially when it is not clear exactly what did happen. Even when a cause is identified, often there is room for self-blame, however unjustified. In almost all cases of stillbirth or neonatal death, it is unlikely that anything you did caused or contributed to your baby's death. While it may feel like a relief to not hold yourself responsible for this loss, it is also extraordinarily difficult to feel so incredibly helpless. You are supposed to be able to protect your baby from harm, and so this loss may call into question your ability to be a responsible parent. As you try to come to grips with what happened, you may find yourself wondering if there was anything that you or your doctor could have done differently.

It may be helpful to meet with your doctor to discuss your baby's death. With this information, you may be better able to understand your experience and to make a coherent story of why and how your baby died. After a stillbirth or a neonatal death, you will be asked if you want an autopsy performed on your baby. Sometimes families elect to forgo this procedure; however, an autopsy can provide you with useful information about what went wrong and whether this problem is likely to occur again. If so, what can you do to prevent it from happening in the future? In addition, having a medical explanation for what happened can help to alleviate feelings of guilt and self-blame and may help you to feel more in control of your situation.

Commemorating Your Loss

After the death of your baby, the hospital staff may encourage you to see and to hold your baby. While it is believed that this practice helps the parents to say good-bye to their child, some women may find this experience emotionally distressing and may decide that they do not want to see or hold their baby. You may instead decide to keep some sort of memento—the blanket your baby was first wrapped in, a lock of his or her hair, or an imprint of your baby's hand or foot. These special items can be very important and serve as tangible evidence of your baby. Many hospitals bathe and dress the baby and take a photograph. Although you may not want this, most hospitals keep these photographs on file should you change your mind later on. There are many ways for you to acknowledge and to remember the loss of your baby; ultimately, you should do what feels the most comfortable to you.

You will probably be encouraged to set up a funeral or some type of memorial service for your child. Although this process may be extraordinarily painful, many parents find that it is necessary and helpful to bring closure to an important chapter in their lives. Some parents may opt for a traditional funeral; others may choose a more private way to commemorate their baby's death. Again there is no "right" way to handle this emotionally wrenching situation; you and your partner should choose to do what makes the most sense to you.

Resuming Your Life

You have spent months preparing for the arrival of your child. What do you do when there is no baby? You will need time to heal physically, but your emotional recovery will undoubtedly take much longer. As your grief starts to subside, you may start picking up more of your usual activities. You may think of meeting up with some of your friends. Eventually you may think about returning to work or your other activities. But everything is different now, and it may be difficult to imagine getting back into the stream of things.

One of the most difficult things about resuming your life is figuring out how to tell others what happened. People's reactions will vary. You will probably find some friends and family members who understand your grief. However, most people have a hard time discussing death, and particularly the death of a child. They feel overwhelmed and do not know what to say or do. Unable to find the right words to comfort you, they may back away, change the subject, or say the wrong thing. Friends or family who are expecting or have recently had a child may not be able to tolerate hearing about your situation. While it is difficult to talk about your loss with your close friends and family, it may be impossible to imagine sharing this most private and personal experience with neighbors, more distant acquaintances, or coworkers. Not knowing you as well, these people are likely to assume that you've been busy taking care of your new baby, so their well-meaning comments may seem especially intrusive and insensitive.

A caring and compassionate environment is essential. This is why many women find it helpful to join a support group. Although it may be your first instinct to bottle up these painful emotions, it may help tremendously to meet and to talk with other women who have had a similar experience. Sharing your emotions with others who can understand the magnitude of your loss can go a long way toward your recovery.

Pregnancy After Stillbirth or Neonatal Death

After experiencing a stillbirth or a neonatal loss, it may take some time to feel that you are ready to attempt another pregnancy. There is no need to rush. Although you may feel some pressure to quickly try again, it is important to allow yourself enough time to recover both emotionally and physically. A recent research study found that women who became pregnant less than a year after a stillbirth were more likely to have problems adjusting to the subsequent pregnancy and experienced more symptoms of depression and anxiety than women who waited longer to conceive.

Going through a pregnancy following a stillbirth can be an emotionally challenging experience. Because there is no point at which you can feel "safe" about the pregnancy, it is difficult to reassure yourself that the pregnancy will end with a healthy child; you are likely to be more vigilant and on the lookout for any type of problem. Under these circumstances, you may notice that it is more difficult to invest in this pregnancy and to let yourself be happy and excited about having a child.

If you are experiencing anxiety, it may come in many different forms. You may worry only about your pregnancy, or the anxiety may spread into all domains of your life and you may find yourself feeling tense or on edge. One recent study from St. George's Hospital in London indicated that, among women who have experienced a stillbirth, 1 in 5 suffers from posttraumatic stress disorder (PTSD). With PTSD, not only do you experience generalized feelings of anxiety, you repeatedly reexperience the traumatic event. The symptoms of PTSD might include flashbacks of the event, panic attacks, nightmares, and difficulty eating or sleeping. These PTSD symptoms seem to be particularly common in those women who conceive sooner (within one year) after having a stillbirth. Reassuringly, these symptoms seem to disappear almost completely after the birth of another child.

Unresolved Grief and Depression

Though emotional distress in pregnancy loss is normal, some women may develop more persistent or disabling psychological symptoms. While these symptoms typically start to subside, at least to some degree, within a few weeks of the loss, others may experience a more prolonged or intense reaction. Some women experience what is called pathological, or unresolved, grief. In this situation, a woman will have a more protracted period of mourning and is unable to separate her loss from other aspects of her life. She may feel intensely guilty about the loss, convinced that she did something to bring about the event or that there was something she could have done to prevent it. She may also spend more time thinking about death and may wonder what the purpose of living is. She may feel worthless. Although any woman may suffer from unresolved grief after the loss of a pregnancy, it is more likely to occur when a woman has planned a pregnancy for a very long time or if it has taken a long time or a great deal of effort to get pregnant. It is also more likely to occur if a woman has had other losses in the past.

Depression may also complicate the picture. One study found that during the six months following a miscarriage, about 10 percent of women showed signs of depression. Based on a study conducted by Dr. Richard Neugebauer and his colleagues at the New York State Psychiatric Institute, it appears that any woman can develop depression after a miscarriage; however, women who have a history of depression prior to pregnancy and women who do not have adequate social supports are more likely to develop depression as a consequence of miscarriage. Not surprisingly, women who already had children seemed to fare much better than those who were childless. Experiencing a stillbirth or a neonatal death probably puts you at even higher risk for depression; one study indicated that a mother's risk for depression after a stillbirth is about seven times higher than a woman who has a live birth. The symptoms of depression and anxiety generally subside following the loss, but 10 percent to 20 percent continue to experience significant symptoms at eight months after the loss.

It is often beneficial to talk to a counselor or therapist who has experience in working with women who have had similar experiences. You should consider meeting with a mental health professional if:

- you are concerned that you may be depressed.
- your symptoms interfere with your ability to function at home or at work.
- you are having problems in your relationship with your partner.
- you are experiencing intense feelings of hopelessness or suicidal thoughts.
- you find yourself using alcohol or recreational drugs to make yourself feel better.

When depression is severe or the symptoms do not respond to support or counseling, you may want to consider antidepressant medication. Although antidepressants are highly effective and relatively well tolerated, many women are reluctant to take antidepressants after a pregnancy loss, particularly if they are planning to attempt another pregnancy. Some women may defer a pregnancy so that they may get treatment for their depression, but more often women do not get adequate treatment in this situation. After a loss, many women are more apprehensive about pregnancy and understandably have concerns about taking a psychotropic medication while pregnant or attempting to conceive, although there is data to support the reproductive safety of certain antidepressants. (In chapter 13, you will find more information on the treatment of depression in women who are pregnant or attempting to conceive.)

How to Make the Grieving Easier

Try not to blame yourself. It is very easy to blame yourself when you lose a pregnancy, especially when you are not sure exactly why it happened. However, blaming yourself is not productive and will only hinder the grieving process. Remember that everyday emotional or physical stressors do *not* cause pregnancy loss. It is very unlikely that you did anything to harm your pregnancy. Remind yourself that a pregnancy loss typically occurs when there is something wrong with the baby or when the pregnancy is unlikely to come to term. It is not your fault.

Allow yourself to express your feelings.   There are many barriers that stand in the way of your emotional recovery. In the short run, suppressing your feelings may seem like the easiest, most comfortable option. However, when you take this approach, the feelings never really go away and may start to interfere with other aspects of your life. When you allow yourself to experience these feelings, you may wonder if things will ever get better. Although the pain is very intense in the beginning, it becomes easier to bear and subsides in its intensity over time.

Build a support network.   It is important to find people you feel comfortable talking to. Although we tend to function with the assumption that those who are closest to us are the best able to recognize and respond appropriately to our sadness, this is not always true. While some friends and family members may be very sensitive to your loss, others may not know how to respond or how to comfort you. You may need to find other sources of support.

- As clearly as you can, let others know what you need from them. You may just need a shoulder to cry on, not words of advice or encouragement.
- Let others know when they are making you feel worse rather than better.
- Join a support group. This is an opportunity to meet other women who have experienced the same type of loss.
- If you need more individual support, consider meeting with a therapist.

Read.   There are many books that deal with miscarriage, stillbirth, and neonatal loss. Reading about the emotional experiences of others may help you to feel less isolated. In addition, learning more about what causes pregnancy loss and other types of complications may help you to free yourself of unnecessary blame.

Establish a ritual to commemorate the loss of your baby.   Rituals are extremely important and help bring closure to a painful loss. Unfortunately, we do not have a culturally sanctioned way to commemorate the loss of an unborn or newborn child in our society. Many couples find it helpful to create their own ritual to mourn this loss. Although you may choose a traditional funeral or memorial service, there are many different ways to remember this loss: lighting a candle, writing in a journal, planting a tree. You should choose some way to commemorate the loss that feels right to you.

Depression Should Never Be Ignored

Many different types of complications can occur during pregnancy and childbirth, and many women do not have the healthy child they had dreamed of. When such a devastating loss occurs depression is a common response. There is an unfortunate tendency to think of depression as a natural or predictable consequence of pregnancy loss, and many women who become depressed after such a loss do not receive adequate attention. However, depression is never normal and it can impede the process of recovery, making it impossible for you to move on with your life.

Chapter 6

A Not-So-Rosy Blush
Depression During Pregnancy

While you may have intense feelings of happiness and excitement during your pregnancy, you may also experience less expected emotions, including anxiety and sadness. Pregnancy is a bit like a roller coaster; it is a time of tremendous change, both physical and psychological. While life transitions may bring happiness, they also have the potential to cause enormous stress. During these times of transition women are most vulnerable to emotional problems. Superimposed upon the psychological transition you must undergo during pregnancy are the dramatic hormonal shifts that may also make you more susceptible to depression and anxiety. While most pregnant women describe at least some mood changes, about 10 percent to 15 percent of women suffer from clinical depression during their pregnancy, a condition known as *antenatal depression*.

Hormonally Driven Mood Changes

Within several weeks of conception, even before a pregnancy test is positive, you may begin to appreciate some subtle physical changes that indicate you are pregnant. Fatigue and morning sickness are typical. You may also notice breast tenderness or unusual cramping. Very early on in the pregnancy, you may experience a change in your appetite and may find yourself having unusual food cravings or aversions. During the first trimester, long before your body starts to show obvious signs of the pregnancy, you may also experience some mood changes. Your emotions may seem unstable or more intense, and feelings of joy and excitement may be mingled with other more unexpected or distressing feelings. Sometimes you may find yourself crying without any clear reason, and it may be difficult to explain why you feel so upset. When you are pregnant, you may feel exquisitely sensitive to rejection or criticism and you may feel that those around you, especially your partner, are uncaring, unsupportive, or unable to comprehend what you are going through.

The mood changes a woman commonly experiences during pregnancy may be caused, at least in part, by dramatic shifts in her hormones. During pregnancy, estrogens are produced by the placenta and their levels increase about a thousandfold; progesterone rises to about four hundred times its pre-pregnancy levels. While these hormones are normally produced—albeit in smaller quantities—by the ovaries in nonpregnant women, this tremendous escalation in estrogen and progesterone levels early in pregnancy may be mood altering.

That said, keep in mind that we cannot blame *everything* on hormones. Even fathers, who obviously do not experience the same hormonal changes, are vulnerable to mood swings during their partner's pregnancy. Needless to say, pregnancy is a time of immense change and uncertainty. While there is the sense that something wonderful is about to happen, not being able to predict exactly what the future holds and how you will respond may feel overwhelming. You may feel that you are being pulled in many different directions.

The intense feelings you experience during pregnancy may be complicated and sometimes difficult to navigate. Almost all women carry some ambivalence about their pregnancy. Even women who have wished for and carefully prepared for the pregnancy may find themselves having second thoughts. Was this the right decision? Was this the right time? When you are pregnant, you will find yourself focusing on the future and how your life will change after the baby is born. You may be looking forward to having a child, yet at the same time, you may also be aware of the many things you will have to leave behind and the sacrifices you will have to make. Ambivalence is expressed by many pregnant women, but it is a sentiment that causes anxiety, guilt, and sometimes despair.

For some women, this level of emotional upheaval is particularly unsettling; it feels uncomfortable to be so out of control. While these mood swings may take a toll on your sense of stability, they are usually relatively short-lived and absolutely normal. Although this first trimester often feels like a roller coaster, most women seem to fare a bit better during the second trimester. When people refer to that rosy glow, it is the second trimester they are talking about. It is during this time that many of the uncomfortable physical symptoms of early pregnancy subside and most women begin to feel more energized and optimistic.

Many women describe feeling more calm and contented during the middle portion of their pregnancy. As you pass into the second trimester, the risk of miscarriage diminishes, and you may find that, with these worries about losing the pregnancy behind you, it is easier to fully invest in and to be excited about the pregnancy. With a more obvious bulge in your belly and the baby beginning to move around, the pregnancy begins to feel real. While this shift in your outlook may help to relieve anxiety, levels of the steroid hormone progesterone also rise significantly, and it has been shown that progesterone and its metabolites, pregnanolone and allopregnanolone, have a Valium-like effect on your brain and help you to feel more relaxed.

During the last weeks of pregnancy, as you anticipate the birth of your child and all the changes this will bring, you may experience more anxiety. As your due date approaches, you will probably discover that you have less energy, and it may become more difficult to be productive. At this point it may also be especially difficult to concentrate, and distractibility and forgetfulness are common complaints during the third trimester. It is almost impossible to sleep comfortably during the last few weeks of the pregnancy. After about nine months of pregnancy, most women are quite ready to have a baby.

Depression Is a Common Problem

Pregnancy is most commonly described as a time of joy and excited anticipation. It seems that as soon as someone notices you are pregnant, they start to gush: "How wonderful! You must be so happy." Every pregnancy and parenting magazine is full of images of smiling and rosily blushing women, their hands resting calmly on their pregnant bellies. Yes, this is a happy and exciting time. However, not every pregnant woman is happy all the time. In fact, a surprising number of women become significantly depressed during pregnancy. So why don't we ever hear about them?

Although most women and the physicians who care for them have some awareness of postpartum depression and approach the postpartum period with heightened vigilance, they rarely consider pregnancy as a time when women may be at risk for emotional problems. Several recent studies have challenged our conception of pregnancy as a time of constant emotional well-being and have demonstrated that women are highly susceptible to depression both before *and* after birth. In a recent study published in the *British Medical Journal*, researchers surveyed more than 12,000 women during pregnancy and after childbirth. What they discovered surprised many health care professionals. A significant proportion of the women were identified as being depressed during pregnancy: 11.8 percent were depressed at 18 weeks of pregnancy, and at 32 weeks 13.6 percent showed signs of depression. Most striking, 25 percent of the women had symptoms suggestive of depression at some point either during pregnancy or after delivery.

Another study from Dr. Sheila Marcus and her colleagues at the University of Michigan yielded similar findings. In this study, among 3,472 women screened in an obstetrics clinic, 20 percent showed signs of depression. Both of these studies clearly indicate that depression is a problem that affects an astonishingly large number of childbearing women.

While this research has attracted a great deal of media attention, that significant numbers of women suffer from depression during pregnancy is not news. In the late 1980s, Dr. Ian Gotlib in Great Britain reported that in one study about 10 percent of pregnant women had significant symptoms of depression. In 1990, Dr. Michael O'Hara at the University of Iowa confirmed these findings and identified several risk factors for antenatal depression. It is surprising that many studies have demonstrated that women are at risk for depression during pregnancy, yet no matter how many times this finding is replicated, women and the doctors who care for them are often unaware or unwilling to accept that depression may occur during pregnancy.

Why Is Depression During Pregnancy So Frequently Overlooked?

Though we know that depression is relatively common among women during pregnancy, only a fraction of the women who suffer from depression are ever diagnosed, and even fewer ever receive any type of treatment. Probably one of the most significant barriers to the recognition of depression during pregnancy is the stigma attached to the condition generally and to the cultural idea of a "normal" pregnancy being a happy one. Women and their families are reluctant to label any pregnancy-related mood changes, even when relatively severe, as depression. Although now we have a more sophisticated understanding of depression as a biological or medical illness, many women still feel that being depressed reflects some sort of weakness or character flaw.

Health professionals also seem to overlook depression during pregnancy. In the vast majority of cases, depression during pregnancy goes undetected and untreated. In the study from Dr. Sheila Marcus described above, only 13.8 percent of the pregnant women who were depressed received any type of formal treatment, despite regular visits with an obstetrician. Many obstetricians, like other health care professionals, have received only the most rudimentary training in the area of mental health and are unable or uncertain how to diagnose depression or similar problems in their patients. Frequently when a woman turns to her doctor to share her concerns about her emotional well-being, she receives support and reassurance. Too often her complaints are downplayed, the implication being that depression is a transient and relatively benign experience, something that will pass with time. Unfortunately, this is *not* usually the case.

How to Recognize Depression

Part of our failure to recognize depression during pregnancy may reflect our inability to fully understand the condition. What exactly is depression? At one point or another, everybody has thought or said, "I'm depressed" or "I'm feeling really down." However, as discussed earlier, clinical depression is not merely having a bad day or feeling upset about a specific something. Depression is a more pervasive, persistent feeling of sadness that does not seem to lift and lasts for weeks or months at a time. Depression affects how you think, how you act, and how you interact with others. Although all types of depression share common features, what makes depression so difficult to recognize is that it may be described in so many different ways. To make the diagnosis, doctors must rely on identifying a constellation of symptoms characteristic of depression. (In chapter 2 you will find a detailed description of the many signs and symptoms of depression.) A woman who is depressed may describe herself as feeling sad or blue, or she may notice that she is more negative or uncharacteristically critical of herself and everything around her. She may merely complain of feeling apathetic, that she is no longer able to enjoy things the way she used to. Sometimes it is difficult to precisely define the problem.

Anita was thirty-two years old and pregnant for the first time. She was very excited about the pregnancy; she and her husband had been trying for some time. Unfortunately, the first few weeks of the pregnancy were horrible. She had such severe morning sickness that she could barely function. By the end of the first trimester, the nausea and vomiting had stopped, and Anita started to feel that she had a little bit more energy, though she just did not feel right. Usually Anita enjoyed her work, but now she found it totally overwhelming. Several times each day she found herself crying, usually for no clear reason. At the end of the day, she returned home expecting to feel better, but she felt even worse. Even relatively simple tasks, like making dinner, seemed too difficult. She tried to do things to make herself feel better but nothing interested her and nothing seemed exciting or worth pursuing.

Her friends called, but she often found it difficult to answer the phone. She dreaded telling her friends and family about the "good" news. She just couldn't bear the thought of them being so excited about her pregnancy when she felt so miserable.

Anita even started avoiding her husband. He was excited about the pregnancy and spent a good deal of time talking about the baby. She couldn't understand why she felt down and disconnected from her pregnancy. For as long as she could remember, she wanted to be a mother. Now she felt ashamed about her feelings of uncertainty, and her husband's enthusiasm about the pregnancy annoyed her and made her feel worse. She just wanted to go back to the way things used to be. She was not happy and, at some level, felt that the pregnancy was to blame for her misery.

Every time Anita looked at another pregnant woman, she was envious. They looked healthy, happy, and excited. She joined a yoga class for pregnant mothers but had to quit after only a few sessions. Among the other women she felt like "the bad mother." Sometimes she would look at her husband and think, *Do you know what you've gotten yourself into? I don't think I can be the mother you expect me to be.* Pregnancy was something she had hoped for, yet she felt she had made a terrible mistake and, worst of all, there was no going back.

When depression occurs during pregnancy, it may elicit intense feelings of shame or guilt. How can you understand or explain feeling depressed at a time when you are expected to be happy? Depression is so commonly viewed as a sign of weakness that you may think that something is wrong with you, that you are unsuited or unprepared to be a mother. You may find it difficult to be around others because you do not feel that you can share in others' excitement about your pregnancy. Worst of all, you may start to believe that your feelings are so alien and unacceptable that you cannot share them with others, not even your partner.

If the depression is very severe, you may feel hopeless. While you may not entertain thoughts of killing yourself, you may find yourself thinking about being in a serious accident or succumbing to a life-threatening illness. People who suffer from depression often have thoughts of death or dying, and expectant mothers are no exception. Understandably you may feel quite ashamed to talk about feelings that seem so contrary to how you are expected to feel during pregnancy. However, under no circumstances should suicidal thoughts be considered a normal consequence of pregnancy. If you are having these thoughts, this is a serious problem you should discuss with your physician immediately.

When depression occurs during pregnancy, you may look back and recognize that you were feeling much better and happier before you became pregnant; under these circumstances, you may find yourself thinking, If only I weren't pregnant, I would feel so much better. Believing that they have no other options, some women find the depression so unbearable that they come to the conclusion that the only way to solve the problem is to terminate the pregnancy. This is a tragedy, as depression is a treatable illness, and even women who are severely depressed may go on to have healthy and happy pregnancies when they get the treatment they need and deserve.

Are You Depressed or Just Pregnant?

It is often difficult to identify depression when it occurs during a pregnancy. If you have suffered from depression in the past, you may be better able to interpret the emotional changes you are experiencing and to label them as depression. However, if you have never experienced depression before, you are more likely to downplay your symptoms or to attribute them to your pregnancy, unless the depression is particularly severe. Especially if this is your first pregnancy, it may be difficult to distinguish what is just part of a "normal" pregnancy from a more serious problem.

Many of the physical symptoms of depression—including fatigue, loss of libido, appetite changes, and sleep disturbance—also occur in pregnant women who are *not* depressed, further confusing the picture. In addition, certain medical conditions commonly seen in pregnancy may produce symptoms that mimic depression. For example, anemia (or a low red blood cell count), when severe, may cause extreme fatigue, lethargy, and loss of libido, as well as feelings of depression. During pregnancy, about 1 in 50 women also suffers from hypothyroidism, a deficiency of thyroid hormone. The most common symptoms associated with hypothyroidism are fatigue, weight gain, loss of libido, and depression. Both of these conditions are serious but easily treated medical problems. If you come to your obstetrician with complaints of depression, you need more than reassurance and a referral to a therapist. You deserve a thorough medical examination to exclude any medical problems that may be masquerading as depression.

So how can you tell if you are depressed? What may help distinguish clinical depression from the normal mood changes that take place during pregnancy are the negative patterns of thinking and behavior that often come along with depression. If you are depressed, you are less able to take pleasure in your usual activities and you may have to push yourself to do things. It is often difficult to think positively about the future, and you may find yourself dwelling on your current problems and worrying about others that may arise in the future. On the other hand, if you are experiencing what would be considered a "normal" pregnancy, you may feel tired and a bit slowed down, but you are able to function relatively well. You want and are able to do the things you usually enjoy. And, although at times you may not feel so well, you can focus on the more positive aspects of your life and can look with optimism to the future.

Pregnancy may generate many worries, and it is absolutely normal to have questions about how things are going to work out in the future. You may wonder if the baby will be healthy or if there will be any problems during labor and delivery. Will you be able to handle everything? How will you be able to afford having a child? How will having a child change your life? These worries are all normal and do not necessarily signify that you are depressed. In general, if you feel these anxieties are manageable and that somehow things can be worked out, this is a good sign. However, if these concerns seem overwhelming and if they interfere with your ability to function or to enjoy yourself, depression may be an issue.

How Depression Can Affect Your Pregnancy

While depression may not make a pregnancy "high risk," it is clear that being depressed during pregnancy may have serious consequences for the mother and her pregnancy. Depression may affect how a woman cares for herself during pregnancy, and what a woman does or does not do may have an impact on the well-being of her developing child. For example, when a woman is depressed, she is less likely to comply with her obstetrician's recommendations. She may find it difficult to follow a well-balanced diet or to exercise. She may miss or delay some of her prenatal visits. Even a woman who is normally conscientious about her health may not have the energy or the motivation to properly care for herself when she is depressed.

Depression and anxiety may significantly affect appetite. While most women experience increased appetite and food cravings during pregnancy, women with severe depression or anxiety often complain of loss of appetite. This is even more of a problem for women who suffer from significant nausea or vomiting during the first trimester. In severe cases, a woman may actually lose weight during pregnancy. When the mother does not gain sufficient weight during pregnancy, her infant develops more slowly and tends to be underweight at birth. There is evidence to suggest that women with depression and anxiety may give birth to babies who are smaller and who weigh less. While these smaller babies tend to catch up relatively quickly within the first few months after delivery, they may be more vulnerable later to other health problems that are more common among low-birth-weight babies.

Women with depression are also more likely to smoke. Tobacco use, particularly when heavy, is associated with lower than expected birth weight and prematurity. Sudden Infant Death Syndrome (SIDS) is also more common in infants whose mothers smoke while pregnant. Despite well-publicized campaigns to reduce alcohol and drug use during pregnancy, pregnant women who are depressed are at risk for abusing alcohol and recreational drugs. Even small quantities of alcohol consumed during pregnancy—as little as one glass of wine each day—can lead to significant problems in the baby, including fetal alcohol syndrome, developmental delays, learning disabilities, and behavioral problems. Similarly, using illicit drugs also places the pregnancy at risk. Lower than expected weight gain is observed in infants exposed *in utero* to marijuana, heroin, cocaine, and amphetamines. Premature delivery is more common in women who have used cocaine during pregnancy. The long-term consequences of these exposures are complex, with several studies demonstrating developmental delays and learning disabilities in children whose mothers used various recreational drugs while pregnant.

It is clear that depression may result in behaviors that place the pregnancy at risk; however, many experts feel that depression itself may actually bring about certain physiological changes. For example, several studies suggest that women with depression may be at greater risk for preterm labor and delivery. In a recent study conducted in France, of 634 pregnant women, those with higher levels of depression were twice as likely to have preterm labor (defined as labor occurring before 37 weeks of pregnancy) than non-depressed women. Similarly, higher levels of anxiety were also associated (although to a lesser extent) with preterm labor. The link between depression and/or anxiety and preterm labor was strongest in women who had other risk factors for preterm labor (for example, women with low weight prior to pregnancy or a history of preterm labor). However, not all studies have demonstrated higher rates of preterm labor in women with depression. In addition, certain pregnancy complications, including preeclampsia, may also be more common. Women with depression during pregnancy are more likely to give birth to newborns with lower birth weight and smaller head circumference, even when the pregnancies are carried to term.

Depression may also have more subtle effects on the baby. One of the most interesting studies comes from Boston University, in which Dr. Barry

Zuckerman and his colleagues examined 1,123 women and their infants. They observed a strong correlation between depression during pregnancy and newborn irritability. Women who had been depressed during pregnancy were more likely than women who were not depressed to have infants that were inconsolable or cried excessively. The more severe the mother's depression, the more likely it was that their infant would be irritable. This finding is interesting for several reasons. There is plenty of evidence that maternal depression negatively affects a child after he or she is born (discussed in detail in chapter 3); however, this is the first study to show us that mood changes that take place *during* pregnancy may also have an impact on the infant's well-being and behavior. The results of this study also suggest that early childhood problems, which are common in women with depression, may be triggered much earlier than suspected.

The mechanism by which maternal depression can lead to these problems is not yet fully understood, but depression may be associated with certain physiological changes that negatively affect the pregnancy. In patients with depression, these effects on physical well-being are probably mediated by changes within the hypothalamic-pituitary-adrenal (HPA) axis, the system that governs the body's response to stressful situations and controls the fight-or-flight response. When a person is depressed, the HPA axis is activated, not just for a few minutes or hours, but for months at a time. The high levels of stress hormones, including cortisol and adrenaline, produced may affect the placenta, decreasing the flow of nutrients to the developing fetus. High cortisol levels may also play a role in preterm delivery. Furthermore, there is evidence from both animal and human studies that exposure to these high levels of stress hormones *in utero* may lead to long-term changes in the architecture of the developing fetal brain and may alter a child's sensitivity to stressful stimuli in the environment long after he or she is born.

What Causes Depression During Pregnancy?

While other illnesses associated with pregnancy—such as gestational diabetes or hypertension—are viewed with relative neutrality, it is frequently assumed that depression is a reflection of a mother's willingness or capacity to be a mother. Indeed, early psychoanalytic theories tended to view depression in childbearing women as an outward manifestation of a woman's negative or ambivalent feelings regarding motherhood. These early theories helped to foster the view of the depressed mother as unprepared, uncaring, or, at the worst, unwilling to be a mother. It is no wonder that most women who suffer from depression during pregnancy end up feeling ashamed and guilty about how they feel and are hesitant to share their thoughts with others.

All too often, women believe that their ambivalent feelings about their pregnancy may have caused their depression. In fact, many pregnant women have ambivalent, or even negative, feelings about their pregnancy and about becoming a mother; these feelings are absolutely normal and are not necessarily a precursor to depression. Even those women who are unwaveringly positive and excited about their pregnancy can become depressed. What you need to know is that, while these less than elated feelings may be quite unsettling or upsetting, they do not necessarily interfere with your becoming a capable and caring parent.

So why do women become depressed when they are pregnant? Probably the factors that lead to depression in a pregnant woman are similar to or the same as the factors that cause depression in a woman who is not pregnant: genetic makeup, early childhood experiences, and stressful life events. Stress plays an important role here. For example, having a pregnancy that is either unexpected or unwanted may cause significant distress for the mother and her partner. Although it is not necessarily a recipe for depression, some studies do suggest that depression may be more common among women who have unplanned pregnancies. In an unplanned pregnancy where both partners ultimately come to accept and cherish their new situation, the outcome may be much better than when the pregnancy is not welcomed by either the woman or her partner.

Women who complain of marital problems or dissatisfaction are more likely to suffer from depression during pregnancy, and women who suffer from depression during pregnancy more frequently describe having inadequate social supports. Victims of domestic violence are clearly at high risk for depression. Also vulnerable are those women who are young and unmarried. Not only are single women forced to contend with the demands of having a child without the support of others, they are more likely than their married counterparts to take on this challenge while being economically disadvantaged.

Similarly women who have experienced stressful events during pregnancy, such as the loss of a loved one, unemployment, or financial difficulties, are more likely to develop symptoms of depression. Although most studies have focused on stressful events unrelated to the pregnancy, there is evidence that pregnancy-related events may also cause significant stress and place a woman at risk. Women who have medical complications during pregnancy are probably at higher risk for depression than those women who have uncomplicated pregnancies.

In many cases, a combination of factors seems to contribute to the depression. It may be difficult to indicate a specific factor as a precipitant; it seems that merely being pregnant is enough to trigger an episode of depression in some women. Probably the most important risk factor for depression during pregnancy is a history of depression *before* pregnancy. Although a pregnancy may be a welcomed and joyous event, it may act a physiological, hormonal, or psychological stressor that triggers depression. At highest risk are those women with a history of severe or *recurrent* depression. But even when a woman has experienced a long period of emotional well-being prior to her pregnancy, she is more vulnerable to depression than a woman who has never suffered from depression.

One population that appears to be particularly vulnerable to depression during pregnancy is women who have had more severe or more recurrent forms of depression and who have taken antidepressants on a long-term basis. In a recent collaborate study from Dr. Lee Cohen at the Center for Women's Health, Dr. Zachary Stowe of the Women's Mental Health Program at Emory University, and Dr. Lori Altshuler of the Mood Disorders Research Program at UCLA, 201 women with histories of depression were followed throughout their pregnancy. About 68 percent of the women who stopped their medication developed depression during pregnancy. Many women who have taken antidepressants struggle with the decision of whether or not to continue their antidepressant medication during pregnancy and, given the limited data regarding the reproductive safety of these medications, are advised by their doctors or ultimately choose to discontinue treatment. However, this study tells us that women with severe or recurrent depression are particularly vulnerable to depression when they stop their medication. And even when a woman has experienced a long period of emotional well-being prior to her pregnancy, she is more vulnerable to depression than a woman who has never before suffered from depression. Fortunately, there are antidepressant medications that may be used during pregnancy (see chapter 13).

Any woman may develop depression during her pregnancy, but if you answer "yes" to any of the following questions, you may be at higher risk for depression during pregnancy. Keep in mind that while these questions may help to indicate who is more susceptible to depression, it remains difficult to reliably predict who will suffer from depression during pregnancy and who will do well.

Are You at Risk for Depression During Pregnancy?

Do you have a history of depression or bipolar disorder?

Do you have a history of anxiety disorder, such as panic disorder or OCD?

Do you have a family history of mood or anxiety disorder?

Have you had any problems with alcohol or substance abuse?

Do you have a history of childhood sexual or physical abuse?

Have you been a victim of domestic violence?

Are you experiencing difficulties with your partner?

Are you unmarried, separated, divorced, or widowed?

Was this an unplanned or unexpected pregnancy?

Do you have a history of miscarriage or fertility problems?

Have you had any significant medical complications during your pregnancy?

Is your baby at risk for any medical problems?

Have you recently experienced any stressful life events, such as unemployment, financial
  difficulties, or the loss of a loved one?

Helping Yourself

There are many things you can do to feel better if you are depressed. The first step is coming to grips with how you feel. Every day there is somebody asking you how you feel and expecting an upbeat answer. What you really want to say is "rotten," but nobody wants to hear that. So what can you do? First of all, recognize that depression is not a sign of weakness and does not indicate that you are unfit to be a mother. Depression is a biological illness, just like diabetes or high blood pressure, and occurs because you probably have inherited some genes from your parents that make you more vulnerable.

When you are feeling depressed, it may be particularly helpful to seek out emotional support. Some women find it helpful to pursue activities specifically directed to pregnant women, such as exercise groups or childbirth education programs. While these activities may go a long way to reduce the isolation that some women feel so keenly when they are depressed, this approach may not work for every woman. When you are feeling so horrible, it may be too uncomfortable to socialize with a group of pregnant women who seem to be doing well emotionally. You need someone you can speak to honestly and openly. When you are depressed, things feel out of control, making it easy to feel hopeless and helpless. You may feel like retreating and waiting for things to get better; however, there are steps you may take that will help you take more control of your life and will also help alleviate the feelings of depression. Chapter 11 outlines a program for managing these symptoms of depression and can help you regain a satisfying and productive life. Remember: depression is not a permanent condition and you *will* start to feel better. But you must also remember that you need not tackle this problem on your own; you may need others, including professionals, to help you out of your depression. In chapter 12, you will find information on how and when to seek professional help.

Getting Treatment

Obviously, treating depression during pregnancy is a complicated matter. Many women never seek professional help because they believe their symptoms are not severe enough. Or they are convinced that nothing can be done about their depression because they are pregnant. However, there are many different options available. For some women, joining a support group may be helpful; individual psychotherapy may help to alleviate the symptoms. These options are very attractive because they do not require the use of any medication during pregnancy, but what happens when your depression is very severe or does not respond to these treatments?

Kay was pregnant for the second time. Her first pregnancy had gone relatively well, but about a month after the birth, Kay fell into a deep depression. Although she probably had had at least a couple of bouts of depression in her teen years, this was the first time she had ever received any treatment. She started taking the SSRI Zoloft and within a few weeks was feeling much better. She continued on medication for about a year and a half. At this point she and her husband were planning to have another child, and Kay felt that she was doing well and no longer needed the Zoloft.

Kay felt well for a few months, but then she discovered she was pregnant. Although she and her husband were very excited about the pregnancy, she started to feel depressed again. She found it difficult to sleep at night, and she frequently woke up in a panic with her heart pounding. She felt miserable and was hardly able to enjoy anything, not even spending time with her husband and daughter. She had no appetite and was trying her best to keep her weight steady.

At about 8 weeks, the depression was quite severe and Kay started having such problems functioning at work that she was on the verge of losing her job. Her obstetrician referred her to a therapist. Although meeting with the therapist was helpful to some degree, Kay continued to feel very depressed and anxious. She asked her obstetrician about starting the Zoloft again but was told that it would be better to avoid taking a medication. Her obstetrician tried to reassure her that things would get better in the second trimester, but things did not improve. Kay began to feel increasingly despondent; she could not imagine lasting another day, much less seven more months. She felt that she had made a huge mistake and did not know what to do about it.

Kay's obstetrician ultimately referred her to a psychiatrist who specialized in the treatment of women during pregnancy. After carefully going over the information provided, Kay decided that she would start Prozac. At first, she felt very ashamed that she had to take an antidepressant during pregnancy, and she was worried that it might harm her baby. But over the next few weeks, her mood improved dramatically and she began to feel like her usual self. She was able to function at work, she was able to take care of her daughter and to be to the mother she wanted to be, and she was finally able to enjoy her pregnancy and look forward to having another child.

Antidepressant medications are highly effective. But you may have been told that it would be better to avoid taking an antidepressant during pregnancy. On the surface, this is a reasonable approach, given that our information on the reproductive safety of many medications is incomplete. Many women, fearful that they may affect the well-being of their child, end up avoiding antidepressants even when their depression is very severe. But if other types of treatment fail, and if you really need medication, avoiding medication is not always the best—or safest—option. Failing to treat depression may place both you and your family at risk.

Over the last decade much research has focused on the use of antidepressants during pregnancy, and we now know that at least some types of antidepressants pose no significant threat to the fetus. Unfortunately, this information has been neither well disseminated nor universally accepted. The result is that most often women who develop depression do not receive any treatment whatsoever, convinced that they must endure their depression until the baby is born. In chapter 13, you will find up-to-date information on the use of antidepressants during pregnancy so that you, in collaboration with your doctor, can make well-informed decisions regarding your treatment during pregnancy.

Depression Should Never Be Ignored

It is acknowledged that being pregnant and giving birth to a child entails some discomfort; however, the message is that a woman must endure and accept these difficulties. Swollen ankles, stretch marks, sleepless nights, and frequent trips to the bathroom are viewed as facets of the normal pregnancy experience. Depression is *never* a "normal" experience and it should not be endured or ignored. Depression is treatable, and there is a wide array of treatments available, many of which can be used during pregnancy. In Part Four you will learn how to take control of your situation and will find many different strategies that will help you combat depression. Taking steps to address this problem is not only important for your own psychological well-being, it is vital to your family.

Part Three

The Postpartum Period

Chapter 7

Crying for No Good Reason
Baby Blues and the Transition to Motherhood

The days and weeks following the birth of a child are filled with intense emotions. It is impossible to predict exactly how you will feel after the birth of a child, and, like many women, you may be surprised and awed by the intensity of the loving feelings you have for your new baby. This is a wonderful opportunity to discover a whole new side of yourself. However, there will also be times when you and your partner may feel overwhelmed, extremely nervous, and sometimes downright frightened about this new dimension of your life. Few first-time parents have encountered anything as exciting and as all-consuming as caring for a child during the first few weeks of life, and many parents, no matter how well prepared they may be, are surprised by the physical and emotional stamina required. Although sleep deprived and physically exhausted, you must find the energy to tend to your baby, to be on call twenty-four hours a day, seven days a week.

The time after a child is born is emotionally charged. Not so long ago, the maternity ward was called the "weeping ward," and for good reason. During the weeks following the birth of a child, about 1 in 10 women suffer from full-blown depression, but *most* women experience some degree of emotional turbulence. If you are a new mother, it is often quite difficult to tell exactly what is happening. With the arrival of a new child, the world is turned on its head. If you are feeling overemotional or distressed, is this just a normal response to having a baby? Is it hormonal? Or is it something altogether different? Most women notice that they are much more emotional—and sometimes they even feel quite out of control—during the days following birth. These women suffer from what is commonly called the "baby blues" or "postpartum blues." This chapter will discuss the baby blues and will also explore the other emotional experiences you may encounter.

What Are the Blues?
"Baby blues" is the term often used to describe the emotional roller coaster that women experience during the first few weeks after birth. Although obstetricians had recognized long ago these short-lived emotional upheavals

that occur immediately after childbirth, it was not until the 1950s that psychiatrists began to study what turns out to be a relatively common type of mood disturbance. Depending on how the syndrome is defined, between 40 percent and 85 percent of women experience the "blues" after childbirth. Rather than feeling depressed or despairing, women with the blues most commonly describe feeling weepy, overemotional, or easily overwhelmed. They cry more easily. They are more sensitive than usual. They may also complain of feeling anxious or worried, particularly about caring for their newborn baby. These symptoms usually are the most severe four to five days after delivery, but they typically last only for a few hours or a couple of days. In most women, the blues disappear completely within two weeks of delivery.

Carolyn was home alone with her one-week-old baby for the first time when her husband went out to get more diapers. The night before had been difficult, and both she and her husband had been up most of the night. After her husband left, the baby finally fell asleep, but then the doorbell rang. And then the dog started barking. And then the baby started crying. Carolyn started sobbing; the sound of her baby's crying felt intolerable. She felt so totally overwhelmed, how would she manage to hold everything together? Would she ever be able to calm her baby? Her husband returned home from the grocery store to find Carolyn and her baby, both crying. However, Carolyn (and the baby) felt much better after a nap.

In some ways, to refer to this phenomenon as the "blues" is somewhat misleading. This implies that what is happening is similar to depression, when, in fact, women with the blues don't really describe feeling depressed or down. Although this experience is often classified as a type of depression, it is clearly distinct from what psychiatrists call clinical, or major, depression. In contrast to those who suffer from depression, women with the blues generally feel positively about themselves and about the future. In fact, women with the blues are just as likely to describe intense feelings of happiness as they are to experience feelings of sadness. More accurately, the blues is not really depression but a heightened sense of emotional reactivity. When you have the blues, events or situations that normally wouldn't bother you seem to affect you more intensely. For example, one mother reported that her baby was born during the winter Olympics. She noticed that whenever she heard the American anthem, her eyes welled up with tears. And it seemed that whenever she saw somebody lose an important event, she cried. She felt somewhat silly about being so emotional, but she just couldn't seem to rein in her feelings. Another woman described that every time she saw her three-year-old daughter holding her new baby sister, she began to weep. She didn't feel sad; she just felt overwhelmed by her good fortune and her loving feelings for her family.

Although the baby blues have been grouped with postpartum depression and postpartum psychosis and labeled a psychiatric illness, it should be understood that the blues are not a pathological state or an abnormal response to having a child. Given the number of women who experience the blues, it is probably more accurate to consider the blues a normal and healthy response to having a baby. In contrast to postpartum depression, where a woman's ability to function may be challenged, the blues do not interfere with a mother's ability to care for herself or for her baby. Although it may be distressing to have such intense emotions and to be unable to control them, it is important to keep in mind that this change in behavior is short-lived and absolutely normal.

What Causes the Blues?

The symptoms women experience when they have the blues are in some ways similar to the emotional changes that some women experience during the few days or weeks before their menstrual period. Women who suffer from premenstrual syndrome (PMS) or the more severe form of this disorder, premenstrual dysphoric disorder (PMDD), typically describe having mood swings, being more tearful, or feeling easily overwhelmed. Women with premenstrual symptoms also frequently report feeling more irritable or tense. The similarity between the symptoms of PMS and postpartum blues has led researchers to hypothesize that the blues, like PMS, may be hormonally driven. During the last two weeks of the menstrual cycle, levels of estrogen and progesterone drop, and it is believed that this rapid fall in hormone levels may trigger mood changes in certain women. Similar but far more dramatic shifts in a woman's hormone levels also occur during the first few days after childbirth. As discussed in chapter 2, estrogen and progesterone interact with the parts of the brain that influence mood, and this may explain why shifts in the hormonal environment trigger mood changes in some women.

But you can't blame everything on your hormones. In fact, mothers are not the only ones who get the blues. Several studies have found that men are almost as likely as women to experience mood changes after the birth of a child, though the blues look a little different in the father. Men are typically not as weepy or overtly emotional as women. Instead, they tend to internalize their feelings, and what you see more commonly is tension or irritability. Men may also complain of sleep problems or fatigue. This is an interesting phenomenon, since obviously men do not experience any significant hormonal changes after the birth of a child, yet they experience what looks like the blues.

It is important to remember that there are other reasons why you may find yourself feeling overwhelmed or uncharacteristically emotional after having a baby. You have just experienced one of the most important and life-transforming events in your life. People find it difficult to hold back the tears at weddings. Parents cry when they watch their children graduate from college. It is normal to experience intense feelings in these emotionally charged settings. When you have a baby, not only are you responding to the event at hand, you are confronted with memories and experiences from your past, as well as your wishes for the future. Why *wouldn't* you be emotional?

Is It Just the Blues or Is It Depression?

Although we like to think of the blues as being distinct from postpartum depression, sometimes it is not so easy to tell the two apart, especially during the first few weeks after delivery. In both cases, women may experience significant emotional distress. Many of the physical symptoms associated with depression—change in appetite, sleep disturbance, fatigue, and loss of interest in sex—are normal aspects of the postpartum landscape and do not help to distinguish depressed from nondepressed mothers. The situation is made even murkier by the fact that, for some women, the blues may actually be the front end of a more severe episode of depression. While we do not have to do anything special about the blues, postpartum depression is a problem that deserves attention and, most important, some kind of treatment.

Several features may help to distinguish the blues from postpartum depression. First, there are the intensity of the emotions expressed and the severity of the symptoms. When you have the blues, you may temporarily lose perspective and find yourself responding with stronger emotions than the situation warrants. Ultimately, though, you are able to think rationally about what is happening. Although things may be difficult at times, you respond within a broader context of knowing that things will eventually improve. With depression, it is much more difficult to hold things in perspective. The negative feelings are much more pervasive, and it is much easier to lapse into feelings of hopelessness or helplessness. Intense feelings of guilt or worthlessness may accompany depression. And in severe cases, life may feel so painful that you may start to think about dying or committing suicide. Depression affects your ability to function and derive pleasure from your life; in contrast, women with the blues, despite feeling exhausted or overwhelmed, want to and feel that they can function and can take care of things relatively well.

About ten months after her son was born, Chinara discovered that she was pregnant again. This was a surprise, but a pleasant one. While her pregnancy went well, after she came home with the new baby a lot of things were easier—breast-feeding, getting the baby to sleep—but she still felt overwhelmed. She was sleep deprived, moody, and she had the sense that she was barely holding things together. She began to feel that she was failing as a mother. Although she was trying to help her older son with the transition, every time he threw a tantrum, she took it personally, feeling that she had disappointed him. Every time the baby cried, she was filled with anxiety. She began to dread waking up in the morning, overwhelmed at the prospect of being alone with her children all day.

Eventually, Chinara began to resent her husband. He left for work every morning and didn't seem to understand how difficult it was for her to care for their children. Every time he asked her to do an errand for him, she would feel anger rise up. How had she ended up with such an insensitive man? Why had she given up her career? Why had she allowed herself to get pregnant a second time?

After the birth of a child, it may take six to twelve months (or even more) to fully adjust, but the moodiness and tearfulness that characterize the blues should not last longer than a few weeks. Sometimes, however, the blues seem to intensify over time. Chinara clearly started out with the blues after the birth of her second child; she was overwhelmed and exhausted. But as time went on, her outlook on her situation became more and more negative, and she began to look more like someone who was suffering from postpartum depression. Although Chinara was not doing well, she had no idea that she was depressed; she thought she just had a bad case of the blues. Unfortunately, many women, as well as the health professionals who care for them, mistakenly believe that the blues may last for several months or even longer. Given this misconception, many women who actually have postpartum depression never receive the care they need.

What's the Cure for the Blues?

There is no real cure for the blues. By definition, the blues should resolve on their own over the course of the first few weeks, although it does help to have a little support and reassurance. You should remind yourself that things *will* get better. However, if your symptoms seem particularly intense or if they seem to be lasting longer than two or three weeks, you may be suffering from postpartum depression. At this point, a more thorough evaluation by a medical professional familiar with postpartum depression is indicated. If your doctor dismisses your concerns, you should get a second opinion.

Breast-feeding Your Baby

The American Academy of Pediatrics now recommends that women breast-feed their children for the first year of life, citing the many benefits to breast-feeding for both mother and child. Human breast milk is by far the best source of nutrition for a growing baby. It also fortifies the baby's immune system and reduces the risk of certain types of childhood illnesses, including diarrhea, respiratory infections, ear infections, eczema, and other types of allergies. Several studies have also demonstrated better cognitive functioning and higher IQs in children who were breast-fed. Many studies also indicate that breast-feeding benefits the mother. Women who breast-feed have fewer problems with postpartum bleeding and anemia and more quickly return to their pre-pregnant weight. They are also at lower risk for hip fractures, ovarian cancer, and breast cancer later in life. In addition, breast-feeding may help to promote bonding between the mother and her newborn child.

Given the many benefits of breast-feeding, many women make the decision to breast-feed their children for at least some period of time. While there are many benefits to breast-feeding, you may decide not to breast-feed. It is not for everyone. You may feel uncertain about your ability to breast-feed and you may be reluctant to ask for assistance. You may find the idea of nursing an infant too uncomfortable or too embarrassing, or it may seem too sexualized. However, deciding not to breast-feed may cause significant distress. Since many women feel a tremendous amount of pressure to breast-feed from their doctors, the hospital staff, and sometimes their friends and family, going against those recommendations may make you feel that you are not being a responsible or caring parent. Under these circumstances it is easy to feel guilty and to worry that you are depriving your child.

Other women find that, despite their best intentions, doing what is supposed to come naturally is not always that easy. Some women have problems breast-feeding and may need the support and guidance of knowledge-able friends or family members or the assistance of a trained professional. Even with help, some women continue to experience difficulties and ulti-mately give up nursing. If this happens, you may feel that you have been de-prived of one of the most meaningful experiences a new mother can have, or you may feel that you have failed as a mother.

It is important to remember that there is more to being a mother than nursing your baby and that breast-feeding is by no means the only way to develop a healthy and satisfying bond with your baby. Although you may feel pushed to do one thing or another, choosing to do something that feels uncomfortable or burdensome to you can take a toll on your emotional well-being. Similarly, if you are having difficulties breast-feeding, you have to take into consideration how this affects you and your baby. If you choose not to breast-feed or if, for some reason, you are not able to breast-feed, you are not a failure. Nor should you accuse yourself of being irresponsible or uncaring. Whatever choice you make, you must take your own well-being into consideration. And keep in mind that a bottle-fed baby with a happy mother is better off than a breast-fed baby with a mother who is unhappy or stressed out.

The Emotional Landscape of the Postpartum Period

For a new mother, having the blues is just the tip of the iceberg. After the birth of a child, a woman must undergo a complicated and often rather pro-longed transition to motherhood. In the context of this transformative expe-rience, you will encounter a wide range of emotions. Happiness and excitement are usually at the top of the list, but not always. After the birth of a child, many women experience ambivalent, or even negative, thoughts and feelings about being a mother. Is this a sign of a problem? Not necessar-ily. Even the happiest of transitions bring with them a significant amount of emotional turmoil. Although you are certainly aware that life will change significantly after the birth of a child, as a new mother you expect to feel happy and positive about having a child. You may not be prepared to deal with the more complicated or negative feelings, and you may end up feeling too guilty or too ashamed to share your experiences with others.

There is the notion that becoming a mother—and knowing what to do as a mother—just happens, like some sort of miraculous instinct. In fact, this transition may be quite difficult, and most women are surprised by how long it actually takes to adjust to motherhood. Long before you have a child, you have a fairly clear idea of how you want or expect things to proceed after your baby arrives. You may expect to slip into your new role as a mother the moment you see your baby for the first time, or you may allow yourself more time to get the hang of things. If you cannot make this transition as smoothly or as quickly as you expected, you may feel inadequate or incompetent, but you need to be patient. Most women describe that, although many things start to feel more manageable and under control after a few months, it may take much longer to feel fully adjusted to being a mother.

Ambivalence

Despite how many people told you that your life would change dramatically after the birth of a child, only through experience can you fully appreciate the magnitude of this change. You will be amazed by the tenderness and intense love you feel for your child and the richness that a child adds to your life. However, when confronted with the emotional and physical demands of caring for your own baby, you may sometimes wonder if you have made a mistake. Was it a good idea to have a child? Did you have a baby for the "right" reasons? Is this what you really wanted? It is totally normal to ask these sorts of questions. Even if the pregnancy was planned and the birth of the child eagerly awaited, you may have ambivalent feelings about being a mother. What happened to the person that you used to be? There are probably a lot of things that you had to give up to have a child and, as a result, you are likely to have some mixed feelings about your new role.

In acknowledging that life has changed so much, you may come to the frightening realization that there is no way to escape from the responsibility of caring for a child, and you may sometimes feel trapped. Although you enjoy being with your new family, you may find yourself feeling jealous of your childless friends who can do whatever they please whenever they want. You may feel resentful that you no longer have the freedom to move about as freely as you once did and that now, with everything you do, you must always consider your child. You may long for life the way it used to be. For many women ambivalence is extraordinarily uncomfortable. Like many mothers, you may equate being ambivalent with being a selfish or unloving mother. You might find yourself looking at other mothers who seem to be enjoying themselves and wondering why you are the only one harboring these complicated feelings. But you are not the only one who has these feelings; ambivalence is a normal feeling, and it doesn't mean you're a bad mother. We have a tendency to view being a mother as a totally wonderful and joyous experience. However, with something as complicated and life-altering as having and caring for a child, it would be unrealistic to assume that you should feel nothing but happiness.

Feelings of Incompetence

In the days and weeks following the birth of your child, will you be able to live up to the expectations you have set for yourself? Probably not. Contrary to popular belief, being a mother is neither totally instinctive nor completely intuitive. You might imagine that as soon as your baby is born, you will know exactly what to do. Unfortunately, this is not what happens. Even things that seem so basic or "natural," like nursing an infant, must be learned, and this takes time. Furthermore, with the disappearance of the extended family in our increasingly mobile society, the first baby most women really get to know is usually their own. With a new baby you have to learn on the job, which may seem like a daunting and sometimes rather frightening experience. There is no gradual or gentle introduction to the art of mothering; you just get thrown into it, ready or not.

During the first few tumultuous months following the birth of your child, you will certainly make mistakes. There are times when you will feel totally clueless. Sometimes you will feel that you cannot do anything right. And just when you think you have the hang of it, your baby will move on to another stage and everything that worked for you in the past will suddenly stop working. Under these circumstances, it is very easy to feel incompetent or inadequate. Even the most confident women are humbled by this experience and are astonished by how hard it can be to take care of an infant. It doesn't help that you will undoubtedly bring to this unfamiliar task preconceptions of what it is like to be a mother. You will want to be the best mother, the perfect mother, the mother who knows exactly what to do and how to do it, without any fumbling or frustration. How can you possibly attain this lofty ideal? When you fall short of your own or others' expectations, it may be a struggle to regain your confidence and to figure out how good is "good enough." It may be very hard to keep sight of all the many things that you do well as you focus on all the things that are not going according to plan.

The problem is exacerbated by the fact that your family, friends, and even people that you meet on the street may feel compelled to give you advice, insisting that they know the "right" way to take care of your baby. Add to this the plethora of magazines and books dedicated to teaching parents how to best care for their children. Although these words of advice may be helpful on some level, they can generate feelings of anxiety and inadequacy. Are you doing enough for your child? What if you do things differently from what others recommend? Although you may not be an "expert," it is important to remember that there is no single formula for being a good mother; you may not know exactly what to do the moment your baby is born, but with time, *you* will find what works best for you and your baby.

Disappointment

Biologically speaking, you become a mother immediately after your child is born. However, long before you have a child, you begin to have a sense of what it means to be a mother. The mother that you hope to be possesses all the positive attributes of your own mother and lacks all those traits that you found troublesome or painful when you were a child. Superimposed upon your image of the ideal mother are the expectations of motherhood dictated by our society and culture. What you eventually come up with is a highly idealized version of a mother, one that is, at the very least, giving without limits, unfalteringly patient, and all-knowing.

Just as you have an idea of yourself as a mother before your child is born, you will also begin to form an image of your baby and to imagine how he or she will look and behave. You will have fantasies about what it will be like to give birth and how you will spend the first hours with your new baby. You will envision the first few years of your child's life. But what happens when things don't work out as you had expected? As discussed in chapter 5, some women experience tragic events that totally transform their experience of childbirth. But even relatively minor deviations from the preconceived plan can bring up feelings of sadness and disappointment. For example, many women expect to have a natural childbirth and feel let down by the experience of having a caesarean section; they feel they have missed out on something essential to the experience of childbirth. If you have had a similar experience, you may feel uncomfortable about sharing your feelings. You might imagine others saying, "How ungrateful can you be to complain about having such a healthy, wonderful baby." Sometimes it may not even feel comfortable to fully acknowledge these feelings of disappointment to yourself, and instead you just feel a sense of sadness or emptiness.

Zoë was thirty-four when she had her son. Although he was healthy, he was a colicky baby and she had to deal with his inconsolable crying every day for several hours. She met frequently with her pediatrician and tried everything that he recommended, as well as every type of old wives' remedy, but nothing seemed to work. She looked at the other (quiet) babies at the park and was envious of their mothers. Zoë felt ashamed; she felt as if she had done something wrong. She felt that other mothers were looking at her, passing judgment on her inability to comfort her own child.

By around twelve weeks, things started to get a bit better, and her son's colic mysteriously disappeared over the next six weeks. Over time, he grew into an absolutely delightful and easygoing baby. Now, years later, when

Zoë looks back on those early days, she still feels sadness and that she missed out on having a good experience that other mothers seem to have had. And despite the fact that her son is thriving, she continues to have doubts about her competence as a mother.

While it may be difficult to voice disappointment in yourself or your experiences with childbirth, most mothers, like Zoë, feel that it is totally unacceptable to say anything bad about their baby. But there is a good chance that the baby that finally arrives is not the baby you imagined. What if the baby is a boy when you wanted a girl? Or if the baby looks different than you expected? Or what happens when the baby does not seem to appreciate you? Of course you will eventually learn to adjust to the situation, but you may feel disappointed or even sad. And what makes the situation worse is that entertaining these thoughts may make you feel incredibly guilty, as if you are being an unloving or uncaring mother.

Guilt

As a mother, you want to do the best for your child, and you probably have fairly high expectations of yourself. While it is natural to enter into motherhood with a well-defined sense of what it means to be a mother, problems may arise when you feel that you are not living up to this perfect image of yourself as a mother or when you feel that you are falling short of other people's expectations.

Jean had her first child at twenty-seven and her second at the age of thirty. She had no problems with her first pregnancy, but the second time around it was much more difficult. Shortly after delivery, she had to have an emergency operation to remove her gallbladder. She tried to keep up her milk supply while in the hospital by pumping, but several days later when she was back at home, breast-feeding did not go well. Her baby seemed to prefer the bottle, and every feeding was a struggle. And after the surgery, she just did not have the stamina to continue with the nursing and made the decision to wean her baby from breast to bottle.

Jean felt horrible. She nursed her first child for a little over a year and felt that it was a really positive experience. She could not stand seeing other mothers nursing their new babies and felt guilty that perhaps she had abandoned it too early. Although she knew intellectually that she was not to blame, she felt badly that she was not able to do what she thought was best for her child. She also felt that she had let her kids down because she had been so sick and exhausted following the birth; she just did not feel that she had the energy or emotional resources to pay full attention to them.

Mothers seem to have a natural penchant for guilt, and there seems to be no shortage of situations that inspire the feeling. Many new mothers feel that they must adhere to a certain code of behavior and often believe that their abilities as a mother are being measured and judged by others. When you cannot do what you want or are supposed to do for your child, you feel guilty. If anything happens to your child or if anything goes wrong, you are likely to feel responsible.

Today's mothers feel a great deal of pressure to be constantly available to their children—to stimulate and entertain them every minute of the day. However, even though you might want to give your children everything they need—including all of your time and energy—it is simply not possible. When something interferes with your ability to care for or spend time with them, guilt may arise, especially when you feel that you must put your own needs ahead of your child's. For example, you may feel guilty about taking time out to exercise or to visit with friends when it feels as if these activities are taking time "away" from your children. When you are physically ex-hausted at the end of the day, you may feel horrible if instead of entertaining your child, you need to take some time out to rest. Although you may feel that you should devote all of your time and energy to your children, each and every day, you will have to make uncomfortable decisions about what you do and how to spend your time.

Feeling Out of Control

Before you had a child, life had a certain rhythm. After the birth of a child, ordinary divisions of time are lost; you operate on baby time, not adult time. You may find yourself taking your shower at three in the afternoon. You may leave the house for the first time only after your baby is down for the night. What you have is a perpetual cycle of feeding, diaper changing, baby soothing, cleaning up, and sleeping. This cycle repeats itself over and over again, and this job seems to have no end.

Over time, things seem to settle down and you will be able to establish some routines. However, life with children retains an element of unpre-dictability; especially with a baby, you never know exactly what the day will bring. Under these circumstances, it is impossible to feel totally prepared and confident. It takes a tremendous amount of resilience and resourceful-ness to respond to the many different things that may come your way, and this can leave you feeling emotionally exhausted. If you are accustomed to living with a certain degree of order in your life, it may be difficult to tolerate the chaos that comes with caring for children, and you may find yourself struggling to impose structure on your family's life.

Sleep Deprivation and Exhaustion

Every new mother seems to talk about sleep. Some babies seem to sleep better than others, but it is usually takes three to six months for a baby to develop a regular pattern of sleep; some children take even longer. Most newborns sleep sixteen to eighteen hours a day, but their schedules do not necessarily conform to our own. While adults prefer to sleep in one uninterrupted shift, newborns sleep in two- to three-hour shifts throughout the day and night. Unless you have round-the-clock help, a soundproof sleeping chamber, and the ability to put all anxieties regarding your new baby out of mind, you are bound to suffer from some degree of sleep deprivation during your child's early years. The first month (or so) can be extremely difficult when your baby is waking up three to four times during the night and needs your undivided attention. Obviously, caring for a new baby is the most common cause of sleep disruption in new mothers, and you may face other demands on your time—caring for other children, domestic responsibilities, or work outside of the home—that may further compromise your pursuit of a good night's sleep. Not only is sleep deprivation a significant problem for mothers, it is one that may last for many months or even years.

So what does this mean for the mother? In new mothers, total sleep deprivation (missing a whole night of sleep) is unusual; however, partial sleep deprivation, usually defined as sleeping less than six hours a night, seems to be common. Although how much sleep is needed varies from individual to individual, most women of childbearing age require seven to eight hours of sleep each day for optimal functioning. Those who consistently have disrupted sleep may accumulate what researchers call a "sleep debt," becoming progressively more fatigued as the days pass. In these situations, a single night of "catch-up" sleep does not reverse the effects of chronic sleep deprivation.

Although some mothers seem to tolerate this disruption of their sleep fairly well, sleep deprivation, especially over a long period, is not good for you. It may leave you feeling chronically exhausted and overwhelmed; it may affect your memory and your ability to concentrate. In some cases, the degree of impairment may be significant. One study assessing the negative effects of sleep deprivation found that it can cause declines in cognitive performance similar to those observed in persons who are intoxicated. Chronic sleep deprivation may also have a negative impact on mood. It may make you more irritable and less patient with your children, and some researchers have speculated that sleep deprivation may make some women more vulnerable to postpartum depression.

Isolation and Loneliness

One of the most challenging aspects of caring for young children is the social isolation. In traditional cultures, a woman's family gathers around the mother after the birth of a child. They help her learn how to care for her child; however, probably one of the most important aspects of this tradition is to provide companionship. Nowadays most women with young children spend most of their time at home, alone.

Before your child is born, you have some sort of social network. After you have your baby, your may be separated, either in part or completely, from that world. As your attention is focused on caring for a new child, it is difficult if not impossible to keep up with old friends and connections. You may not have the time, energy, or emotional resources to nurture those relationships. Furthermore, it is likely that before having a child, you probably spent much of your time socializing with people who, like you, did not yet have children. Your old friends may not exactly abandon you, but it may be difficult for them to understand and share in your new experiences. It may also feel awkward for you, with your new life so focused on your new child, to connect with your old friends.

You may find your social life lacking. You probably spend most of your time talking about your baby to other people who have babies. With one half of the brain you are participating in a conversation, but with the other half you are watching over your child and attending to his or her needs. With your partner, you may feel that you tend to the practical aspects of taking care of your children and your home and have little time to talk about other things. With your family clearly at the top of the list of your priorities, you may find that other aspects of your life are unattended, unnourished, and in the process of withering away.

Adjusting to Your Baby's Personality

Babies are not all alike. Some babies are easygoing, and nothing seems to bother them. Some are more cautious and take a long time to warm up and feel comfortable. Others are more intense, more difficult to please, and require a great deal of attention. Although you probably have a good sense of the mother you would like to be, being a mother is a two-way street, and your baby's personality will have a powerful influence on how you parent. What you do as a mother is, in part, influenced by how your baby behaves and responds to you. If you do something that makes your baby smile or laugh, you do it again (and again and again). If you do something else and your baby cries, you quickly learn to do things differently. This dynamic process is the earliest form of communication between mother and child; your baby learns how to make his needs known, and you learn how to respond.

Problems may occur when there is not a good match between a mother and her child. For example, a mother who is more outgoing may have a hard time understanding and responding to a child who is more cautious or more anxious. She may feel frustrated by her child's discomfort in certain settings, and she may find it difficult to understand exactly what her child needs in order to feel more comfortable. In contrast, a mother who is very emotional may have difficulty with a child who is less expressive. She may struggle to understand her baby's more subtle forms of communication, or she may feel rejected when her child does not respond to her as positively or as enthusiastically as she had expected.

Parenting a baby with an even temperament is usually uncomplicated and very rewarding. These babies seem to accept everything you do and are easy to please. Having a baby with a difficult temperament is another story. If your baby is difficult to soothe or becomes easily frustrated, parenting can seem less rewarding. One of the ways you know you are doing the right thing is seeing your baby smile or calm down in your presence. With a difficult baby, you may not always get this kind of feedback. And it is easy to feel incompetent or inadequate with a demanding baby.

Confronting Feelings About Your Own Childhood

As you care for your own baby, you will probably spend a fair amount of time thinking about your own experiences as a child. As you think about the type of mother you would like to be, you are likely to evaluate and reflect on the parenting skills of the parents you know the best—your own. You may also have the opportunity to see your mother or father interacting with your baby, and this also may shed some light on how you were cared for when you were a child. Thinking about your own childhood may bring back pleasant and reassuring memories; however, it may often generate more complicated feelings.

After the birth of her first child, Sarah asked her mother to stay with her for a few weeks to help out. Sarah noticed that her mother always seemed anxious around the baby and often on the verge of hysteria. She hated the way her mother hovered over her daughter; it made Sarah remember how overbearing and protective her mother had been when she was a child.

When her mother was around, Sarah found herself trying to protect her daughter and was reluctant to leave the baby alone with her mother. She became incensed when her mother fussed too much about the baby, raised any type of concern, or tried to give Sarah advice. When Sarah spent time with her baby, she cringed every time an anxious thought or worry floated into her head. She was terrified of becoming like her mother. Her mother had never given Sarah an opportunity to be an independent adult. She did not want her daughter to suffer in the same way.

If you have had a more conflicted or difficult relationship with your parents, your feelings may be more intense or painful. Often women are surprised by the intensity of the emotions that arise as they reflect on their own childhood and sometimes find that these thoughts and feelings affect how they interact with their own child. For example, women who feel that they were neglected as children may find themselves taking heroic measures to attend to their child's needs and may feel guilty if they fall short of their own expectations. Women who have been physically or verbally abused as children may, after the birth of a child, find themselves plagued by painful memories. They are often very fearful that they will repeat the misdeeds of their parents.

Balancing Work and Family

In our society, most women work. But after having a child, about half of all new mothers make the decision to stay at home with their children. For most women, deciding to be a stay-at-home mom represents a dramatic change in lifestyle. While being at home to take care of your children brings many rewards, it is hard work, and being at home may feel isolating as you try to establish a network of other women in a similar situation. Many stay-at-home moms comment that it takes time to adjust to the rhythms and routines of life at home with young children.

Other women make the decision to return to work. For some, this decision is relatively easy; for others, it is more complicated. Working outside the home has many benefits; it can give you a sense of confidence, financial independence, camaraderie, and intellectual stimulation. If you have a career that you enjoy, it may seem difficult to give these things up after having a child. While going back to a job you enjoy and find stimulating may be a very positive experience, returning to a job that you do not like or find satisfying is a very different experience.

For many women, having to return to work after having a child is not easy. First, there is anxiety. Will your baby be okay without you? Will other caretakers be able to understand what she needs? What if something bad happens? With your baby changing so quickly, you may worry that you will not be around when your child says his first word or takes his first step and that somebody else will get to have that experience. Though you may worry that your child will learn to prefer a new caretaker over you, it is important to remember that, even if you do work, you are still the most important person in your child's life.

Working mothers may carry a tremendous amount of guilt. Putting your own needs ahead of your baby's often feels very uncomfortable. And when you see other women, even those who have had successful professional careers, choose to be full-time moms, you may wonder if you have made the right decision. While there are plenty of studies that suggest that child care outside of the home can be a positive and nurturing experience, there remains a social stigma attached to day care.

It is possible, although never easy, to balance work and family. Probably the most important aspect of making this balance work is finding quality child care. If you are worrying all day about the welfare of your child, you cannot work productively. Having some degree of flexibility in your work life is also helpful, so that you can find a schedule that works best for you and your child and have the capacity to change things around if you are needed at home. Obviously this is not always possible, and many working mothers feel overextended and overwhelmed as they try to juggle home and work life with their own personal needs. Even in the best of situations, working mothers may be ambivalent about working. They derive satisfaction and self-confidence from their work, yet they miss being at home with their children. There is never a perfect solution.

Being an Older Mother

Although there is no firm age at which one becomes an "older" mother, there is a clear consensus that age does have an impact on you as a mother. Older mothers may have less energy and physical stamina, but they may bring certain advantages, too. You may feel more confident and secure than you did when you were younger. You may also be at a different stage of your life where you have more resources and more options and are not feeling such intense pressures related to your financial situation or career.

Nonetheless, parenting as an older mother has its challenges. Many older mothers complain about not having enough energy to do everything they would like to do. With a new baby, you may find that missing a few hours of sleep is harder on you than it used to be, or you may feel chronically exhausted. If you have older children, you may sometimes feel too tired to run around with them or to engage in physical play. While this may be extremely frustrating and disappointing to you, the most important thing is that you spend time with your child; you will be able to find other, less physical activities—like cuddling up to read a book or sitting on the floor to do a puzzle—that are entertaining and nurturing.

Probably one of the most startling experiences for older mothers is realizing how different your life is with a child. If you have led a childless life for several decades, you may have a hard time adjusting to your new situation. The idea that somebody else is depending on you 100 percent of the time may be quite unsettling, and you may find yourself longing for the days when you had to worry only about yourself. You may miss the person that you used to be and feel a bit lost. You may feel like you do not fit in with your old friends because they are either childless or have older children, yet you may feel somewhat awkward and out of place among younger mothers.

Being a Single Mother

In the United States there are over 12 million single mothers, and single-parent households are on the rise. Women become single mothers for many different reasons. Most women end up being single mothers when a relationship fails; others are single mothers by choice. No matter how you come to this situation, being a single mother is often very challenging and emotionally demanding. Single mothers must go through all the emotional turmoil that mothers with partners do, but they also face other unique challenges. Probably one of the most difficult aspects of being a single mother is that you have to navigate this difficult transition to motherhood on your own. Although you may have family and friends for support, there is nobody else you can rely on completely when it comes to the day-to-day demands of taking care of a child. When the baby wakes up in the middle of the night, there is nobody else to take care of him but you. If your baby is sick, you are going to be the one staying home. It is this enormous and often frightening responsibility that is difficult for many single parents to handle.

In addition, most single mothers experience significant financial pressures, and about one-third of families headed by single mothers live below the poverty line. Many single mothers are forced to work outside the home, and managing the delicate balance between work and family without a partner can be a real struggle. Even with good work, you may find it difficult to support your family. You may end up feeling that there is no safety net. If your work becomes intolerable, you are hesitant to leave your job because your family depends on you, and if something happens to your child, you can't quit your job, because you need the money. It may feel as if you have very few options.

Single motherhood also carries its own emotional baggage. If you are now single because a relationship fell apart, you may be left struggling to figure out what went wrong. As you are caring for your new baby, you may also be trying to work out problems with the father of your child and may be trying to put the relationship back together again. You may feel jealous of other mothers who have partners. Or you may be trying to figure out if you want the father to play any role in your child's life. Even when the father is involved, negotiating the complexities of shared child care can be cumbersome. Too often these battles are negotiated in the courtroom.

Some Strategies for Surviving the Postpartum Period

Although the months following the birth of your child may be difficult, ultimately the tough times will pass and, along the way, there are many things you can do to make things easier for yourself.

Remember to take care of yourself. When you are so focused on caring for your child, you may forget to take care of yourself. If you do not take care of yourself first, you cannot possibly have the emotional and physical resources needed to care for your baby.

Give yourself time to rest. Remember that your body has gone through a tremendous physical ordeal. You cannot survive without sleep, and you need to rest so that your body can recover. Ask your partner to help with nighttime or early-morning feedings so that, at least on some nights, you can get a longer uninterrupted chunk of sleep. If you are a single mother, try to have a family member or friend spend a few nights with you. Especially during the first few weeks of your baby's life, rest when your baby is resting. Although you may feel compelled to use this time to do other tasks, you need to set aside nonessential household chores or get additional help.

Find a routine that works for you. Life with a young child is unpredictable. Find a good routine for you and your baby and try to stick to it. This will help you to feel more relaxed and in control, and having a regular routine will also help your baby to feel more comfortable.

Try to manage your time realistically. New mothers often have unrealistic expectations of what they can accomplish and they typically underestimate how much time child care really takes. By being more realistic about time management, you will feel less overextended and will be more productive and in control of your life.

Learn to be flexible. With a new baby, it is impossible to feel totally in control, and things often do not go according to plan. It is important to learn how to tolerate these disappointments, come up with new alternatives, and move on.

Learn to accept and express your negative feelings. The reality is that motherhood is always challenging, frequently frustrating, and sometimes not particularly rewarding. Not being able to let go of negative feelings can interfere with your ability to enjoy the more positive aspects of mothering and can generate feelings of shame and guilt. Finding somebody who is willing to talk honestly and openly about these uncomfortable aspects of motherhood can be immensely helpful.

Learn to be a "good enough" mother. While you may want to strive for perfection, there is such a thing as a "good enough" mother. What this means is setting realistic expectations of what is important to you and what you are capable of doing. It also means learning to accept your shortcomings.

Build up your support networks. One of the most common complaints that mothers have is lack of support. Cultivating a strong support network, one that includes one's partner but also other sources of support, is vital to your well-being and may also help to prevent or alleviate depression.

Ask for help. Mothers have received and internalized the message that they should be able to take care of everything on their own. In reality, being a mother is not a one-person job, and it is important to ask for help whenever you feel that you need it. You don't have to wait for a disaster. Help may be getting your partner to do the cooking. It may be hiring a babysitter or someone to clean house now and then. You may need more emotional support. This may mean talking more openly to friends or joining a new mother's group; many women also find it helpful to talk to a mental health professional.

Give Yourself Time to Adjust

Adjusting to a new baby is more than just knowing how to change a diaper or to prepare a bottle. Even if you have other children at home and feel relatively comfortable with taking care of children, giving birth is a physically and emotionally demanding experience. The transition to motherhood is complicated. It may generate feelings of joy and contentment, but it may bring up feelings of disappointment, sadness, and loneliness. What is so important to remember is that all of these feelings, even the negative ones, are absolutely normal. Although you may feel that there is little room for these less than joyous feelings and you may feel reluctant or ashamed to share this side of your experience with others, you need not feel embarrassed or ashamed about the way you feel. Although many new mothers are reluctant or ashamed to ask for help, caring for a new baby is a job too big for one person to handle alone.

Chapter 8

Beyond the Blues

Postpartum Depression and Anxiety

Although most women experience some degree of emotional upheaval during the few weeks after delivery, about 10 percent to 15 percent of women suffer from postpartum depression, a more serious and potentially disabling form of mood disturbance. A significant proportion of women may also suffer from significant anxiety during the postpartum period. In contrast to the blues, where the symptoms are relatively mild and short-lived, postpartum depression can be quite severe and may significantly affect a mother's ability to function and to care for herself and her child. There is good evidence to indicate that depression in the mother may have long-term effects on her child's well-being.

Despite an increasing public awareness of postpartum depression, this disorder often goes unrecognized and untreated. Many women feel ashamed or guilty about how they feel and are often reluctant to talk to others about it. Even when the symptoms are severe, it may be difficult for a mother to acknowledge that she is depressed. Even worse, all too often when a woman turns to others for help, her concerns are downplayed and she is told that this is the normal stress a women experience after having a baby and nothing to worry about. The bottom line is that most women with postpartum depression never receive any type of attention or treatment, and this is a tragedy. When a mother is depressed, she cannot attend to herself or to her baby, and she cannot fully participate in the important early months of her child's life.

Is It Really Depression?

The weeks following the birth of a child are tumultuous. Because these first weeks (or months) of your baby's life may be chaotic, it may be difficult to get a good sense of exactly how you feel. You may be sleep deprived and overwhelmed by the demands of caring for a new baby. You are unable to pursue the activities that you normally do to take care of yourself. There is no extra time to do the things that you enjoy. Especially if you have never had a child before, you may not have a good sense of what is "normal" or expected after the birth of a child. It is *not* normal, however, to feel depressed. As discussed in the previous chapter, most women experience some type of "moodiness" or "mood swings" during the first few days or weeks after the birth of a child. These relatively benign mood changes are usually just the blues. Depression is different. With depression, the negative emotions you experience are more intense, more pervasive, and more persistent.

> Kris felt well prepared for the birth of her first child. Her two older sisters had already had children, and she had helped them to care for their babies. Kris was surprised that the first month after the birth of her child was so difficult, although with the help of her husband and her family she was able to manage.
>
> She expected that things would get better as the baby got older. But even though she always felt exhausted, and her baby was sleeping for longer and longer stretches, it was difficult to sleep. She just couldn't relax. Every time she tried to close her eyes, she found herself listening for her baby's cries. Whenever her baby woke her up, she was in a panic and it was almost impossible to fall back asleep again.
>
> Kris's days were not much better. After a night without enough sleep, even the simplest tasks felt overwhelming. She found herself lashing out at her husband. She knew that her responses to his efforts to help were often out of line, but she just couldn't help it. She was disappointed that things were not working out better for her. Sometimes she felt depressed and was convinced that things would never get better.

Typically, the symptoms of depression are relatively mild at first—kind of like the blues—but they worsen over time. At first, you may know that you do not feel right or as good as you expected to feel, but it is often easy to blame the way you feel on your circumstances: "If only my baby was sleeping better, I would feel much better." "Things would be going a lot better, if only my husband were more helpful." It may be true; there may be a lot of things that could make your life easier, but when it's depression, nothing really helps to lift your spirits.

Although there is a tendency to think of postpartum depression as being distinct from other types of depressive disorders, the only thing special about postpartum depression is its timing. Postpartum depression typically emerges gradually over the first two to three months after the baby is born, although some women describe a more sudden onset of depressive symptoms after delivery. Some women may actually start to experience some milder symptoms of depression late in the course of pregnancy. After childbirth, these symptoms seem to worsen and look more like a full-blown episode of depression.

The symptoms of postpartum depression are really no different than what one would expect to see with any other type of depression and are described in greater detail in chapter 2. At the very core are feelings of sadness or the inability to derive pleasure from your life, but depression comes with other symptoms, including sleep problems, fatigue, change in appetite, and poor concentration. You may feel less confident and have doubts about your ability to care for your child. When depression occurs after the birth of a child, you may also find it difficult to enjoy or to bond with your child; this inability to connect often brings intense feelings of shame and guilt.

Milder cases of postpartum depression may be especially easy to miss because many of the symptoms of depression (such as sleep disturbance, change in appetite, and fatigue) also occur in new mothers in the absence of depression. There are several ways for you to tell the difference between depression and what women typically experience during the postpartum period. Although many women feel more emotional or "moody" during the first few weeks after delivery, these mood changes, compared to an episode of depression, are relatively benign and short-lasting. Depression is more than being overwhelmed or teary-eyed. With depression, the negative emotions are much stronger and more pervasive, and it is often easy to lapse into feelings of hopelessness or helplessness. You may be plagued by intense feelings of guilt or worthlessness; you may also feel inadequate or incompetent as a mother. Depression permeates every aspect of your life: your capacity to function, your ability to enjoy yourself, and your interactions with your baby and others around you.

Tiffany was from a close-knit family, the youngest of three daughters and the last to have a child. As long as she had remembered, she had envisioned the day she would have her own children, and she and her husband anxiously awaited the arrival of their baby.

Labor and delivery went well, and their baby boy was healthy and full of life. Tiffany was so excited during the first few weeks after the birth of her child, but after her husband returned to work she felt herself sinking into despair. Despite having her family nearby, she felt sad and lonely. She loved her son, but she just felt that she was missing out on something. She expected to feel an intense bond with him, but it wasn't there. When she went out for a walk, she looked at the other mothers and wondered what she was doing wrong. Why wasn't she enjoying herself more? What was wrong with her?

As Tiffany watched her own mother care for her son, she often felt inadequate. She felt guilty about the times when she did not understand what her son needed or was unable to soothe him. She felt that she could never be as good a parent as her mother, and sometimes she thought her son would be better off without her. She had never before thought of killing herself, but sometimes she thought it would be okay if she died. She knew her son would be well cared for and loved.

In severe cases of postpartum depression, life may feel so painful that you may start to think that you would be better off dead or you may even contemplate committing suicide. Uncertain how others will respond to these distressing feelings, you may feel uncomfortable or afraid to talk to others about how bad you feel. Many women fear that, if they share these thoughts, they will be "locked up" or their child will be taken away. It is important to recognize that suicidal thoughts are a relatively common complication of depression. Fortunately, the vast majority of women with postpartum depression do not act on these thoughts, and recent research indicates that, despite the high prevalence of depression and anxiety after the birth of a child, new mothers are at low risk for suicide or other self-injurious behaviors and only those with the most severe forms of illness require hospitalization. However, suicidal thoughts should never be ignored, and if you are having these sorts of thoughts, you should discuss them with your doctor. If you feel that your doctor is not taking your complaints seriously, then you should contact a mental health professional. If you feel that you cannot wait to talk to somebody or if you worry that you may act on your impulses, you should go to the nearest emergency room or call 911.

Postpartum Depression and Sleep Deprivation

Women who suffer from postpartum depression often complain of difficulty sleeping. Their sleep is frequently interrupted and they complain of constantly feeling exhausted. Although sleep disruption is a symptom of depression, it's also a problem common to all women caring for infants or young children, whether or not they are depressed. Some women can cope with long periods of sleep deprivation, but most start to have some problems when their sleep is disturbed night after night. When you are sleep-deprived, everything is more difficult. It is harder to concentrate, and performing certain tasks or making even the simplest of decisions may seem totally overwhelming. You may also feel more anxious, more irritable, or overly emotional. It is no surprise that during the early weeks after the birth of a child, many women may not be able to tell if they are depressed, stressed, or merely exhausted. It may not be until things start to settle down a bit that you are able to clearly evaluate your situation.

But there are some signs that may help you to distinguish depression from the aftermath of chronic sleep deprivation. With depression, sleep issues are not the only problem. You are likely to have feelings of sadness, worthlessness, or excessive guilt; these sorts of feelings are not the usual consequences of losing sleep. Furthermore, if you are just sleep-deprived, you are tired and should have no problem falling asleep. However, if you suffer from postpartum depression or anxiety, you may find yourself lying awake for hours despite feeling totally exhausted. Or you may find yourself sleeping so lightly that you wake every time your baby stirs or makes a sound.

While sleep disturbance may be a manifestation of depression, some experts wonder if chronic sleep deprivation may actually *cause* postpartum depression. There is some data to suggest that sleep deprivation can have a negative impact on mood and may increase one's vulnerability to depression. A study published by Dr. Ken Armstrong and his colleagues at the Royal Children's Hospital in Queensland, Australia, indicates that among mothers whose babies had significant sleep problems, 40 percent had symptoms suggestive of postpartum depression. The good news, according to Armstrong, is that interventions that improve infant sleeping patterns also lead to a significant improvement in the mother's mood.

Postpartum Depression and Obstetric Complications

While some studies have shown that having any type of obstetric complication increases the risk of postpartum depression, others have shown no connection. It has been my experience, however, that while having some sort of medical or obstetric complication does not always cause depression, it certainly makes the postpartum period more stressful. Clearly, some women are more vulnerable to depression when this happens.

Having complications during pregnancy or delivery is like starting out on the wrong foot. Sometimes it is relatively easy to bounce back; however, for many women the days and weeks ahead may seem daunting. It is difficult to be the mother you had wanted or expected to be when you must tend to your own physical condition in addition to your new baby.

Not only is it difficult to heal physically, you may have to allow yourself some time to recover emotionally. When things do not go as expected, it can be extremely unsettling or disappointing. When you are so emotionally invested in something—like the birth of your child—a deviation from the expected may feel like a tremendous loss. You may feel like you lost the earliest moments of your child's life and that this precious time can never be recaptured.

Postpartum Depression and Breast-feeding

As we discussed in the previous chapter, there are many benefits to breast-feeding, and some experts believe that breast-feeding may also protect you from postpartum depression. While there is some research to indicate lower rates of depression among breast-feeding women, not all the research supports this view. Furthermore, these studies may be somewhat difficult to interpret, because women who have postpartum depression often experience more problems with breast-feeding and are more likely to abandon breast-feeding earlier than nondepressed mothers. The truth is that both breast-feeding and bottle-feeding mothers are at risk for postpartum depression. You should not use your worries about postpartum depression to determine whether or not you should breast-feed, nor should you assume that your breast-feeding protects you from postpartum depression.

Experts have also raised the question of whether weaning or discontinuation of nursing may bring on postpartum depression. This is a good question, but one that has not been well researched. From a theoretical standpoint, it makes sense that weaning may trigger an episode of postpartum depression. After a woman stops nursing, there is a fall in the levels of certain hormones, including estrogen and prolactin. If hormonal fluxes do play a role in causing postpartum depression, weaning may trigger a depression. Clinically, it seems that some women do experience the onset of their depression after weaning. More commonly, however, these symptoms begin long before breast-feeding is stopped and what seems to happen is that women feel more comfortable pursuing treatment after they have given up nursing.

If you are depressed and are planning to take a medication to treat your depression, you may be counseled to wean before initiating treatment. This is a highly charged issue, and many women struggle with this decision. Because of your depression, you may feel less confident and unsure of your abilities as a mother. You may believe that breast-feeding is something you are doing well and that it helps bolster your self-confidence. To give up what may be a deeply satisfying experience would be a tremendous loss, and you may decide, despite your depression, to continue breast-feeding rather than receive treatment. However, as we will discuss in the chapter 13, you don't have to make this sacrifice; it is possible to continue breast-feeding *and* to receive treatment for your depression safely at the same time.

For other women, breast-feeding, despite its many benefits, feels like torture. For whatever reason, it is not going well, yet you may feel a considerable amount of pressure to persist, in order to avoid intense feelings of inadequacy and incompetence. Breast-feeding is not for everyone. Especially when you are depressed, it may be difficult to sustain the physical demands of nursing. Being the one who is always responsible for the feeding may feel like an unmanageable burden, and if you are having problems sleeping, waking up to nurse your baby every few hours may push you over the edge. Keep in mind that, in the long run, a bottle-fed baby with a calm, contented mother is likely to do better than a breast-fed baby with an unhappy or stressed-out mother.

Bipolar Disorder and the Postpartum Period

Although most women with postpartum depression suffer from the most common sort of depression, unipolar depression, some women may have bipolar disorder (also known as manic depression). Given the massive hormonal shifts and prolonged sleep deprivation that occur after the birth of a child, women with histories of bipolar disorder are very vulnerable to mood changes during the postpartum period. Most commonly, women with bipolar disorder experience depressive symptoms; pure mania (feelings of euphoria or elation) is actually quite uncommon during the postpartum period. Women also present with symptoms that are a mixture of depression and mania; these include agitation, irritability, profound sleep disturbance, and severe anxiety. (You can find more detailed information on the symptoms of bipolar disorder in chapter 2.)

It is important to distinguish between unipolar and bipolar depression because the treatments for the two are quite different. If you have symptoms suggestive of bipolar disorder or if you have had manic symptoms in the past and became depressed after pregnancy, it must be assumed that you have bipolar disorder. Although antidepressants are typically used to treat depression, they may actually make your condition worse if you have bipolar disorder. The treatment for bipolar disorder is much more complicated than for unipolar depression but relies upon the use of a mood stabilizer, a drug that can treat symptoms of both depression and mania. You can find more information on the treatment of bipolar disorder in chapter 13.

Postpartum Anxiety

While we have been focusing mostly on depression, it is important not to ignore the symptoms of anxiety women frequently experience during the postpartum period. Caring for a new baby is a tremendous responsibility. Even if you have a lot of experience in caring for children, you are likely to have worries about your baby and his well-being. All new mothers experience at least some anxiety, but for many, the anxiety is severe and sometimes debilitating.

> Lisa had always been a worrier. As soon as she discovered she was pregnant, she started to worry about everything. She was most afraid of having a miscarriage or finding out that there was something wrong with the baby. After the first trimester, and after seeing her perfectly formed baby on the ultrasound, she began to feel more confident that the pregnancy was going well.
>
> Unfortunately, her anxiety resurfaced soon after delivery. Her baby girl was strong and healthy, but Lisa was worried that something bad was going to happen. Her baby looked so fragile that she was almost afraid to hold her. Every time she tried to nurse her, Lisa felt tense and panicky. While she was in the hospital, she felt comforted by the nursing staff which was always there to help her when she had questions or concerns. However, her first night home, Lisa was terrified. The baby was having problems nursing, and neither Lisa nor her husband could get the baby to stop crying. Lisa called the pediatrician, who tried to reassure her, but Lisa was sure that there was something seriously wrong. The next day was better, but Lisa was filled with dread, and she tensed up every time the baby cried. Lisa had more and more problems nursing; her milk supply was not adequate and she was instructed to wake the baby every hour to feed her. She felt so overwhelmed and guilty that she just wanted to give up.
>
> As time went on, Lisa became more and more afraid to be alone with the baby. After putting the baby to rest, she lay awake waiting for her to cry again. If the baby didn't cry, she had to go into the nursery to check on her, terrified that the baby would die of SIDS. Whenever she nursed the baby, she was worried that she would fall asleep and drop the baby. Her pediatrician suggested that she try nursing in bed, but Lisa was convinced that she would roll over and smother the baby. After a few weeks of sleepless days and nights, Lisa felt exhausted and emotionally distraught. She just wanted to enjoy being with her baby, and this seemed impossible.

Many women who develop postpartum anxiety recognize that they have struggled with anxiety long before having children, but the anxiety they experience during the postpartum period is often more intense. Anxiety may come with or without depressive symptoms. Many women start out with anxiety alone, but when the symptoms persist week after week, they may start to feel more depressed. Unfortunately, postpartum anxiety disorders are often missed because it is believed that anxiety is a normal experience for all new mothers.

During the postpartum period, the most common type of anxiety disorder is a form of **generalized anxiety disorder** (known as GAD). Women with generalized anxiety are plagued by worries about their baby and are unable to keep these fears under control. They can't seem to shake these fears, even though they usually realize that their anxiety is more intense than the situation warrants. It is almost impossible to reassure them that everything will work out okay. They are edgy, often irritable, and restless; they often find it difficult to fall or stay asleep. With generalized anxiety disorder, a woman may also experience physical symptoms: muscle tension, frequent headaches or muscle aches, upset stomach or nausea, diarrhea, and sweating or hot flushes.

For some women the anxiety is even more intense, and they suffer from **panic disorder.** In this situation a woman has panic attacks, which are recurrent, unexpected episodes of fear and anxiety accompanied by physical symptoms linked to the body's normal response to danger. When a panic attack strikes, your heart may pound or race, and you may have chest pain or shortness of breath. You may feel sweaty, weak, or dizzy. You may feel tingling sensations or numbness in your arms and legs. These feelings are so intense that you may feel like you are going crazy, losing control, or are on the verge of death. Most attacks last a couple of minutes, but they may last much longer. Since panic attacks usually occur without warning, most women who suffer from panic disorder experience considerable anxiety between attacks. They live in fear of the next episode and often become fearful of leaving their house or being in a place where it would be difficult or embarrassing to have a panic attack. Everyday situations like driving, riding on a train, or being in a crowd may seem totally overwhelming. In extreme cases, the anxiety is so severe that a woman becomes agoraphobic and is actually unable to leave her home.

Although anxiety is a normal response to a stressful situation, it is not entirely clear why some women develop such severe symptoms during the postpartum period. It is likely that many women have a biological predisposition toward anxiety; indeed, anxiety disorders are incredibly common among women, with about 1 in 3 women suffering from an anxiety disorder at some point during their lifetime. Many women with postpartum anxiety disorders recognize that they have had problems with anxiety in the past, although most of them managed the anxiety on their own and have never received any treatment. It seems that the physical and psychological stress of having and caring for a new baby may help to unmask this tendency, and the hormonal changes of the postpartum period may also act as a trigger. Whatever the cause, anxiety emerging during the postpartum period may be severe and may cause significant distress.

Another Symptom of Anxiety: Intrusive and Disturbing Thoughts About Your Baby

Anxiety may also take the form of recurrent, intrusive thoughts or obsessions. We all have random, sometimes really disturbing, thoughts pop into our minds, but usually they last for a few seconds or so and then vanish. With an obsession, no matter how hard you try to erase an upsetting thought, it keeps coming back. Although you realize that your obsessions are irrational or excessive, you cannot control these thoughts. Women with postpartum depression may have these sorts of obsessions, and what can make these obsessions so unsettling is that they often involve the baby.

Sandra had been an anxious kid, and she never really grew out of her worrying. After her baby was born, her anxiety seemed to intensify. Was her daughter eating enough? Was she gaining enough weight? Did she have enough wet diapers? She often found herself checking on her baby at night, sometimes waking her to make sure that she was okay. Her husband tried to tell her that everything was going well, but she was always worried that something bad would happen to the baby.

About three weeks after her daughter was born, Sandra was preparing dinner and her baby was in the kitchen in a bouncy seat on the floor. As she was cutting the vegetables, an awful image flashed through her head, an image of herself stabbing her baby with a knife. She was horrified. How could she have had this thought? And what was worse, she couldn't get the picture out of her head.

Over the next few weeks, this image kept coming back to her. She was so afraid that she might accidentally stab the baby that she took all the sharp knives out of the kitchen and locked them in a closet upstairs. But she started to have other thoughts. She was afraid to carry the baby down the stairs or next to an open window, because she was afraid she would throw the baby down the stairs or out the window. She asked her husband to give the baby her bath because she was convinced that she would accidentally drown her.

Sandra felt frightened and confused. Where were these thoughts coming from? She loved her daughter and would never, ever do anything to cause her harm, but she wondered if one day she might lose control. She was reluctant to tell anybody about these terrifying thoughts; she was convinced that they would take her baby away from her. But she was frightened to be alone with the baby and tried her best to make sure that somebody was with her at all times.

Sandra has what we call **postpartum obsessive-compulsive disorder** or **postpartum OCD.** Although there are many different types of obsessive thoughts, usually the mother with OCD is preoccupied with thoughts of possible harm to her baby and is vigilant of threats posed by other people or situations. New mothers with postpartum OCD also worry that they themselves might harm their baby. These thoughts, which are so out of character and seem so inconsistent with the loving feelings they have for their child, are very disturbing and very frightening.

Although it is called obsessive-*compulsive* disorder, obsessions may occur with or without compulsions. A compulsion is a behavior or ritual that is repeated over and over again in an effort to reduce the anxiety generated by a particular obsession. For example, a mother who worries that her child will become ill compulsively washes her child or engages in various cleaning rituals in response to this fear. Another example is a mother who worries that her house will burn down; over and over again, she goes to the kitchen to check that the stove is turned off. The urge to carry out these rituals is so intense that the person feels unable to resist them. Common compulsions include checking, rearranging things, or putting things in a certain order and cleaning or washing hands. Sometimes the compulsions verge on the superstitious, like having to say a certain phrase or word before doing something or going someplace. If the person does not say this phrase, she is convinced that something bad may happen. Although these compulsions are often frustrating, interfering with one's ability to complete tasks or interrupting one's daily activities, they may be relatively benign when compared to the disturbing obsessions that some postpartum women have.

About 3 percent of all people in the United States have OCD, but nobody really knows how often postpartum OCD occurs. Many women with postpartum depression may have some type of obsessions but may not have the full-blown syndrome described here. While symptoms of OCD sometimes appear for the first time after the birth of a child, more commonly women with postpartum OCD have had mild OCD symptoms long before pregnancy. In most cases, they are not aware of their illness until they develop more severe symptoms after the birth of a child.

Many women with postpartum OCD are concerned that they may lose control and act out their thoughts. You probably have heard horrible stories in the news where a mother has killed her own child and you may worry that you will become one of those mothers. However, women with postpartum OCD, while they may have disturbing thoughts, are in touch with reality and know that these thoughts do not make any sense. In contrast, women who try to harm their own children often suffer from *postpartum psychosis*; they may also have thoughts about harming their children, but these thoughts are not grounded in reality. For example, a woman with postpartum psychosis may believe that her child is possessed by the devil and that she is saving others from harm by killing her baby. Women with postpartum OCD do not have these bizarre or psychotic thoughts and exhibit no other behaviors to suggest their children are at risk; in fact, they tend to be hypervigilant about their children and go to great lengths to ensure their children's safety.

It is easy to imagine how having these distressing thoughts on a daily basis may affect how you interact with your baby. Certainly it would be more difficult to relax and feel comfortable around your baby if you must always be on guard against yourself. In fact, many women who have these intrusive thoughts feel as if they are bad mothers. Like Sandra, many women become afraid to be with, and start to avoid being alone with, their children. Not surprisingly, having these symptoms may lead to or exacerbate feelings of depression.

Women with postpartum OCD symptoms often do not let others know that they are suffering. They are alarmed by and ashamed of their thoughts and often fear that their baby will be taken from them. If you are having these symptoms, you should discuss them with your obstetrician, primary care provider, or a mental health professional. It can be an immense relief to share these disturbing thoughts with another person, and there are many highly effective treatments available that can help alleviate these distressing symptoms.

Who Is at Risk for Postpartum Depression and Anxiety?

Any woman who has had a child is vulnerable to depression, regardless of age, marital status, or economic class. Experienced mothers are as susceptible as first-time mothers. That said, some women seem to be more vulnerable. Although it is difficult to predict exactly who will develop postpartum depression, certain risk factors have been identified, including:

- previous episode of postpartum depression
- depression during pregnancy
- anxiety during pregnancy
- history of depression or bipolar disorder before pregnancy
- history of anxiety disorder
- history of physical or sexual abuse
- history of premenstrual mood symptoms
- recent stressful life events
- inadequate social supports
- marital problems

Unfortunately, postpartum depression tends to be a recurrent problem. If you have had an episode of postpartum depression after a previous delivery, your chance of having another episode of postpartum depression is about 50 percent. The risk is especially high if your next pregnancy comes soon after the first. In this situation, many women report that the depression is more intense the second time around. One of the strongest predictors for postpartum depression is depression *during* pregnancy. If you have had postpartum depression in the past or are experiencing any depressive symptoms during pregnancy, it is important that you discuss this with your obstetrician or a mental health professional, so that you can be monitored more closely during the postpartum period. There may also be ways to decrease your risk for postpartum depression.

Also at high risk for postpartum depression are women who have suffered from a mood disorder prior to pregnancy. If you have had depression before, especially if you have experienced recurrent episodes, your risk for depression is about two to three times higher than a woman who has never before been depressed. If you have been diagnosed with bipolar disorder, the risk is even higher, with most studies indicating that at least half of women with bipolar disorder experience worsening of their illness during the postpartum period. Because the risk of postpartum illness is so high in women with recurrent mood disorders, it is often recommended that they receive some type of preventative treatment during the first few months after delivery to minimize the risk of postpartum depression. This is a topic that will be discussed in greater detail in chapter 13.

The risk factors for postpartum anxiety are less well defined. Certainly, women who have had a history of any type of anxiety disorder—generalized anxiety disorder, panic disorder, or obsessive-compulsive disorder—are at risk of worsening of anxiety symptoms during the postpartum period. It also seems that women with these anxiety disorders are more vulnerable to postpartum depression.

There may be other factors that help to *reduce* your risk of postpartum depression. One of the most important factors is having adequate help and support. Although most new mothers expect that they should be able to do everything on their own, having enough help for the first few months after your baby is born is extremely important and may help to reduce your levels of stress. If you are having marital problems or if your husband and family are unsupportive or unavailable, this time may end up feeling like a lonely struggle. Conversely, having an understanding partner and a helpful family and friends can go a long way in improving your mental well-being.

Why Is Postpartum Depression So Frequently Overlooked?

Although postpartum depression is a relatively common complication of childbirth, it is alarming to note that most women with postpartum depression never receive any type of treatment. Part of the problem may be that many women are not aware—or are unable to admit—that they are depressed. If you are experiencing depression for the first time in your life, it may be difficult to understand exactly what is happening to you. The situation is complicated by the fact that the first few months after the birth of a child are emotionally charged. How are you supposed to tell what is normal or abnormal? Furthermore, many women are not informed about postpartum depression before having a child; this is a topic that may be touched upon in childbirth preparation classes, but far too often no real discussion of this issue comes from the obstetrician or the other medical professionals a woman encounters. What obstacles may stand in your way of getting the help you need and deserve?

You may convince yourself that the depression is not "bad enough" to ask for help. When you think of somebody who is depressed, you probably imagine somebody who is totally debilitated by their depression, unable to function, get out of bed, go to work. Or you may think that depression is severe only when you start to think about harming or killing yourself. When you look at yourself, you see something different. You get up every day to take of your baby. You may feel sad and you may not enjoy yourself as much as you used to, but you do what needs to be done. Is this depression? It could be. Depression may be severe or it may be relatively mild. Do you have to wait until it gets worse to get help? Of course not. Many women who have postpartum depression do not come in for help because they believe that their depression is not bad enough to merit professional attention. However, there is no need to wait; even when the depression is relatively mild, you can help yourself and your family by getting treatment.

You may tell yourself that the depression will go away on its own. Many women believe that postpartum depression will eventually go away on its own. They may be told by their obstetrician that they have "the blues" and that things will get better over time. This does happen sometimes; a depression can resolve on its own without any intervention. But for many women, the symptoms of depression persist for months and months. In one study, about one-third of women with postpartum depression were still depressed *one year* after the birth of their child! And that is way too much time to lose.

You may feel too ashamed or embarrassed to ask for help. Despite many advances in the treatment of depression and an increasing awareness of the problem, depression retains a stigma. Being depressed at a time when society says you should be happy may make you feel like a failure as a mother and too ashamed to ask for help. Having caring and supportive family members and friends may help you to overcome this obstacle. However, if those close to you do not fully understand depression or are suspicious of the mental health profession, it may be even more difficult for you to seek help.

You may not have the time or energy to take care of yourself. Most new mothers remark that it is difficult to find the time to do even the most basic things, like getting a bite to eat or going to the bathroom, let alone having time or energy to take care of their emotional well-being. Although you may recognize that something is wrong, it may seem easier to just keep pushing ahead. And depression itself may make the situation worse, sapping you of your energy and making it difficult to take action and to find help for yourself.

Even when you ask for help, you may not get what you need. Too often, women in this situation face a lack of understanding, even among health professionals, regarding their condition. Unfortunately, doctors receive little training on postpartum depression. In fact, many physicians and other health professionals are misinformed about the problem, nor do they really know how to evaluate a woman for postpartum depression. Despite the fact that women in one study saw their doctors several times during the first few months after their child was born, *less than 10 percent of cases of postpartum depression were detected.* Later in the postpartum period, doctors were better able to identify postpartum depression; still it appeared that nearly half of the cases were never identified.

Because it has been so difficult to identify women with postpartum depression, researchers have developed tools to help doctors and other health professionals to screen for it. In the appendix, you will find the Edinburgh Postnatal Depression Scale. This ten-item questionnaire can identify women who may have postpartum depression. If you score a 12 or higher on this scale, there is a good chance you have postpartum depression and should contact your obstetrician, your primary care provider, or a mental health professional for a more thorough evaluation. If you answer yes to question 10, indicating that you are having suicidal thoughts, you should contact your doctor immediately. Although this questionnaire may be a useful tool, it is important to remember that this is not a substitute for a thorough evaluation from a trained professional. If you—or somebody who knows you well—thinks that you may be suffering from postpartum depression, you should discuss this with your doctor.

What Causes Postpartum Depression?

If you're depressed, you want to understand what is happening and you want to find a reason for it. This is especially true for the new mother. Having a child is supposed to be a joyful experience, and there seems to be little room for being sad or depressed. Many women find it difficult to understand why they are depressed under these circumstances. If you have a new baby who is healthy and doing well and a husband who loves you, there seems to be no good reason for feeling sad. Unable to find a good reason, you may end up trying to construct an explanation for the depression, blaming somebody or something for how you feel. You may tell yourself, "If only my husband were more helpful, I wouldn't feel so depressed." Or, "The baby is colicky. Who *wouldn't* feel depressed?" But often it's not that easy to find an explanation; it may seem as if your depression has no obvious cause.

Rebecca and her husband were married six years. Rebecca was working as a corporate lawyer; she loved her career even though it was demanding. But she also wanted to have children, so after her thirty-fifth birthday, she and her husband decided to try. Very quickly she became pregnant. She was happy but also very frightened. How would things change? How much would she have to give up to have this baby? Over time, she felt reassured by her husband, who was so excited about being a father and who clearly would do everything he could to help her.

The first few weeks after the birth of the baby were difficult for Rebecca and her husband, as they learned to care for their new baby. Eventually things started to settle down, and Rebecca felt more comfortable and competent as a mother. Still it was not entirely enjoyable for her; she felt lonely during the days, and every time she saw her husband leave for work, she felt a pang of jealousy. Sometimes she just felt so trapped. She had planned to take off six months for maternity leave but found herself wanting to go back earlier. Every time she had these thoughts, she felt like a bad mother. She looked at other mothers with their new babies and was convinced that they were better mothers than she could ever be. She tried so hard to enjoy herself and to be happy being a mother, but when she was not able to feel content with her new situation, she felt like a failure. She had succeeded at everything else she had tried; why couldn't she make this work?

Often, women and their families believe that postpartum depression occurs when a mother is unhappy about being a mother or when the pregnancy was unwelcome or unwanted. This is simply not true. Like Rebecca, many women feel tremendously guilty about feeling depressed and blame themselves for their depression. However, it is important to keep in mind that postpartum depression is an illness that may affect *any* woman after the birth of a child. It does not mean that a mother is unprepared, unwilling, or unable to be a good mother.

Postpartum depression is an illness that may have many different causes. For all women, the postpartum period—with its intense physiologic changes and psychological demands—has the potential to be a uniquely potent stressor. A landmark study from Dr. Robert Kendell and his colleagues at the Edinburgh University in Scotland indicates that during the first month following childbirth, a woman is more likely to develop a serious psychiatric illness than at any other point in her lifetime. As we discussed earlier, if you have a history of depression or other psychiatric problems, you may be at even greater risk for postpartum depression. However, *all* women are at risk. Whether or not you become depressed after delivery is influenced by many different factors—hormonal, psychological, social, and cultural. Despite much study in this area, our understanding of exactly what causes postpartum depression remains incomplete.

Hormonal Changes

The postpartum period is characterized by rapid fluctuations in your hormone levels. During pregnancy, levels of estrogen and progesterone rise to 200 to 1,000 times their pre-pregnancy levels. Since the primary source of these hormones is the placenta, estrogen and progesterone levels drop precipitously at delivery when the placenta leaves the body. Within three to five days estrogen and progesterone drop to their pre-pregnancy levels and remain relatively low until menstruation resumes.

As we discussed in chapter 2, estrogen, progesterone, and other steroid hormones interact with multiple neurotransmitter systems within the brain and may play an important role in regulating mood. Given this important interaction, it has been hypothesized that postpartum depression may be triggered by the decline in estrogen levels and that women who develop postpartum depression have lower levels of estrogen after birth. While the estrogen deficiency hypothesis makes a great deal of sense from a purely scientific standpoint, several studies failed to identify any consistent difference in estrogen levels between depressed and nondepressed women. Other researchers have attributed postpartum depression to a progesterone deficiency. In fact, progesterone is sometimes used to treat women with postpartum depression in Europe, though there appears to be little evidence to support this approach. Studies have demonstrated no difference in progesterone levels between depressed and nondepressed women.

While these studies indicate that measuring blood levels of estrogen and progesterone may not be particularly useful in making a diagnosis of postpartum depression or in identifying women at highest risk for this disorder, these findings do not exclude a role for reproductive hormones. We suspect that certain women may be particularly sensitive to the normal hormonal changes of the postpartum period and more likely to experience mood changes in response. Similar although less dramatic hormonal shifts occur during the premenstrual phase of the menstrual cycle, and some researchers contend that women who have more intense premenstrual symptoms may be more vulnerable to postpartum depression. These women show no overt evidence of a hormonal imbalance or abnormal levels of these hormones, yet what they experience is an abnormal response (i.e., depression) to normal hormonal fluctuations.

Research has also focused on the role of other hormones in postpartum depression. For some women, abnormalities in thyroid hormone levels may play a role. This theory makes a great deal of sense scientifically, since thyroid hormones regulate the body's metabolism and level of activity. Hypothyroidism, or a deficiency in thyroid hormone, causes a variety of symptoms, including fatigue, weight gain, loss of libido, and depression. Women are at high risk for thyroid abnormalities during the first six months following the birth of a child. However, it appears that only a small number of cases of postpartum depression can be attributed to thyroid dysfunction. Since thyroid function abnormalities may cause postpartum depression and are easily treated, it is important to screen for thyroid dysfunction if you develop depressive symptoms during pregnancy or the postpartum period.

Psychological and Social Factors

After the birth of a child, you are faced with many new situations and unfamiliar emotions. Although this transition may bring much joy, it also comes with a significant amount of stress. Early psychoanalytic theories held that postpartum depression was a disorder driven by a woman's unconscious rejection of motherhood; it was thought to be more common among women with a distorted perception of motherhood or conflicted relationships with their own mothers. While these theories are interesting and merit some discussion, it is important to recognize they are not based on systematic research. While postpartum depression in some women may be associated with negative or ambivalent feelings about being a mother, it cannot be assumed that *all* women with postpartum depression have similar feelings. You should be reassured that having postpartum depression is not an indication of your unwillingness or inability to fulfill your role as a mother.

Recent research takes a more systematic approach to understanding the role of psychological factors in postpartum depression, and it does appear that these factors play an important role in determining vulnerability to depression during the postpartum period. Some studies suggest that unmarried women and women who report marital discord or dissatisfaction are at higher risk for postpartum depression than happily married women. Postpartum depression is also more common among women who report that they have insufficient support from their partner or their family.

Several studies have also demonstrated that stressful life events occurring either during pregnancy or near the time of delivery appear to increase the likelihood of postpartum depression. Being exposed to physical abuse seems to be one of the most potent stressors; one study indicates that postpartum depression occurs in about 25 percent of women who are victims of domestic violence. Other life events that have been strongly associated with postpartum depression include loss of employment by the mother or her partner, financial hardship, and the serious illness of or death of a loved one.

While it is apparent that one or two stressful events may increase a woman's vulnerability to depression after delivery, it is also clear that the risk is even higher when a woman experiences multiple stressors. In a recent study, women who reported six or more significant stressors were almost five times as likely to develop postpartum depression than women who reported no significant stressors. Unfortunately, stressful life events tend to occur together. While postpartum depression affects all women regardless of class or socioeconomic status, we know that women living in poverty are particularly susceptible. In addition to suffering extreme economic hardship, these women may be exposed to multiple stressors associated with poverty including teenage pregnancy, single parenthood, domestic violence, alcohol and drug abuse, and poor physical health.

Only a few studies have looked at the impact of stressful events specific to pregnancy. Rates of postpartum depression appear to be similar between women who have had a caesarean or uncomplicated vaginal delivery, though a prolonged or difficult labor may increase the risk of postpartum depression. Anything that may complicate or slow the process of physical recovery after the birth may make a woman more vulnerable to depression. Another factor that clearly increases risk for postpartum depression is having a premature infant or a baby with significant health problems; these women experience at least a twofold to threefold increase in risk for postpartum depression. Caring for and attending to a baby's multiple medical problems puts a significant strain on the mother.

Cultural Attitudes

Postpartum depression has been observed in cultures throughout the world, but early studies suggested that postpartum depression was more common in industrialized countries than in less developed or non-Westernized cultures. Although there may be several ways to interpret this discrepancy, one explanation is that non-Westernized cultures practice certain customs related to childbirth and the transition to parenthood that protect a woman from postpartum depression. In more industrialized countries like the United States, although a great deal of attention is paid to the mother during her pregnancy, the focus shifts dramatically after the baby is born. All nurturing is directed toward the baby, and the mother is expected to provide attentive caregiving, while also taking care of herself, her partner, the rest of her family, and her household. Even when family members are involved, they typically gravitate to the newborn. Contrast this situation to the Latin American custom called *la cuarentena*, or "the quarantine," referring to the period of rest a woman takes after giving birth.

The practice of *la cuarentena* allows the new mother to rest for forty days while female relatives take over her domestic chores. She is given special foods to promote her healthy recovery (chicken soup, tortillas), while other foods that are believed to be unhealthy for a new mother are avoided (pork, beans, and chiles). During this period, the woman avoids certain activities including bathing and walking barefoot, which may result in exposure to *male de aire* (literally the "bad wind") and may make her more vulnerable to other health problems. In China there is a similar practice of "doing the month," or *Zuo Yue*, which allows the mother to rest while she is cared for by her extended family for a month after delivery. In Japan, this practice is called *Satogaeri bunben*. One to two months before her child is due, the mother returns to her family of origin, and there she is cared for by her mother and other family members. When the baby is two months old, she returns to her husband.

Although modern cultures have strayed from many of these time-honored traditions, these rituals serve an important function for the new mother and her family. While they may not be driven by scientific evidence, their benefits cannot be ignored. First, these customs all recognize that a woman and her child are particularly vulnerable during the postpartum period and need protection. They maintain the integrity of the family and allow the mother to assume her new role within a nurturing and supportive environment where she is allowed to rest and recover. At the same time she is given the opportunity to learn to care for her infant from those who are more experienced, and she is allowed to give her full attention to her baby. It is interesting to note that among immigrants to the United States, those who continue to practice *la cuarentena* have lower rates of postpartum depression than women who give up this custom.

Infant Temperament

When a new mother is depressed, her ability to form and to maintain a connection with her child may be affected. While this disruption has been considered a by-product of maternal depression, some researchers, such as Drs. Lynn Murray and Peter Cooper at the University of Reading in Great Britain, believe that disruption of the relationship between mother and child may actually *cause* postpartum depression. We know that the infants of depressed mothers are less content, more tense, and more difficult to soothe than the infants of nondepressed mothers. While it is typically assumed that these infant behaviors occur *in response* to the mother's depression, it is possible that these difficult infant behaviors may actually cause depression in the mother.

In one study, mothers and infants were observed ten days after delivery, before the onset of depression, and again two months later. Dr. Murray and her colleagues observed that two infant factors could be used to predict which mothers would be depressed at two months postpartum: first, depression was more common in women whose infants had poorly regulated physical activity. These infants either had poor muscle tone and were limp, or they were tense and rigid. Second, women with infants who were more irritable or fussy were more likely to become depressed. These infants were more sensitive to changes in their environment, appeared to be distressed or tense, and were very difficult to soothe. If both poor motor functioning *and* irritability were present, the risk of postpartum depression was particularly high.

How certain infant behaviors may increase a mother's vulnerability to depression is not entirely clear, but caring for a "difficult" child can certainly create significant stress. Routine caretaking activities, such as feeding and bathing the infant, place considerable demands on the mother. When a baby is not easily comforted, it may be difficult for a mother to feel competent and in control. Furthermore, these kinds of behaviors may impede communication between mother and child, and, as we discussed in chapter 3, it is these earliest forms of communication that are so important for maternal bonding. If during the earliest weeks of her life, a baby is hard to read and difficult to comfort, it may contribute to long-lasting disruption in the interaction between a mother and her child.

Recognizing the Effects of Postpartum Depression on the Family

We know that depression affects a woman's ability to function and to derive pleasure from her life. It colors her relationships with everybody around her, and may have a pronounced ripple effect, affecting her children, her husband, other family members, and even her friends. Even a relatively mild episode of postpartum depression may have a pronounced effect on a child's development and well-being, since depression interferes with a mother's ability to attach to and attentively care for her infant and to enjoy and derive satisfaction from her role as a mother. This early disruption in attachment may result in developmental delays and behavioral problems as the child grows older.

Many women who suffer from postpartum depression worry about the scars their depression may leave on their children. They wonder whether things would have been different if they had been able to engage more actively with their child and to be more emotionally available. And long after the depression subsides, they are often left with tremendous feelings of guilt and regret, believing that they have missed out on many aspects of their child's early life and struggling with the fear that they cannot get that time back. This is why it is important to recognize depression early and get good treatment. In fact, if a woman is at risk for postpartum depression, there may actually be an opportunity to intervene before the baby is born, and to avoid the devastating effects of this illness. In chapters 12 and 13, we will discuss how to find treatment and strategies that may be used to treat or prevent postpartum depression.

Chapter 9

No Sense of Reality

Postpartum Psychosis

Postpartum psychosis is a rare event, affecting only 1 in 1,000 women after childbirth. What distinguishes postpartum psychosis from other types of postpartum illness is not only the severity of its symptoms, but also the presence of psychotic symptoms, or *psychosis*, a pronounced detachment from reality. This is a horrible and frightening experience for the mother and her family, and, what's worse, postpartum psychosis may make a mother behave in inexplicable and potentially dangerous ways. Within the warped context of her psychotic thinking, a woman with postpartum psychosis is able to justify inappropriate, bizarre, and, sometimes deadly behaviors. Especially terrifying are the strange or violent thoughts and feelings a mother may have regarding her children. In the summer of 2001, the public was shocked and horrified by the actions of Andrea Pia Yates. In this case a loving mother, under the influence of her psychotic beliefs, was motivated to drown her five children. Although Yates now sits in prison, we must accept that this was not the deranged behavior of an evil or immoral woman but rather the misguided actions of a mother with postpartum psychosis.

Until very recently, most people were totally unaware of this form of psychiatric illness; many books about postpartum depression don't even mention it. Despite the media's recent attention to this topic, there continue to be many misconceptions regarding postpartum psychosis. Although it is a relatively rare complication of childbirth, it is imperative that women, their families, and their doctors be able to recognize the symptoms of this very serious illness. *Postpartum psychosis is a psychiatric emergency, a situation that under no circumstances can be ignored.* Although this can be a dramatic and devastating illness, with early intervention it is highly treatable, and the vast majority of women recover completely.

What Exactly Is Postpartum Psychosis?

Postpartum psychosis is, in some ways, a rather nonspecific term that tells little about the underlying disease. Psychosis is not a disease: it is a symptom. Psychosis—a loss of contact with reality—may occur in those suffering from a wide range of different psychiatric illnesses. Many people worry that psychotic symptoms necessarily imply a psychotic disorder, like schizophrenia. However, these symptoms may also be seen in patients with severe depression or bipolar disorder.

So what exactly is postpartum psychosis? Is it a psychotic illness like schizophrenia? Or is it more like a mood disorder? Or is it something entirely different? Some experts have argued that postpartum psychosis is a disease that is distinct from all other psychiatric disorders, having its own characteristic symptoms and course of illness. However, most now believe that the majority of women with postpartum psychosis suffer from a mood disorder—either major depression or bipolar disorder. About 5 percent of women with postpartum psychosis most likely have either schizophrenia or a similar type of chronic psychotic illness. In general, the prognosis for women with postpartum psychosis is very good. The vast majority of women recover from this illness and return to a high level of functioning.

What we typically see in women with postpartum psychosis is a spectrum of symptoms that most resembles the manic symptoms observed in women with bipolar disorder. In addition to psychotic symptoms, sleeplessness, agitation, rapidly shifting moods, and erratic behavior are prominent in both. A handful of studies has evaluated the long-term course of illness in women with postpartum psychosis and suggest a link between bipolar disorder and postpartum psychosis. In a recent follow-up study of women with postpartum psychosis, it was observed that about three-quarters of the women had another episode of psychiatric illness. Most went on to have a course of illness that was most consistent with bipolar disorder, having recurrent episodes of either depression or mania. Most often, these other episodes were not related to pregnancy or childbirth.

Early Signs of Illness

The symptoms of postpartum psychosis are usually quite severe and tend to emerge very early after the birth of a child, usually within a few days of delivery and sometimes while the mother is still in the hospital recovering from childbirth. In almost all cases, the symptoms are evident within the first two weeks after delivery. Postpartum psychosis affects a woman's emotions, her behavior, and her capacity to think rationally. However, in its earliest stages, a woman may not be aware that anything is wrong, and even women with severe symptoms may have limited insight into their condition. Especially in the early stages of illness, a woman with postpartum psychosis may not reveal any significant changes in her mood or her ability to think rationally; however, the way she behaves is usually quite different from her usual self or deviates markedly from what one would expect of a new mother, and this is what family members often notice first.

SYMPTOMS OF POSTPARTUM PSYCHOSIS

Insomnia or decreased need for sleep

Increased energy, restlessness, or agitation

Racing thoughts

Elated or euphoric mood (mania)

Sadness or despair (depression)

Rapidly shifting moods

Irritability

Grandiosity (thinking one is special in some way or has special powers)

Talkativeness

Depersonalization (feeling detached from one's surroundings or others)

Distractibility or confusion

Paranoia or bizarre behavior

Auditory or visual hallucinations

Delusions (false beliefs)

Inability to care for self or baby

Thoughts of harming self or baby

Initially, a woman with postpartum psychosis may have problems sleeping, especially if she is getting up frequently to feed the baby. Even when the baby is asleep, the mother may be unable to settle down and rest and, despite the lack of sleep, she may not feel tired. She may even seem agitated or restless, pacing back and forth, seemingly unable to stay still for any length of time. In some cases, a mother may describe feeling energized or "hyper"; it is impossible to slow down. She moves fast. She talks fast. When she is unable to sleep, she tries to find things to do with all her extra energy, like cleaning the house, rearranging her closets, or sending e-mails to all of her friends and family.

As with postpartum depression, anxiety may be one of the earliest symptoms of postpartum psychosis. Although every new mother is likely to have some worries about her child, when anxiety is part of a psychotic illness, it often has a very different flavor: it is more intense and all-encompassing. A mother with postpartum psychosis may also have worries that seem unusual or even bizarre to others. For example, she may be convinced that her child has a life-threatening illness, or she may be afraid that somebody is trying to harm or to take her child away from her.

Extreme Mood Changes

A woman with postpartum psychosis experiences significant and rapid shifts in her mood. Over the course of a few days, or even hours, she may move from a state of excited exuberance to intense irritability and despair. While this may sound somewhat like the emotional roller coaster described by women with postpartum blues, it is definitely *not* the blues. Again, the tell-tale difference is that a woman with postpartum psychosis cannot recognize that she has little perspective on what is going on around her or that her perceptions of the external world may be fantastically distorted. Women with postpartum psychosis may appear elated or euphoric, even manic. They feel excited and extraordinarily confident of themselves. They talk rapidly with great intensity, moving from one topic to another. Their thoughts move through their head so quickly that with this "flight of ideas," their thinking may become muddled or chaotic. They are excessively and frenetically active, although they may end up being so disorganized or distracted that they cannot complete even the simplest of tasks.

> Cara was thirty-five when she and her husband had their first baby. She was ecstatic when the baby was born. She was so excited that she could barely sleep, and a few days after she returned home from the hospital, she decided to have a party for her friends and family so that they could all celebrate together. She had always been an active and dynamic person, but everybody was impressed—even shocked—by her energy and enthusiasm. Cara just felt like she could not stop; she had so many things that she needed and wanted to do.
>
> About a week later, Cara crashed. She found herself crying all day long and barely able to think straight. Although only a few days earlier she had felt so confident about her skills as a mother, now she felt totally incompetent. She repeatedly asked her husband for reassurance and help. She was afraid to leave the house, fearful that somebody would comment on how she was caring for her baby and convinced that her baby would be taken away from her. Despite her husband's attempts to comfort and reassure her, she could not shake these worries. She even started to be suspicious of her husband and refused to let him or his mother be alone with the baby; she was certain that they were planning to take the baby away from her.

Cara continued to have trouble sleeping even though she felt totally exhausted. She could barely eat, and within a few weeks of delivery had returned to her pre-pregnancy weight. She felt tense and edgy and just couldn't let go of the fear that something bad was going to happen to her or her baby. Every time she listened to the radio or television, Cara listened for some type of message—a certain word or phrase—that would tell her what was going to happen and when. When the baby was about four weeks old, she started going to a nearby church. She felt that she and the baby would be safe from harm there.

As was the case with Cara, depression may follow on the heels of a manic phase. When a postpartum psychotic episode is depressive in nature, a woman feels sad and despairing; she is unable to derive pleasure from her life. She withdraws from others. Many women exhibit what are called "mixed" symptoms, where they have features of both mania and depression. This is an uncomfortable condition where the agitation and irritability of mania are mingled with the pessimism and despair of depression. A woman with mixed symptoms lashes out at others with little provocation. She may become irrational and overemotional, responding to events with unpredictable intensity. At the same time she may be plagued by intense feelings of hopelessness and may find it extraordinarily difficult to motivate herself or feel positive about the future.

Women with postpartum psychosis frequently have thoughts of their own death. The depression may seem so very deep and dark that it appears there is no way out of it. When women experience this level of despair and hopelessness, suicide may seem like a viable option; it may feel like the only means of escaping from what seems a horrible nightmare. Delusions may cloud a woman's ability to think clearly. Some women have an unswerving belief that they are going to die in the immediate future. They believe that they have a life-threatening illness or that something bad will happen to them. It must be emphasized that women who are in this state are at very high risk for suicide; in the midst of a psychotic episode, they are not rational. Furthermore, when these women think about taking their own life, they tend to choose very lethal or violent methods—like jumping from a building or shooting or stabbing themselves. This is *not* just a cry for help.

The tragic story of Melanie Stokes, a mother from Chicago, helps to highlight the seriousness of this problem. Soon after the birth of her first child, Melanie became deeply depressed. Although she had always wanted to be a mother, she felt that her baby had ruined her life and she feared that her husband would leave her. As the depression worsened, she stopped eating and drinking. Her behavior became more erratic. She wandered out of her house in the middle of the night and was found at the lakefront. She asked a neighbor if he owned a gun. She started having paranoid thoughts about her neighbors, convinced that they were sending her messages telling her that she was a bad mother. During the first three months of her child's life, she was hospitalized four times. Despite the attempts of her family to watch over her, when her daughter was three months old, Melanie disappeared from her home. Four days later she committed suicide by jumping from a twelfth-story hotel window.

Losing Touch with Reality

In all women with postpartum psychosis, the ability to think clearly and rationally is impaired or distorted, although the degree to which this happens may vary considerably. Often women with postpartum psychosis describe feeling very "fuzzy" or confused. They may sit and stare into space for hours or may wander around aimlessly. One of my patients described hearing the phone ring but not knowing that she was supposed to answer it. Another woman walked around for hours with her baby in a stroller and ended up miles from her house, with no idea of where she was going or how to return home. At worst, a woman may actually feel disconnected from what she is doing and from her child. Some women experience "depersonalization" or "derealization"; they describe the experience of being a detached onlooker. This feeling may begin at the time of labor and delivery. Some women actually describe watching the entire delivery from above, as if they are floating above the scene. They feel no pain whatsoever; it is as if they are watching a movie.

In the earliest stages of postpartum psychosis, it may be difficult to distinguish psychosis from postpartum depression or anxiety. However, as the condition progresses, a woman usually begins to exhibit more overtly psychotic symptoms. While a woman with postpartum depression is able to make more or less correct interpretations of the events in her life, a woman with psychosis has lost touch with reality. She is likely to misinterpret or distort many of the events in her life. She may have delusions, which are strongly held beliefs with no basis in reality; she cannot separate fact from fiction. Frequently the delusional thoughts are focused on the baby. For example, she may be paranoid and convinced that somebody is trying to harm her or her baby. Sometimes women believe that their baby has an incurable illness and is going to die. Another relatively common delusion is that the baby is not their own, but a changeling that was secretly exchanged for their own baby. It is impossible for the new mother to put things back into perspective. Even when others try to point out what is real, she clings to these beliefs.

For Karen, the pregnancy went smoothly, although she had some problems at delivery and her baby was admitted to the special care nursery for a few days. Early on, it seemed that her son was having some breathing problems and occasionally would stop breathing for a few seconds. Although the doctors were not able to explain exactly why this happened, the problem seemed to disappear entirely. After the baby did not have any of these episodes for forty-eight hours, he was discharged and went home with Karen.

When she left the hospital Karen was worried. It was difficult for her to leave the baby alone for fear that he would stop breathing. At night, she and her husband took turns watching their son. But even when her husband was keeping an eye on the baby, Karen could not allow herself to rest; she was so terrified that he would die. As she lay awake, she wondered if maybe her doctors were keeping something from her. Maybe there was something horribly wrong with their child.

Over time, she became more and more suspicious about what had happened when the baby was in the nursery without her. When she was alone with him, she looked for signs that her baby had been harmed in some way. She wondered if one of the nurses or doctors had tried to poison him. On several occasions, she called the hospital to inquire if there had been any unusual deaths in the nursery. She called the medical licensing board, as well. Although she trusted her husband, she did not feel comfortable leaving the baby alone with anybody else. She was worried that others, including some of her friends and family members, may also be trying to hurt her son. Because she was so fearful, she refused to leave the house, and she stopped answering the phone.

While some delusions have some hint of plausibility, others have no connection to reality. One mother was convinced that she was the Virgin Mary and that her child was the baby Jesus. She took her baby to church several days after his birth; at the end of the service, she announced, "Here is the Son of God." Some women may fear that their child has evil powers or is possessed by the devil or a malicious spirit. It is especially unsettling that these strange thoughts can emerge so suddenly; one day everything is fine, and then the next the world feels upside down.

A woman with postpartum psychosis may also have unusual sensory experiences. She may have auditory hallucinations—sounds or voices that others do not hear. Sometimes these are just sounds, like footsteps, a floorboard creaking, or a baby crying. Some women may also hear voices when nobody else is around. One woman described hearing voices making derogatory comments about everything she did: "You are a horrible mother; your baby will never love you." "You don't deserve your baby." Sometimes a mother hears her baby talking to her. A woman may also have what are called *command* auditory hallucinations, voices that tell her what to do. This is of particular concern, because sometimes the mother acts on these voices that may be telling her to harm herself or her baby. Less commonly, visual hallucinations may occur. They are most often shadows or hazy images, rather than fully formed, Technicolor apparitions. Nonetheless, hallucinations of any sort are a warning sign and should never be ignored.

While some women may discuss these experiences with others, many women keep these thoughts to themselves. Often women with postpartum psychosis suspect that their thinking is not normal and they fear that their thoughts or actions may be misunderstood or misinterpreted by others. They are understandably concerned that they will be committed to a psychiatric hospital or that their child will be taken away if they are honest about their thoughts and feelings. But other women have less insight into their situation. They do not ask for help because they are not even aware that they are suffering from an illness. In some instances, they become so paranoid of others that even when questioned directly by someone who is empathic and outwardly understanding, these disturbing thoughts and symptoms may remain a secret.

Children at Risk

Unable to sleep and feeling totally depleted, a woman suffering from postpartum psychosis may not have the energy or strength to take care of a new baby. While we tend to focus on the welfare of the baby, it is important to remember than the whole family is at risk. A woman with this debilitating illness may not be able to fully attend to the needs of any of her children. In addition, she may be so haunted by disturbing thoughts that she may be unable or afraid to take care of her children, or her behavior may be so erratic and disorganized that even the simplest tasks seem confusing or overwhelming to her. A mother may feel detached from her new baby. So preoccupied with the chaos of her internal world, she may seem unresponsive to her child's cries. In this situation, the child may be neglected or left to the care of others. This behavior may also be motivated by delusional thinking. For example, if a mother believes that her baby is going to die, she may not want to care for her child. If she believes that her child is possessed by the devil, she may reject him.

Of grave concern is the possibility that the baby is the focus of a complicated delusion. While some women with postpartum depression think about harming their infant, they recognize that these thoughts are irrational and wrong and so do not act them out. In contrast, a mother in the midst of a full-fledged psychosis may temporarily lose the ability to make appropriate decisions regarding her child; she may be motivated to act in accordance with these delusions and behave in a way that poses a threat to her child. Her inability to provide her baby consistent care may place the baby at risk, but the situation can be even more extreme. For example, a mother who believes that a child is not her own may abandon her baby. A mother who thinks her baby has an incurable illness may decide to kill the baby herself, to put the baby out of his misery. A mother who believes her baby is possessed by the devil may kill her baby, fearful that the baby may harm her or the rest of her family. It is for this reason that postpartum psychosis represents a psychiatric emergency.

It is hard to imagine how a mother can possibly think about harming or killing her child. Although this act by a mother is incomprehensible, there are literally thousands of reports of mothers who have killed their children while in the grip of a psychotic episode. Although there are many different reasons why a mother may kill her child, experts agree that severe psychiatric illness is a factor in many of these cases. When a mother thinks that killing her child is the right thing for her to do, what is unimaginable to others makes sense within the context of her delusional thinking. She is not a criminal but someone who is gravely ill, and she desperately needs treatment.

What Causes Postpartum Psychosis?

Despite considerable research, there is still no clear medical consensus as to what causes postpartum psychosis. The illness sometimes runs in families and it is believed that many women have an underlying genetic or biologic vulnerability to this disorder. Recent studies have shown that about 65 percent to 75 percent of women with postpartum psychosis will go on to have another episode of illness. For the majority of women, postpartum psychosis is not an isolated event but rather the manifestation of an underlying and recurrent mood disorder. Even when this is the first episode of illness, women with postpartum psychosis are likely to go on to have other episodes of illness.

It appears that the postpartum period acts as an extraordinarily potent trigger for psychiatric illness, and various studies have estimated that, during the weeks following childbirth, women are 20 to 30 times more likely to develop a serious psychiatric illness than at any other point in their lifetime, so it is not surprising that women with an underlying mood disorder, such as depression or bipolar disorder, may experience a recurrence or a more severe episode of this illness after childbirth. So what is it about the postpartum period? Many investigators point to the dramatic hormonal changes that take place after delivery. Others blame the extreme sleep deprivation that often occurs around the birth of a child, particularly for women with bipolar disorder or an underlying vulnerability to this illness.

Who Is at Risk for Postpartum Psychosis?

Postpartum psychosis is so rare that much of what we know about this devastating illness is gleaned from case reports and a few small studies. As a result, our understanding of the risk factors for postpartum psychosis remains unclear. What we *do* know is that postpartum psychosis, like postpartum depression, can affect any woman, young or old, married or single, wealthy or poor. Several studies indicate that postpartum psychosis may be more common among single mothers; first-time mothers may also be more vulnerable. Some researchers have proposed that these women are under greater stress than married women or women in a stable relationship. Other researchers have questioned whether postpartum psychosis may, in fact, be an abnormal response to a stressful situation; however, most studies fail to show any association between stressful life events and postpartum psychosis.

A woman's vulnerability to postpartum psychosis may be hereditary, and the literature is speckled with reports of families in which many women, across several consecutive generations, have been afflicted with this illness. It appears that if a woman has one close female relative with a history of postpartum psychosis, her risk of developing the same illness is increased. In some families, postpartum psychosis appears to cluster together with bipolar disorder (manic depression), and recent studies demonstrate a high risk of postpartum psychosis among women who suffer from bipolar disorder. If you have bipolar disorder, your risk of developing a psychotic episode in the first month after delivery is about 25 to 30 times greater than other women.

Even if you have had only one episode of illness and have been well for many years, you should be aware that you are at high risk for illness during the postpartum period.

Although certain women may be at greater risk for this illness, many of the women who develop postpartum psychosis have never had any type of psychiatric illness prior to pregnancy. It is for this reason that *all* women, as well as their families and health care professionals, should be able to recognize the signs and symptoms of this potentially devastating illness. If there is *any* concern that a mother is suffering from severe postpartum depression or psychosis, professional help should be sought immediately.

How Is Postpartum Psychosis Treated?

Unfortunately, there is little consistency in how postpartum psychosis is treated, and practices vary widely. This is in part due to the lack of well-designed studies to guide clinical practice and is complicated by the fact that postpartum psychosis may encompass a bewildering array of symptoms. What is clear to all, however, is that postpartum psychosis represents a medical emergency in which both the mother and her child (and possibly other children) are at risk. Although with careful monitoring it may be possible to manage this illness while the mother remains at home, most women who develop this illness are hospitalized. This ensures the safety of everyone and allows doctors to see how the mother responds to medication.

In the vast majority of cases, antipsychotic medications (also known as neuroleptics) are used as the first line of treatment. These medications are specifically used to treat psychotic symptoms, including delusions and hallucinations. While the older antipsychotic agents, including haloperidol (Haldol) and chlorpromazine (Thorazine), are very effective, they are fraught with multiple side effects, including certain types of movement disorders. The newer generation of antipsychotic medications are highly effective and extremely well-tolerated. (More information on these antipsychotic medications can be found in chapters 12 and 13.) Olanzapine (Zyprexa) is commonly used in women with postpartum psychosis; it is effective for psychotic symptoms and may also be helpful in promoting sleep in women who have severe insomnia. Within a few days or weeks of treatment, the psychotic symptoms typically begin to improve, although it usually takes longer for the symptoms to disappear completely.

Because most women with postpartum psychosis have an underlying mood disorder, more than one type of medication may be needed. For women with symptoms suggestive of bipolar disorder, a mood stabilizer should be considered. This type of medication is helpful for alleviating both manic and depressive symptoms. The conventional mood stabilizers include lithium and several antiseizure medications, carbamazepine (Tegretol) and valproate (Depakote or Depakene). Lamotrigine (Lamietal) is a newer antiseizure medication that appears to be quite helpful for women who have predominantly depressive symptoms. Olanzapine (Zyprexa) is also considered to be a mood stabilizer and may have an advantage over other medications in that it treats psychotic symptoms as well as mood symptoms. Given the strong link between postpartum psychosis and bipolar disorder, antidepressants should be used with caution. In a patient with bipolar disorder, an antidepressant may bring on an episode of mania or may cause agitation or irritability.

Electroconvulsive therapy (also called ECT, or electroshock therapy), although not used very commonly, is a highly effective and safe treatment for women with postpartum psychosis and depression. (See chapter 12 for more on ECT.) Usually a patient will receive between six and twelve treatment sessions, one every other day, and improvement may be seen within the first week of treatment, compared to the two to four weeks it may take a woman to respond to a conventional mood stabilizer. Women who are nursing may also find this a more attractive option because it avoids exposure of the baby to medications secreted in the breast milk.

A research group from Finland has also explored the use of estrogen in women with postpartum psychosis. In this study, women with psychosis were treated with estradiol, a form of estrogen, and noted improvement in their symptoms within the first week of treatment. While this is an interesting study and suggests a link between postpartum hormonal changes and psychosis, other studies do not support the effectiveness of estrogen. Estrogen remains an experimental treatment, and conventional treatment with antipsychotic medications and mood stabilizers should be considered the primary forms of treatment.

Whatever type of treatment is chosen, it is of utmost importance to control the symptoms quickly. While some countries, including the United Kingdom, have mother-baby inpatient psychiatric units where the mother can be hospitalized along with her baby, we usually do not have this option in the United States. When the mother is hospitalized, she may be separated from her child for at least several days or even a few weeks. Although women with severe psychiatric illness may feel relieved to be in a hospital so that they can focus on their own recuperation without having to care for a new baby, being separated from one's child at this early stage may be particularly traumatic. It is important that postpartum psychosis be recognized early and treated aggressively so that the mother can return home and care for her child.

Exactly how long to continue treatment varies. Although antipsychotic medications are usually discontinued at some point (typically after three to six months of treatment), women with an underlying mood disorder will require long-term maintenance treatment with an antidepressant or a mood stabilizer to prevent recurrent episodes. In cases of postpartum psychosis where the woman recovers quickly and has no history of psychiatric illness prior to pregnancy, the decision may be made to discontinue treatment after six to twelve months. However, given the high risk of recurrence in this population, cessation is an option that should be pursued with caution and close monitoring.

How Long Does It Last? Will It Ever Go Away? Will It Return?

Just how long an episode of postpartum psychosis lasts is unclear. In the literature, there are reports of very brief periods of illness, lasting only a few days. However, most cases, when left untreated, may be quite protracted, lasting several months or longer. Medical texts dating from the turn of the century report cases of women who were institutionalized after the birth of a child and remained so for many years. This may give us some idea as to what happens with severe postpartum illness in the absence of treatment; however, with effective treatments now available, even the most extreme symptoms can be controlled within a few weeks, although it may take longer for *all* the symptoms to clear completely.

Although postpartum psychosis is usually severe and quite dramatic, most women with this disorder go on to do very well after receiving treatment. About 5 percent of women have a very complicated course of illness and have difficulty returning to their previous level of functioning, but the vast majority of women with postpartum psychosis do quite well over time. As discussed earlier, most women with postpartum psychosis have some type of mood disorder and will go on to have other episodes of either depression or mania. As a result, many women who have postpartum psychosis will require some sort of maintenance treatment and monitoring. For those with a diagnosis of bipolar disorder, long-term treatment with a mood stabilizer, such as lithium or lamotrigine, is indicated.

Some women have a less common form of postpartum psychosis where their episodes occur *only* after childbirth; at other times they are well and show no signs of illness. This postpartum-only pattern appears to be more common in women for whom postpartum psychosis occurs very early after delivery and is the first ever episode of illness. Even when the illness is very severe at its onset, women with this "pure" form of postpartum psychosis recover quickly and completely and remain healthy and symptom-free, even after discontinuing medication.

Probably the most important question that women ask is that regarding their chance of developing psychosis after another pregnancy. Postpartum psychosis is such a frightening experience that many women who have suffered from this illness choose never to have children again. Given the existing data, it is difficult to reassure women planning to have another child. While some studies show modest rates of recurrence, in the range of 25 percent to 35 percent, others demonstrate a recurrence risk as high as 90 percent. Although the risk is high, it is important to recognize that certain interventions reduce a woman's risk of developing postpartum psychosis in subsequent pregnancies.

How to Prevent Postpartum Psychosis

In many cases, it may not be possible to prevent postpartum psychosis. For many women, this represents the first episode of illness, and they enter into the postpartum period unaware they are at risk. In these situations, the best we can hope for is to identify the illness early and to make sure that the appropriate treatment is initiated. But it is possible to identify, long before the baby is born, certain women who are clearly more vulnerable to postpartum psychosis—women with histories of bipolar disorder or postpartum psychosis after a previous pregnancy—and there is solid evidence indicating that it is possible to prevent postpartum psychosis from occurring.

In several studies, lithium has been used in women who have had a prior episode of postpartum psychosis and is initiated during the third trimester of pregnancy. Although one would expect very high rates of recurrent illness in this group of women, the risk of illness was reduced to about 10 percent. A similar study was carried out in women with histories of bipolar disorder by Dr. Lee Cohen and his colleagues at the Massachusetts General Hospital. This study showed similarly good results. Only 1 in 14 women with bipolar disorder receiving prophylactic treatment with lithium became ill after delivery, as compared to 8 out of 13 (62 percent) of the women who received no preventative treatment. Although other mood stabilizers or antipsychotic agents have not been studied for this purpose, they may be a better option for women who are not able to tolerate lithium or who have not responded to lithium in the past.

This type of pharmacologic intervention is clearly beneficial; however, there are many other things that should be in place if you believe that you are at high risk for postpartum psychosis.

- Early in your pregnancy or ideally before you plan to conceive, you should meet with a psychiatrist to discuss your risk of postpartum psychosis and determine if you are a candidate for some type of prophylactic intervention.
- If possible, bring your partner or another family member with you so that they can learn about the signs and symptoms of postpartum psychosis and learn whom to contact in case of emergency.
- Arrange for frequent check-ins with your doctors during the first few months after delivery.
- Be sure to inform your obstetrician or midwife of your situation. They will be in a position to monitor you during the first few days after delivery.
- Discuss with your partner how you can minimize your levels of stress during the postpartum period. It is especially important for you to protect your sleep. Arrange for extra help if you feel that you may need it.

The Importance of Early Intervention

Postpartum psychosis is a rare event, but its destructive potential is immense. Unfortunately, many women with postpartum psychosis do not seek help. They are either too debilitated, or they and their families are not aware that postpartum psychosis is an illness for which effective treatments are available. This is why it is so important for women, as well as their families and their health care providers, to be aware of the signs and symptoms of postpartum psychosis. You can never ignore postpartum psychosis or assume that it will go away on its own. By intervening early, we have the opportunity to spare the woman and her family from the potentially devastating effects of this illness.

Part Four

Minimizing the Impact of Depression

Chapter 10

Life After Children
Partners As Parents

The moment you discover you are pregnant, your relationship with your partner changes. This shift may be subtle or quite extreme. After your child is born, the relationship continues to shift. For better or for worse, children forever change the landscape of your life. The transformation from a couple to a family is viewed by most people as a deeply satisfying and meaningful experience. Having children often helps to deepen and strengthen a relationship, but this transition to parenthood does not always proceed smoothly.

While sharing this new responsibility with a partner may enrich the quality of your lives, other important aspects of the relationship may fade into the background. When children become a priority, the sense of having a romantic, sexual, spiritual, or intellectual partner may wane. Exhausted and overextended, couples often complain that it is difficult to find the time and energy to nurture the nonparental aspects of their relationship. As attention shifts to the children, it is common for one, or even both, members of the couple to feel neglected or abandoned. For other couples, having children serves only to increase friction within the relationship. Problems that existed before the children are exacerbated, and resentments continue to build.

In this chapter, we will discuss how to recognize problems and will outline some basic skills for improving the quality of the relationship. Although having children may strain even the healthiest of relationships, this is also a chance to make positive changes. For many couples, having children provides an opportunity to renew their commitment to each other and to their family. With children in the picture, a couple may become more aware of their conflicts and more willing to resolve these problems so that they do not affect their family. Partners committed to each other can learn to modify old patterns of behavior and can learn to communicate more effectively. Working to improve the quality of your relationship with your partner not only benefits the two of you, it may help to ensure your children's emotional well-being.

The Decision to Have Children

Whether or not to have a family is a question most women consider long before they find the right partner, but within the context of a relationship, the focus on this issue intensifies. When men and women discuss whether or not they want to have a family, the question at the forefront is how having a child will change their lives. They imagine how having a child will enrich their lives, but they also consider the sacrifices they will have to make and they wonder how a child will affect their relationship. In many instances, both partners feel very similarly about their desire to have a family. However, this is not always the case, and the issues surrounding the decision to have a family may cause significant strain within a relationship. While couples may be able to compromise in many different areas, this is an issue so important and so highly charged that differences of opinion on this question may lead to intense conflict and, in the worst of cases, the dissolution of the relationship.

Also emotionally loaded is the decision of *when* to have a child. Is there a "right" time? So many different factors feed into this formula—age, satisfaction with the relationship, financial security, and career—that it is probably impossible to find a time when everything is lined up perfectly. While a couple may have very similar views on their desire for a family, agreeing upon the right time may be much more complicated. Imagine a situation in which one partner feels established in his or her professional life and would like to start a family, while the other partner is still in the midst of starting a career and feels that having a child would be disruptive. Whose needs should prevail in this situation? Obviously, there is no easy answer.

As more people now marry at a later age, many couples have little time to carefully and thoroughly work through this decision together. Instead, their decision is influenced by the biological clock. They may be forced to have a child when other aspects of their life feel very unstable or unpredictable, and this may make the transition to parenthood more difficult. Some couples circumvent taking this decision-making step altogether; about one-half of all pregnancies are unplanned. While this approach may make certain decisions easier, in most cases an unplanned pregnancy generates significant stress.

Carolyn and Philip Cowan are psychologists from the University of California at Berkeley who in the 1970s began to work with and study couples who were becoming parents for the first time. One of the areas addressed in the Becoming a Family Project was how partners decide to become parents. The Cowans observed four different types of couples. Half of the couples were identified as Planners, while the remainder fell into three other categories: Acceptanće of Fate, Ambivalent, or Yes-No. Not surprisingly, the Cowans found that how couples approached the decision to have children had a significant impact on their later transition to parenthood and their satisfaction in being parents.

The Planners spend a significant amount of time deliberating whether or not to have a child and when. At the outset of this process, all Planners are not necessarily certain about their decision to have a child, nor are all Planners entirely in agreement on this topic; however, they are able to engage in a process of negotiation. By the time conception occurs, they both feel relatively comfortable with the decision they have made together.

The Acceptance of Fate Couples are those that become pregnant unexpectedly and, although surprised at first, begin to view the pregnancy relatively quickly as a favorable event. They have very positive feelings about their marriages and feel that a baby will not only enrich their personal lives but also enhance their partnership. The Ambivalent are those couples who, even after becoming pregnant, continue to struggle with mixed feelings about becoming a parent. In the Yes-No couples, there is unresolved conflict about becoming a family, with one of the partners strongly in favor of this decision and the other opposed.

It is these early attitudes toward parenthood that determine how a couple adjusts to parenthood and whether or not this transition will be successful. While all couples describe some deterioration in the quality of their partnership after the birth of a child, the Planners and the Acceptance of Fate couples seemed to fare the best while the Ambivalent and Yes-No couples experienced much higher levels of dissatisfaction. In fact, in the Cowans' study, all the Yes-No couples separated or divorced by the time their child was eighteen months old. It seems that these couples were already having difficulties with communication and negotiation that persisted into parenthood, ultimately causing significant stress and the dissolution of the relationship.

The bottom line is that it helps to prepare for parenthood. You will never be *fully* prepared to have a child, but this process of planning and preparation is critical and helps to solidify your relationship with your partner. Even if you become pregnant unexpectedly or much sooner than anticipated, this is a chance for the two of you to discuss what life will be like after the birth of your child. What are your expectations? Your fears? Are you and your partner on the same page? As you and your partner go through this process, you have the opportunity to develop better communication and negotiation skills, and these will undoubtedly help you as you transition into parent-hood.

The Transition to Parenthood

Most couples look forward to being parents, but even when a child is de-sired and planned for, they are often unprepared for the strain that children may place on their relationship.

> After the birth of their daughter, Abby made the decision to return to work part-time. She wanted to spend more time with her family, but she did not want to give up her career as a pediatrician. The first few months back to work were rough: her days at work were intense and her days at home were not any easier. She took care of the baby, plus the cooking and the cleaning and all of the errands.
>
> As time went on, Abby felt more and more resentful of her husband. George—also a physician—worked long hours. When he was at home, he was tired and spent a few hours each day watching TV or reading the news-paper. Abby was tired too, but she had so many things to do at home that there was no time for her to take care of herself; she was always taking care of somebody else—her baby, her husband, or her patients.
>
> And there was always the sense that George's work was more important. When their daughter was sick, it was Abby who had to miss work. When the baby woke up at night, Abby stayed up with her because George had to be well rested for work the next day. It felt as if her efforts—both inside and outside of the home—were not fully appreciated.

What Abby and George are experiencing is relatively common. Before children, most marriages function as an equitable partnership. The partners have more or less equal footing, sharing domestic and financial responsibil-ities, and even when things are not so equitable, there often seems to be an acceptable reason for the disparity. After a child arrives, however, very often the partners tend to gravitate toward more traditional roles. One parent, usually the mother, takes on the primary responsibility for the child while the other parent takes on responsibility for affairs outside of the house. Even when couples try to share things equitably, there is almost always an un-equal division of labor and this inequality places a considerable amount of strain on the relationship.

While these more traditional roles may work well for some, they do not suit every couple. As the primary caretaker, you have a never-ending and all-consuming occupation and you may feel that your partner does not value the work you do. You may feel that you partner does not appreciate how demanding it is to take care of children, especially when this job is combined with other responsibilities. On the other hand, if you are the member of the couple who is working outside of the home to support the family, you may also feel intense pressure. As you focus on being a good provider, you may worry that, if you do not perform well at work, you may be putting your family in jeopardy. You may feel that you are not allowed to pursue the things you enjoy. In addition, this sort of pressure may drive you to spend more time at work and to be less active in the daily tasks of parenting, a shift which may leave your partner feeling abandoned and overburdened. When this sort of traditional family structure is not working well, you or your partner — or maybe even both of you — may end up feeling that you are bearing too heavy a load, and that your partner is not helping you enough. And over time, this breeds anger and resentment.

Another big problem is that you may not have the time to set aside time for your partner and to nurture your relationship. Most parents are not able to engage in the recreational and social activities that they pursued before they had children. For many couples, these activities are integral to maintaining a healthy relationship; when a couple pursues an activity together, they have the opportunity to cultivate their friendship and to stay involved in each other's lives. Without them, a couple must find other ways to stay connected. Unfortunately, many parents complain that, because they spend so much time focused on their children, they lose touch with their partners.

Melinda and Michael had been married for about a year before having children. They were both working for an investment bank when they had their first child. After the second child, they both agreed that Melinda would leave her job. Melinda was relieved; her job was becoming increasingly stressful and was not particularly family-friendly. She knew she would ultimately go back to work but she looked forward to having time with her young children.

The first six months after the second child arrived went very well; Melinda enjoyed being at home with her children. Initially she felt lonely but she was working to make connections with other stay-at-home mothers. Michael worked long hours and when he came home spent most of his time playing with the children. Melinda was happy to have an involved husband, but she really wanted the chance to talk to him. She worried that he was bored with her. But she also felt a bit resentful. Since she was at home, she was in charge of all the cooking and cleaning. She wanted to ask for help but felt that she could not bother Michael because he was so busy at work. Over time, she felt more and more distant from her husband. She used to ask him about work, but now there was less time to have these conversations. And he didn't seem to ask her about her daily activities. It just seemed as if she had her world, and he had his.

Michael and Melinda both felt that the romantic side of their relationship had almost completely disappeared. When Michael saw how affectionate Melinda was toward the children, he sometimes felt jealous and missed the attention she used to lavish upon him. Melinda felt that Michael was less attentive to her than he used to be; he seemed to be much more interested in the children than in her. They both felt neglected.

Figuring out how to maintain your relationship with your partner *and* pay attention to your children is not always easy. Most parents tend to their children better than to their own relationship. You may find that you have put your relationship with your partner on hold, and you may inadvertently end up shutting out the person to whom you are closest and who is most likely to be supportive.

Although many couples hope and expect that children will improve the quality of their relationship, the research indicates quite the opposite. In fact, most marriages become *less* satisfying after the birth of a child, and this downturn in marital satisfaction may persist for many years. In one long-term study of marital happiness, sociologist Mary Benin of Arizona State University tracked 6,785 couples with and without children over a period of many years. Benin discovered that marital satisfaction tends to follow a U-shaped curve over time. Marital satisfaction is at its highest in couples before having children and seems to plummet in the years following the arrival of the first child. In couples with teenage children, marital happiness is at its lowest, though things begin to improve after this tumultuous time, and marital satisfaction returns to its prechild levels only after the children have left the home. In contrast, marital satisfaction among childless couples tends to improve steadily over time.

While it seems that marriages are particularly vulnerable after the birth of a child, not all marriages seem to suffer to the same degree. What helps to protect marriages during this transition? Researchers John Gottman and Alyson Fearnley Shapiro at the University of Washington found that certain couples manage to keep their relationship strong and healthy despite the demands of parenthood. They point to three things: having affection and respect for your partner, being aware of and engaged in what is going on in your partner's life, and approaching problems as something you and your partner can solve together as a couple. While having a child may place a considerable amount of stress on your relationship, the good news is that when a couple is able to confront and work through these problems in a mutually agreeable way, your marriage can actually become stronger and more satisfying.

Sexual Intimacy

Sex, when it goes well, is a mutually satisfying emotional and physical experience. It is an important part of your relationship that helps to generate positive feelings toward your partner and a sense of connectedness. It is easy to think of making love as something that comes naturally, but sometimes things don't always run smoothly. Sexual intimacy is a sensitive barometer of what is going on in the relationship and in the external world, and having children may have a profound impact on this important aspect of a couple's relationship.

Most couples describe the greatest satisfaction in their sex lives early on in their relationship. Although most consider sexual intimacy to be an important part of their relationship, sex becomes less frequent over time. The average couple who has been married five years or so makes love once or twice a week. About 10 percent of the population has sex only a few times per year. When taking a look at these statistics, it is important to remember that every couple is different. You may be having sex less often than the "average" couple, but this is not necessarily a sign that your relationship is any less satisfying. It should be recognized that it is quality that counts here, not quantity. The question you should be asking yourself is whether or not you feel satisfied with your sex life.

Recently more and more married couples are expressing dissatisfaction with their sex lives. About 70 percent of married couples report feeling satisfied with their sex life, meaning that about one in three couples are unhappy with their situation. Many experts blame the stressed-out lives we lead, where there is little time to relax and to enjoy ourselves. Others put the blame on the children.

Pregnancy clearly has an impact on sexual intimacy. Many couples worry about having sexual intercourse during pregnancy, fearful that it will put the pregnancy at risk. In general, if your pregnancy is healthy and uncomplicated, sexual intercourse is considered to be safe. There are only a few situations in which your obstetrician may advise against sexual intercourse. If you have any questions or concerns, you should discuss them with your obstetrician. But just because sex is safe during pregnancy doesn't mean you'll necessarily want to have it. Many expectant mothers find that their interest in sex waxes and wanes during the course of pregnancy. Many of the symptoms that occur during the first trimester, including fatigue, nausea, and breast tenderness, make sex less appealing. A woman's interest in sex generally improves during the second trimester but again diminishes during the last trimester, when intercourse may be awkward and physically uncomfortable. During the last weeks of the pregnancy, many women also find they are preoccupied with the impending arrival of the baby and the excitement of becoming a new parent. Frequently couples avoid intercourse toward the end of pregnancy because they are worried about inducing premature labor, and many doctors recommend that women hold off on sexual activity during the last few weeks of pregnancy for this reason.

Obstetricians usually tell their female patients that sexual activity may be resumed six weeks after delivery. Many women, however, find that it may take much longer to return to their regular sex life after the birth of a child. Early on, many women experience discomfort on sexual intercourse or complain that it feels different. This generally improves over time; however, if you have had a traumatic delivery, you may need more time to fully recover. In addition, if you are breast-feeding, you have high levels of the hormone prolactin, which may diminish your libido. Although these physical factors may play a role, probably the most important reason new parents give for their lack of sexual intimacy is exhaustion. Given the demands of caring for a new baby, many parents prefer sleep to sex. For many couples, sexual intimacy seems to improve as their children get older, but this is not always the case, and a significant proportion of married couples continue to experience sexual difficulties. Problems with sexual intimacy may be a reflection of other problems in the relationship. If there is conflict or tension, this is likely to be felt in the bedroom.

Depression in either partner may also exacerbate this problem. If you are depressed, you may be less interested in sexual activity. It may be more difficult to relax and to enjoy sex, or you may feel uncomfortable with this degree of vulnerability and intimacy. Furthermore, many of the medications used to treat depression may have sexual side effects. Not only do some of these medications diminish libido, they may make it more difficult to have an orgasm.

How Depression May Affect Your Relationship

The people who are closest to you are the ones most likely to feel the negative effects of your depression, and it is often a woman's partner who bears
the greatest burden. Even if you feel that your relationship with your partner
has remained strong, being depressed *does* affect the people around you,
and many couples find that when one partner is depressed they have to work
hard to protect their relationship and to make sure it is running smoothly.

Ashley and Robert had known each other for only a year before they got
married, and Ashley was pregnant within a month of their wedding day.
They were both delighted, but as the pregnancy progressed, Ashley became more and more anxious both about the pregnancy and about her relationship with her husband. She tried to conceal her concerns, but she
found herself calling Robert several times a day to ask him questions; although she had always been very independent, she now found it difficult to
make decisions on her own. She felt much more needy and sensitive.
Often when her husband tried to joke with her, she felt hurt and ended up
in tears.

Robert was surprised by Ashley's behavior. When he had first met her,
he was taken by her sense of confidence and courage. He admired Ashley
for speaking out and letting him know exactly what she wanted. Now she
was clearly unhappy, and nothing seemed to please her. As time went
on, he found himself trying to avoid her. The more she needed him, the
more he pulled away. He felt angry. What had happened to the woman he
married?

As Ashley's due date approached, Robert's anger turned to fear that Ashley would disintegrate even further after the birth of a child. How would
she manage? How would *he* manage if she could not? Could he trust her to
be alone with the baby? Would he be able to return to work or would he
have to stay home to take care of the baby *and* his wife? Ashley too was terrified, and she had many of the same questions. Although she had a lot of
experience taking care of babies and young children, she began to doubt
her own skills. To make things worse, she sensed that Robert was pulling
away, and she did not know if she would be able to rely on him.

When you are depressed, your partner may wonder what happened
to the woman he used to know. If your partner has some familiarity with
depression and its manifestations, he may be able to sort things out and understand that it's the depression—and not you—that is the problem. How-

ever, depression can so dramatically alter your personality that your partner may feel that he has lost the person he fell in love with.

If you are depressed, it may be more difficult to stay connected with others, including your partner. You may prefer to be alone, or it may be difficult to talk to or to feel emotionally engaged with your partner. Unfortunately, your partner may take your withdrawal personally or worry that he is to blame. He may think that you are no longer attracted to him or that you have fallen out of love.

Depression may also make you feel more insecure, and you may feel more needy. You may question the decisions you make and find yourself relying more on your partner. Depression also makes you more negative or critical of yourself, and it may be difficult to view yourself as a competent and capable person. You may come to believe that your partner shares those feelings and that he does not respect or value you anymore. You may worry that your husband is no longer attracted to you or that you are too much of a burden. These insecurities can wear down even the strongest relationships.

Although you may feel good about your relationship when you are feeling well, when you are depressed, the relationship you have with your partner may look very different. Everything your partner does may annoy you. The negative aspects of the relationship are blown out of proportion, and it may be impossible to focus on what is good and what holds the two of you together. Many women, in the midst of a depression, wonder if they will be able to sustain the relationship and they may entertain thoughts of separating or divorcing. However, once the depression has resolved they are able to put things into perspective.

How your partner responds to your depression is an important factor in determining how your relationship will fare. You may be fortunate to have a partner who is supportive and willing to help you through a difficult situation. But even though he may offer his support, you may sometimes feel that he does not fully understand what you are going through emotionally. Especially when the depression is very prolonged or severe, you may recognize that your partner is tolerant of your situation but feel that he does not really appreciate the nature of your struggle, and this may make you feel even more isolated and ashamed than you already feel.

In the worst case, you may discover that your partner is not there for you. He may not be able to acknowledge the depression and may act as if everything is going just fine, or he may not be able to accept that depression is a real illness, and he may think that you just need to pull yourself up by your bootstraps. If your partner is unable to understand your depression, he may be emotionally unavailable or distant, or he may be angered by your behavior and may say things that are hurtful or insensitive. When your partner responds to you in this fashion, it may be devastating to your sense of self-esteem and your trust in him. You may end up feeling unwanted, unworthy, and unlovable. At a time when you are in greatest need of support, you may find yourself pulling away in order to protect yourself.

The Importance of Good Communication

Good communication is at the core of every healthy relationship. It means that you are able to express your thoughts and feelings openly and that you encourage your partner to do the same. You feel that your partner is listening to you and making an effort to understand you, and you are willing to make the same effort. Even though problems may arise within the relationship, there is the sense that the couple can work together to resolve the issue. Whereas good communication can strengthen a relationship, poor communication threatens its integrity. If you feel that you cannot talk openly to your partner or you feel that your partner does not understand you, you are likely to feel disappointed and lonely, and conflicts cannot be resolved. If you feel that you are not listened to or not understood, you are likely to feel angry and resentful. Sometimes these feelings may be expressed openly; however, they more often take a more insidious form, manifesting in other ways including sarcasm, silence, uncooperativeness, or emotional withdrawal.

Very early on, couples develop certain patterns of verbal and nonverbal communication and many couples enter into parenthood with preexisting problems. Not surprisingly these problems do not miraculously disappear after the birth of a child. But even couples with relatively good communication skills can stumble into trouble after they become parents. Having children can place a tremendous strain on the relationship and, when a couple is under stress, they may sometimes revert to less healthy or more negative forms of communication. There is less time and energy to resolve the conflicts that may arise. Often unresolved issues carry over from one conflict to the next, and repetitive misunderstandings can lead to anger and resentment that drive the couple apart.

Rachel and Jason had been married for five years before the birth of their first child. They had always thought of themselves as supportive of each other but things seemed to change after the baby. Rachel had decided to leave her job and stay at home after the birth of her second child and was sometimes resentful that her husband had the opportunity to get out of the house and be on his own. She felt that she always had to ask—or even beg—Jason to help her out. He seemed to have little appreciation for how hard it was to care for a new baby and a two-year-old; he always talked about his work and never seemed to be interested in what was happening in her life.

Jason always felt tense around Rachel. Although he hated to admit it, he actually *was* spending more time at work. He didn't feel his efforts to help out at home were appreciated; it seemed that everything he did fell short of Rachel's expectations. He missed the affection Rachel used to have for him. Now he wanted to share with her the joy of having a new baby, just looking at their daughter or playing with her, but Rachel was so busy and so focused on the day-to-day chores—the feeding, the diaper changing, the laundry. Sometimes he got the impression that Rachel felt she would be better off without him, so he put more energy into his work. It was exciting and made him feel good about himself.

Both Rachel and Jason have very specific needs, and they have not been able to communicate these needs to each other. In the end, they both feel hurt and misunderstood. They love each other but are in the process of drifting apart.

If you feel that you and your partner are frequently having conflicts, this is a sign that you need to take some time to tend to your relationship. Many people believe that good relationships can weather difficult times, and there is some truth to this. However, relationships rarely fix themselves. If you are having problems, take a closer look at your relationship. Working on your relationship together may make the transition to parenthood much smoother. It may also give you the opportunity to develop new communication skills that will help you to negotiate the difficult situations you may encounter in the future. The first step in improving communication is to take a good look at how the two of you communicate with each other and to try to identify unhealthy communication styles.

EXAMPLES OF BAD COMMUNICATION

Interrupting	You do not allow your partner to make his point.
Ignoring	You do not listen to or pay attention to what your partner is saying.
Blaming	You blame your partner for the problem.

Scapegoating	Your partner is the one with a problem; you are happy and have nothing to complain about.
Martyrdom	You claim that you are an innocent victim in the situation.
Defensiveness	You are not able to accept any responsibility for the situation.
Sarcasm	Your words or tone of voice convey hostility or contempt.
Name-calling	Rather than focusing on the problem, you criticize or put down your partner.
Bringing up the past	You bring up problems from the past rather than focusing on what is going on now.
Mind reading	You assume what your partner is thinking or feeling without asking, or you expect your partner to know what you are thinking and feeling.
Threatening	You attempt to get your way by using threatening or demanding statements rather than making a request.
Counterattack	When your partner brings up a concern, you respond by criticizing him.
Denial	You do not acknowledge how you feel when you are hurt, sad, angry, or resentful.
Hopelessness	You act as if the problem cannot be resolved; you give up.

Improving Communication with Your Partner
Next, Try Using These More Effective Techniques

Tell your partner exactly what you need. The bottom line is that to get what you need, you have to ask for it. You may not feel comfortable expressing your needs, or you may think, If my partner really cared about me, he would know exactly what I need. I shouldn't have to explain this to him. Unfortunately your partner cannot read your mind. If you do not ask for what you need, you run the risk of not getting it. Furthermore, if you are not specific, you may not get what you want and may end up feeling disappointed or angry. For example, "I need your support," is not a specific request. On the other hand, it may work better to say, "Could you finish up the dishes after dinner? I think I need to go up to bed early tonight." Or, "I have a busy day tomorrow. Do you have time to schedule the appointment with the pediatrician?" These are clear requests, allowing less room for misinterpretation.

Ask for help, don't demand it. Particularly if you feel frustrated or resentful, your request for support may sound more like a demand, and you may not get your desired response. For example, "Could you at least take out the garbage from time to time?" Or, "Why don't you ever want to spend any time with me anymore?" Although this may seem like a good way of communicating your anger or disappointment, this approach is unlikely to yield the support you need. It is important to discuss these feelings; however, when you make these sorts of comments, it forces your partner to take the offensive; he will be busy defending his actions rather than listening and responding to your feelings and to your request for help.

Don't guess. If you don't know what your partner means, ask. You can make assumptions about what your partner wants or needs, but you run the risk of getting it wrong. This may leave your partner feeling annoyed or disappointed, and in turn you may feel angry or resentful if you feel that your efforts were not appreciated. Jason thought that Rachel preferred to have him out of the house so that she could do her own thing. When he increased his time at work, he thought he was just doing what she wanted; he was surprised to learn that she actually wanted to spend more time with him.

Learn to listen to your partner. Just because you hear your partner talking does not mean you are actually listening. Sometimes you may not listen to what your partner is saying because you think you have heard it before. Or you may be so eager to make your point that you are not paying any attention to the other person. Or you may not be able to focus on what your partner is saying because you are busy doing something or thinking about something else. So how can you communicate effectively if you don't know what the other person is saying? You can't. It is essential that you *actively* listen to your partner and make an effort to understand what he or she is saying. Give your partner the chance to speak without interruption. If you don't understand what he or she is saying, ask for clarification. And then repeat back what you heard your partner say. This may seem like a lot of work but if your partner feels listened to and understood, he or she will be more willing to listen to what you have to say.

Resolving Conflicts

Even couples with healthy relationships have conflicts. An occasional argument is not a sign of a failing relationship. It simply means that there is a disagreement, and rest assured that it is possible to negotiate conflicts in a mutually satisfying way. There are many different ways to handle a dispute. The goal is to come to a resolution of the problem that you are both comfortable with. Here are some guidelines.

1. *Find a good time to discuss the problem.* This may sound strange, but settling a dispute works out best when it is planned in advance. Unfortunately, many of us seem to have a knack for starting fights at the worst of all possible times: in the car on the way to work, as soon as your partner walks in the door after work, in front of your in-laws.

Avoid having a discussion when you are tired, hungry, or if you have had too much to drink. Avoid having a discussion if you are distracted or preoccupied. When something happens that displeases you, it may be especially tempting to just say a few words and get it out of your system, but this does not often work out well. When you have children, finding a good time to have a discussion (or a fight) can be particularly difficult. Remember that it's absolutely okay to fight, but it is best not to fight in front of your children.

Never start a discussion when you're angry. This is a recipe for disaster and a good opportunity to say a lot of things you will later regret. Wait until you can think more clearly and rationally. Feel free to express your dissatisfaction with the situation, but agree with your partner on a time to talk when you both can give it your full attention and engage in a meaningful discussion.

2. *Identify a problem and stick to it.* Many couples see a fight as an opportunity to air all their grievances. Using this approach, a lot of unpleasant things are laid out on the table, but, even after the lengthiest discussion, none of the problems are fully resolved. A fight is not a time to bring up all the old issues. With your partner, identify the problem you would like to work on, and discuss *only* that problem. If there are other issues you both want to discuss, set aside another time to tackle those.

Be specific about what is bothering you. It isn't enough to simply say "I'm upset." If your partner refuses to pick up his dirty laundry or change the baby's diaper, and that's what's making you angry, say so. If there is an ongoing problem, select an example to illustrate your point.

3. *Avoid making accusations.* When you say something like, "You never seem to want to spend any time with me anymore," you may not get the desired response. Your partner may feel like he is being attacked. When you talk about what is bothering you, try to make "I" statements rather than "you" statements. Say "I feel," "I need," or "I want." Talk about how your partner's actions make you feel. For example, you might try saying, "When you come home so late, it makes me feel unwanted and lonely."

In addition, try to avoid generalizations or exaggerations. Avoid saying "always" or "never." These statements are usually inaccurate and are likely to make your partner defensive and unable to listen and respond to what you are saying.

4. *Offer some solutions to the problem.* Many people expect their partner to know exactly what they want. However, this is not always realistic and this approach may make your partner feel apprehensive or defensive, if he knows that you will be hurt or angry it the "wrong" solution to a problem is offered. If you need something specific, you have to spell it out.

Try to come up with some suggestions on how to solve the problem. Instead of "You never help me out," say "I am really overwhelmed by the amount of work I have to do. I really need you to help me clean up after dinner." Instead of "You always think of yourself first," say "I would like a little more attention from you. I miss the way things used to be."

5. *Invite your partner to express his or her point of view, and then listen carefully.* Let your partner speak, and try not to interrupt. If you do not understand what your partner is saying, ask for clarification. And when you understand what the issue is, repeat it back to your partner: "What I am hearing is that you have a problem with X." It is important to recognize that there is no such thing as the "right" or "wrong" way to feel. Just as you want your partner to acknowledge and respect *your* feelings, you should extend the same courtesy. You may not feel the same way, but it does not mean that your way is the right way.

6. *Accept responsibility for your own behavior.* Try to understand how *you* may contribute to the problem. Is there anything that you do that makes things worse? Is there anything that you can do to make things better? If you accept some responsibility for the situation, your partner will be more open to negotiation.

7. *Stay calm and in control.* This is a discussion, not a shouting match. When you are having a fight, each partner must feel that this is a safe and secure environment. If the emotions are too strong for you to manage or if you feel that you are about to lose control, ask to take a break, then come back to the discussion at an agreed time.

Resist the temptation to hit below the belt. When you fight with your partner, it's not all about winning. It's about coming to a mutually satisfying resolution of a problem. Everybody has weaknesses or flaws, and this is not the time to bring them up. Remember that your partner is not your enemy; he is somebody you care about. Making hurtful comments undermines this process and may result in battle wounds that are slow to heal.

8. *Be willing to compromise.* If you offer your partner only one way to solve a problem, you may find yourself in an uncomfortable stalemate. Furthermore, if one person always feels that he is giving in to the demands of the other, this can generate feelings of resentment and anger. Remember that this is a process of negotiation, and the goal is to come to a solution to the problem that satisfies *both* of you. If, after a prolonged discussion, no solution has been reached, schedule a time to begin the discussion again.

Warning Signs

When so much of your energy is spent on taking care of your children, you may not be fully aware that your relationship is suffering. Furthermore, you may blame other things: stress at work, sleep deprivation, family issues. While it may be easier to ignore the problems you are having with your partner, it is important to acknowledge them and to work together to try and resolve them. Here are some signs that you and your partner may be having relationship problems:

- You and your partner spend less and less time together.
- You find yourself avoiding spending time with your partner.
- You feel that you are cut out of certain aspects of your partner's life.
- You talk to others more than you do to your partner, especially about important aspects of your life.
- You feel that you have little in common with your partner. Your discussions seem strained or superficial.
- You frequently become irritated by your partner and your discussions frequently escalate into fights.
- You find yourself questioning the relationship and wonder if your partner is the right person for you.

Although many couples having problems think about seeking professional help, most do not. This is unfortunate given that many couples who do seek help find couples counseling to be very helpful. Meeting with a professional may bring to the table many issues that the couple has not been able to discuss or to successfully resolve. It also offers the couple an opportunity to improve their communication skills and to develop new strategies for resolving disputes. It's important to intervene earlier rather than later. When problems persist over a long period of time, it can be difficult to undo the damage.

Protecting Your Family

Sometimes children become the glue that holds the relationship together. A couple's relationship as a twosome recedes to some degree, but they are able to build a new type of partnership, caring for their children and intertwining their own lives with their children's. They approach raising their children as a wonderful and enriching experience. Although sharing this new role with a partner may enhance the quality of the relationship, sometimes other aspects of the relationship may fade. For other couples, children only serve to increase friction within the relationship. It seems more difficult to resolve conflicts, and now there are new issues related to the children that are even more perilous to negotiate.

If you are having problems with your partner, it is not only a problem for you, it affects your children as well. Marital conflict can leave you feeling emotionally depleted and less available to your children and can interfere with your ability to parent effectively. Children who are exposed to conflict within the home are more likely to have behavioral problems and are more likely to suffer from depression and anxiety during their childhood and adolescence.

Protecting Your Relationship

It would be nice if, from time to time, you could just switch your relationship to "cruise control." Unfortunately, there is no such option. Especially after the birth of a child, even the most stable of relationships will undergo some degree of transformation. Although you may feel that your energies should be devoted to your children, it is just as important to take care of your relationship with your partner.

Although your time may be limited, it is important to set aside time to be with and to talk to your partner. Many of your discussions will revolve around your children and the management of your household affairs. It is important to discuss how the two of you want to divide child-care and household responsibilities. And the two of you will have to figure out how work outside the home fits into this puzzle. As you and your partner attend to these important issues, you will be working to find a system that works for you both. Although it may take a great deal of time to find a workable solution, it's worth it. In many families, these issues are often never given the attention they need; bringing these complicated issues to the table will help you to feel that you are working as a team and will help to prevent feelings of resentment.

But talking is more than just agreeing on what chores need to be done; take the time to tell your partner how you are feeling and what is going on in your life. And make an effort to listen to what your partner is saying. You should always treat your partner with respect and kindness. Even if you are stressed and exhausted, this is no reason to let good manners fall to the wayside. If you and your partner take the time to nurture your relationship and make a concerted effort to understand each other, it will strengthen and enrich your relationship.

Chapter 11

Helping Yourself
Practical Techniques for Managing Stress and Depression

One of the most important elements of your recovering from depression is getting good professional help. However, you should not feel that your recovery is a passive process; there are many things that you can do to help yourself to feel better. In this chapter, you will find practical techniques to reduce stress and to alleviate the symptoms of depression. You will learn how to make positive changes in your life. You will also gain skills that may help combat some of the negative thinking patterns that go along with depression: feelings of incompetence, isolation, and helplessness. These techniques may not only help to alleviate the symptoms of depression but may protect you from depression in the future.

Identifying Sources of Stress in Your Life

Although stress can be an energizing and motivating force, it can also cause a lot of problems. Feeling stressed or overwhelmed makes it more difficult to relax and to fully enjoy yourself. Stress can affect how you interact with others and may interfere with your ability to form and maintain satisfying and supportive relationships. It can also have a negative effect on your physical health and sense of well-being, and medical experts believe that many ailments—for example, high blood pressure, headaches, and ulcers—are either caused or exacerbated by stress. The bottom line is that too much stress is bad for you.

Many women recognize that they often feel tense or stressed, yet they do not always have a good understanding of where all the stress comes from or how to make meaningful changes. Contrary to popular misconception, "handling" stress is not learning to tolerate it. Stress is something that you should learn to manage. The first step is identifying the various sources of stress in your life and understanding how stress affects you. Where is the stress coming from? Usually there are many different sources. Taking care of your children? Dealing with other family members? Managing the household? Your career? Like many women, you are probably juggling a number of different activities and responsibilities, and this can leave you feeling totally depleted.

WHERE IS THE STRESS COMING FROM?	
Your Relationship	Disagreements related to pregnancy, parenting, domestic responsibilities
	Poor communication
	Sexual difficulties
Your Family	Caring for family members (elderly parents, children)
	Conflict with family members
	Social obligations
Your Home	Domestic responsibilities
	Unstable or unsuitable living conditions
	Financial difficulties
Your Work	Inflexible or long work hours
	Unrealistic demands
	Conflict with coworkers
	Inadequate pay
	Lack of job security
	Job dissatisfaction

Although having children can be a wonderful and enriching experience, it adds stress to your life. In most families the woman assumes the primary responsibility for caring for the children, even when there is a supportive and involved partner. Unfortunately, women receive far less credit than they deserve for this work they do, and women tend to minimize their accomplishments in this arena. In fact, taking care of a child is a challenging and time-consuming job. While it is often enjoyable and deeply satisfying, it can also be demanding, unpredictable, and unrelenting.

But child care is usually not a mother's only job. All women carry many other responsibilities, such as cooking and cleaning, managing the finances, arranging social activities, or caring for other family members. To further complicate matters, many mothers with young children work outside of the home. Many women feel that they should "have it all" and be able to handle everything on their own, and be an attentive and engaging mother, too. But it is simply not possible to take on all of these tasks singlehandedly. Fighting to live up to these unrealistic expectations, many women end up having little time for themselves and feel exhausted and overburdened.

Although it seems that many women can tolerate a tremendous amount of stress, everybody responds to stress differently. What may seem fairly normal and easy to manage for one woman may be extraordinarily difficult for another. How you respond to the stress in your life is what matters here. Too much stress may manifest itself as physical or emotional symptoms, or changes in your behavior. When you are stressed, do you withdraw or avoid the situation? Do you become angry or irritable? Do you have headaches, backaches, or stomach problems? Do you just feel tired or worn out? Learning to be aware of these emotional and physical signals may help you to recognize stressful situations and help you to make positive changes.

Some Techniques for Managing Stress

Just as there are many different sources of stress in your life, there are many different ways to manage it. You may be able to eliminate some sources of stress, whereas others may be impossible to eradicate. How can you gain more control?

Determine what situations are the most distressing to you. While there are many things on your list of what's bothering you, you do not have the time or energy to address them all at once. Rather than focus on the things that are mildly irritating, try to pick out and address those things that cause you the greatest distress.

Understand how you respond to these stressful events. What seems to make the situation worse? For example, do you feel more tense or irritable when you have not had a good night's rest? What seems to make the situation better? For example, if you are worried about a doctor's visit, does it help to bring your husband or a friend along?

Focus on what you can change. While you probably can't change other people, there are things that *you* can control. Can you do anything to eliminate or avoid certain situations? Or if you find yourself in a stressful situation, can you do anything to reduce the intensity of distress you feel? Is it possible to take a break or to leave for a while? Or would it help to have more support? For example, if you are taking care of an ailing parent, can you enlist the help of other family members or hire someone to help?

Learn how to modulate your reactions to stressful situations. In stressful situations, both your mind and your body react. Gaining control of these responses can help you to feel better and more in control. You may learn that you need to walk away from situations that upset you, or you may find out that exploding in anger only makes the situation worse. You may also be able to use certain relaxation techniques to help you better tolerate those situations you cannot avoid.

Changing the Way You Think

When you're depressed, the way you look at the world is distorted and clouded. In contrast to someone who is not depressed, you are more likely to draw negative conclusions about yourself and to focus on your problems rather than how to solve them. When you are depressed, this may make it more difficult to recover, and patterns of negative thinking may make you more vulnerable to depression in the first place. Working to correct these unhealthy patterns of thinking may facilitate your recovery and may also help to protect you from depression in the future.

Cognitive therapy is a type of psychotherapy that addresses these negative or distorted perceptions, and you may be able to employ many of the techniques employed by cognitive therapists to alleviate the symptoms of depression. The first step in eliminating these negative patterns of thinking is being able to identify them. Although most of us, from time to time, engage in negative or self-critical thoughts, these patterns of thinking can become deeply ingrained in those suffering from depression. They interfere with your ability to accurately appraise your situation and to solve problems effectively. In his book *The Feeling Good Handbook*, Dr. David Burns lays out ten different types of cognitive distortions that are common in those who suffer from depression. They are listed below.

COGNITIVE DISTORTION	RESULT	EXAMPLE
All-or-Nothing Thinking	You look at things in absolute, black-and-white terms. There are no in-betweens or shades of gray.	Robin's two-year-old daughter falls out of her chair while eating lunch. She sheds only a few tears yet ends up with a black eye. Every time Robin looks at her daughter's face, she criticizes herself for not being more responsible and attentive. She feels that she is a total failure as a mother.

(continued)

Cognitive Distortion	Result	Example (continued)
Overgeneralization	You experience a single, negative event as a repeating pattern of defeat.	In the midst of a disagreement, one of Alexa's friends tells her that she is being selfish. Alexa is now hesitant to call other friends because she is convinced that they are also upset with her and that nobody wants to spend time with her.
Mental Filter	You focus on the negatives and ignore the positives.	After a picnic with her family, Kim talks only about the bad weather and the fact that she forgot to bring enough sodas; everybody else seemed to have a great time.
Disqualifying the Positive	Your positive attributes and accomplishments don't count.	Rachel's husband thanks her for preparing a wonderful dinner. Although she spent all day cooking, Rachel has a hard time taking credit for what she does well. She dismisses the compliment, saying, "It wasn't a big deal. Anybody could have thrown it together."
Jumping to Conclusions	You assume that people are reacting negatively to you or that bad things will happen.	Claire calls her friend Linda to arrange for a lunch date. When Claire does not hear back from Linda for a few days, she begins to worry that she has done something to offend her. Claire is convinced that she will never hear from her again, but Linda calls the next day. She explains that she was not able to call earlier because her mother had been in the hospital.
Magnification and Minimization	You blow negative things out of proportion while minimizing positive things.	Liz brings her children to visit her in-laws. Although everybody seemed to enjoy themselves, she feels the trip was a failure because she forgot to bring her camera.
Emotional Reasoning	You give more weight to your emotions than to reality.	Laura is upset that she has to do the bulk of the household chores. She wants to ask her husband for help but feels overwhelmed by the thought of it. This is hopeless, she tells herself. Why should I even try to ask him for help?

Cognitive Distortion	Result	Example
"Should" Statements	You criticize yourself using statements with "shoulds," "musts," and "have tos."	Maura has a long list of things to do: "I should pick up the dry cleaning. I have to do the shopping for my mother-in-law's birthday party. I can't be home later than five to get dinner started." Maura has a demanding job and often resents that she has to use her limited time to take care of all these chores. When she is not able to take care of all of these things, however, she feels guilty.
Labeling and Mislabeling	You label yourself inappropriately, calling yourself "a loser," "a "failure," or other names.	After an argument with her husband, Connie berates herself: "What a witch I am; I can't believe my husband doesn't leave me."
Personalization	You blame yourself for things that go wrong, even if you are not totally responsible.	Jackie received a call from her son's day care center letting her know that he threw up at school and needed to come home. Although he seemed well this morning, she felt that the teachers were upset at her for sending her son to school.

If you always view yourself in a negative light, you may feel that you will never overcome your depression. However, this is not true, and there are many things you can do to help yourself. First of all, train yourself to identify these self-critical thoughts and cognitive distortions. Sometimes it helps to keep a daily log in which you write down situations that are upsetting or difficult for you and record how you responded to them. As you go through this process, you should try to recognize how your thoughts may be distorted. For example, Robin's daughter fell out of the chair. Does that really mean that Robin is a failure as a mother? Obviously not, but this is how Robin often feels about herself. As you identify these distortions, you may be able to find other ways to respond which are less self-critical and more accurately reflect reality. Rather than criticizing herself, Robin might be able to tell herself that accidents happen and that there was nothing she could have done to prevent her daughter's fall. Furthermore, Robin could also make herself feel better by acknowledging that the injury was not serious and that her daughter would likely have no signs of it in a few days.

Although it may appear relatively simple, this process of cognitive re-structuring is often hard work. Because depression distorts the way you think, you may not be able to accurately identify your misperceptions, and when you try to look for more rational ways to respond, you may come up empty-handed. Your friends and family members may be able to help you keep things in perspective. Meeting with a professional may also help you to make some more positive changes in the way you view yourself and your world.

Enhancing Your Resilience

Although you can reduce stress, it is impossible to totally eliminate it. Life is unpredictable, and unexpected changes or events may make you feel stressed or out of control. The following strategies may help to make you feel more in control and better able to handle the curveballs.

Remember to take care of yourself. Especially if you are caring for a baby or young children, you probably have little time to take care of yourself—to eat well, exercise, relax, and get plenty of sleep. And if you are depressed, it may become even more of a challenge to attend to these important aspects of your health. However, if you do not take the time to tend to yourself, you cannot expect to function at your best. Furthermore, there is good evidence that a healthy diet and regular exercise can help alleviate stress and may also have positive effects on your mood.

Learn to have realistic expectations of yourself. Many women expect to achieve the highest standards in many different domains: at home, in their marriage, within their family, within the community, and at work. Striving to be perfect is a noble goal; however, it is simply not possible to achieve perfection in everything you do. Pushing yourself in this manner may leave you feeling depleted, incompetent, and inadequate. Instead, try to figure out what is most important to you and focus on excelling in those areas and learn to live with "good enough" in the others. And keep in mind that perfection in any arena is not a realistic goal.

Manage your time realistically. Women seem to have perfected the art of multitasking. While this skill may be useful in some situations, it is also a recipe for burnout. Oftentimes what a woman feels she can accomplish is unrealistic, and an overburdened schedule does not take into consideration the unexpected. Instead of compiling a mile-long to-do list, establish priorities. Be honest about how long it actually takes to accomplish a given task. By being more realistic about time management, you can learn to feel more in control and less overextended. In the long run, you will be more productive.

Remember to take a break. Most women do not build any time into their schedules to rest or to relax, and mothers in particular often feel that they cannot spare the time to rest. Sometimes taking a break may feel like you are avoiding the many things you have to do, but instead rest and relaxation should be viewed as time to replenish your emotional and physical resources. Learn to say no. Lots of women have trouble declining to be class mother, host the sleepover, book the vacation, coordinate the church fundraiser, arrange the party for a coworker's birthday, etc.

Ask for help. Although it would be nice at times to be totally self-sufficient, we cannot and do not need to be so independent. There are times when you will need the assistance of others, and it is important to recognize that you can ask for help. Women, particularly new mothers, often complain that they do not have enough support, yet they are often reluctant to ask for help.

Bolster your support network. Although being independent is highly valued in our society, having a strong and reliable support network is essential. Furthermore, the companionship and support you derive from others may alleviate stress and protect you from depression. Support may come in many forms and from many different places, including one's partner, family, friends, and neighbors. Later in this chapter, we will discuss how you can start to build a strong support network.

Learn to express your negative feelings. Life can be challenging, frustrating, and sometimes not particularly rewarding. Although you may feel uncomfortable sharing these negative sentiments with others, holding them in may make you feel more stressed out or depressed. Not being able to let go of these negative feelings can also interfere with your ability to enjoy the more positive aspects of your life. Finding somebody who is willing to talk honestly about these uncomfortable feelings can be immensely helpful.

Sleep Is Essential

You cannot live without sleep. Although how much sleep one needs varies from individual to individual, most experts agree that women of childbearing age need around eight hours of sleep each night for optimal functioning, but some women need as many as ten. It is fair to say that most women are not sleeping enough and carry a sleep debt. The problem with sleep debt is that it is impossible to "pay it off." A single night of "catch-up" sleep does not reverse the effects of a chronic sleep debt. Sleeping late on the weekends doesn't make up for the sleep you lost during the week. In fact, on the days when you sleep too much, you may end up feeling more tired. Unfortunately, many things may prevent you from getting the sleep you need, and when you are juggling many different responsibilities, sleep is probably low on your list of priorities.

According to a poll by the National Sleep Foundation, 78 percent of women report disturbed sleep during pregnancy. When you are pregnant, you have to go to the bathroom more often, and some of the physical symptoms common to pregnancy—such as nausea, heartburn, back pain, and sinus congestion—may also keep you up at night. You may find that, especially during the last few months of your pregnancy, you just cannot find a comfortable sleeping position. In addition, about 15 percent of pregnant women also suffer from restless leg syndrome. In this condition, you may have tingling or cramping sensations in your legs, or simply the physical urge to move. The only way to find relief is by moving your legs—stretching, rubbing them together, or walking—and this can make falling asleep at night very difficult (and frustrating).

After delivery you may be even more sleep-deprived. Most newborn babies wake up every one to three hours at night and need to be fed. If you have a baby that feeds quickly and efficiently and then falls back to sleep, you may be able to get enough sleep—albeit interrupted—during the course of a night. Some women choose to cosleep to make these nighttime feedings less intrusive. Nonetheless, these disruptions, however brief, *do* reduce the overall quality of your sleep. Furthermore, if after taking care of your baby, you feel fully awake, it may be very difficult to fall back to sleep and you may feel as if you are getting only a few good hours of sleep each night. When this type of sleep disturbance goes on for a long period, your sense of physical and emotional well-being may suffer.

Many women, even those with the best sleep habits, have problems falling or staying asleep. This may reflect an underlying sleep disorder, but depression and anxiety are common causes of sleep problems among women. If you are depressed, you may find that you cannot fall asleep or that you sleep less restfully than usual. Or you may feel exhausted all the time and find yourself sleeping too much each day. Anxiety may also disrupt sleep; Charlotte Brontë observed: "A ruffled mind makes a restless pillow."

If you suffer from anxiety, you may discover that you have trouble falling asleep because you cannot let your mind rest when you lay down at the end of the day, and you may also wake frequently during the night so that you wake up feeling tired.

People who consistently have disrupted sleep may accumulate a "sleep debt," becoming progressively more fatigued as the days pass. Although some women seem to tolerate disruption of their sleep fairly well, sleep deprivation, especially when it occurs over a long period, is not good for you. It may leave you feeling chronically exhausted and overwhelmed. It may affect your memory and your ability to concentrate, and in some cases, the degree of impairment may be significant. One study found that sleep deprivation can cause declines in cognitive and motor coordination similar to those observed in persons who are intoxicated. Chronic sleep deprivation may also make you feel more irritable and less patient with others, especially your children, and some researchers have speculated that sleep deprivation may make some women more vulnerable to depression.

To figure out how much sleep you need, read your body's signals. If you feel tired after seven uninterrupted hours of sleep every night, it probably means that you need more sleep. Developing good sleep habits—what sleep experts call good "sleep hygiene"—can also make a huge difference in the quality of your sleep and your energy level during the day. Here are some useful tips:

Stick to a regular sleep routine. Your body has its own daily rhythms. Fighting those natural rhythms can leave you feeling exhausted; however, going to sleep and waking up at the same time *every* day (weekday or weekend) can lead to more efficient sleep and less daytime sleepiness. While it may be hard to adhere to a regular schedule if you have small children around, keep in mind that your children also will benefit from a consistent sleep routine.

Remember that your bed is a place for sleeping. When you are in bed, avoid reading, watching television, or working on your laptop. You should learn to associate your bed with rest and relaxation, not with activity and productivity. Make your bedroom a good place to sleep; it should be dark, quiet, and a comfortable temperature.

Allow some time to wind down before you plan to go to sleep. Avoid starting a new task or getting into a big project right before you go to bed, and don't make a lot of phone calls. Choose activities that are soothing—taking a bath, doing some light reading, listening to music.

Avoid naps in the late afternoon or early evening. If you are feeling sleep-deprived, you may desperately want to take a nap during the day. A short nap (about twenty to thirty minutes) can be rejuvenating. However, a longer nap, especially late in the day, may make it more difficult to fall asleep at night.

Avoid large meals and excessive intake of fluids before you go to bed. Having a large meal or having to go to the bathroom in the middle of the night disrupts your sleep. If you need an evening snack, choose something that is small, not too spicy, and low in fat. Foods rich in the amino acid trypto-phan—including bananas and milk—may help to promote sleep.

Avoid drinking caffeinated beverages in the late afternoon or evening. Caffeine is useful if you are sleep-deprived and need to stay awake and feel alert during the day. However, too much caffeine too late in the day can disrupt sleep, making it more difficult to fall asleep and sleep restfully.

Avoid using alcohol before bedtime. A nightcap may make you drowsy and help you to fall asleep; however, the effects of alcohol wear off after two to four hours, and you may find yourself awake again. Furthermore, alcohol disrupts normal sleep cycles such that drinking before bedtime may actually worsen the quality of your sleep. You may awake in the morning feeling even more exhausted and, in the worst case, hungover.

Try to develop a consistent exercise plan. Physical exercise can improve the quality of your sleep and make you feel more energized. Avoid exercising late in the day because vigorous exercise may make it more difficult to settle down before you go to bed.

If you are taking any medications, consult with your doctor. There are many medications that may affect your sleep, including certain antidepressants, stimulants like Ritalin, cold remedies, and asthma medications. Your physician can help you to determine if any of your medications may be disrupting your sleep.

The Antidepressant Effects of Exercise

Many women with depression ask about exercise and wonder if it can be helpful for treating their symptoms. While exercise is unlikely to be a "cure" for severe depression, there is evidence to suggest that exercise may help to relieve stress and improve mood. Studies indicate that those who exercise regularly experience lower levels of depression and anxiety than those who lead a more sedentary lifestyle. A recent study from researchers at Duke University demonstrated that for older adults with mild to moderate depression, regular aerobic exercise (for forty minutes three times a week) was as effective as medication for the treatment of depression.

Some feel that exercise may have direct physiologic effects on the brain. When you exercise, your body releases endorphins and other hormones that may have a calming effect. Exercise may also help to modulate levels of certain neurotransmitters, including norepinephrine and serotonin, which have mood-enhancing effects. Exercise is also a distraction from the stress and strain of everyday life, and feeling fit and looking good may also improve your self-esteem and confidence. In addition, exercise improves the quality of your sleep and may help you feel better rested and more energetic.

Exercise may not be a replacement for standard treatments but it certainly can be combined with traditional techniques for treating depression and can have long-lasting effects on your emotional and physical well-being. The Centers for Disease Control and Prevention have recommended that adults engage in thirty minutes or more of moderate-intensity exercise (including brisk walking, swimming, or bicycling) on five or more days of the week. However, if you have not been exercising regularly, it is important to start slowly and gradually work up to an exercise routine of moderate intensity.

If you are pregnant or postpartum, you should discuss your exercise routine with your physician. While exercise is not prohibited in either situation, some forms of exercise may pose certain risks. For example, pregnant women should avoid contact sports and other activities where there is a greater risk for falls or other injuries (such as horseback riding, skiing, or gymnastics). Vigorous exercise is also not recommended for pregnant women with certain complications, including incompetent cervix, bleeding, and preterm labor.

Many women, especially those with babies or young children, find it difficult to adhere to these recommendations. It is important to remember that some exercise is better than no exercise. While it is unlikely that you have the time and freedom to go to the gym every day, it may be possible to find an exercise routine that fits into your schedule. If you cannot carve out time for a thirty-minute exercise break in your day, you may spread it out over the course of the day—for example, by doing two fifteen-minute intervals. Also choosing an activity that you may pursue with your children, even if it's taking your baby for a walk in the stroller, may make it not only easier for you but also more enjoyable.

The Importance of Good Nutrition

When you are feeling depressed, your diet often suffers. While some women with depression lose their appetite and tend to lose weight, others overeat or eat things that are unhealthy. Unfortunately, these eating behaviors may worsen the way you feel. Not eating enough can make you feel weak and can affect your ability to think clearly, while taking in too many calories can make you feel sluggish or sleepy.

The belief that food affects the way we feel has been around for centuries, and more recently researchers have hypothesized that the taste and smell of certain foods cause the body to secrete hormones that affect mood. For example, researchers from the University of Bristol recently reported that the methylxanthines in chocolate can improve cognitive functioning and wakefulness. Whether or not eating certain foods can relieve depression is still controversial, but food provides the nutrients your body and brain need to function. A balanced diet helps to ensure that you get *all* the nutrients your body needs to work optimally.

Although deficiencies of certain nutrients, including vitamin B_{12} and folic acid, can cause depression, this is unusual in developed countries. Some believe that supplementing the diet with certain vitamins, minerals, amino acids, and fatty acids may be helpful for treating depression. Although taking a good multivitamin with the recommended daily allowances of vitamins and minerals is a sound practice, high doses of certain nutritional supplements are generally not recommended. There is evidence that even natural compounds, including vitamins, may have harmful effects at high doses. For example, some reports suggest that excessive amounts of vitamin A taken during pregnancy have been associated with an increased risk of certain types of birth defects.

The best approach is moderation. You should choose a balanced diet that is healthy, satisfying, and relatively easy to stick to. If you are trying to lose weight or if you are not sure what is the best diet for you, it may be helpful to meet with a nutritionist. Similarly, if you are pregnant or breast-feeding, you may need some help figuring out how to eat to meet the nutritional needs of both you and your baby.

Getting the Help You Need

The relationships you have with other people—family members, friends, coworkers, and acquaintances—are vital. Not only do these important social connections help you to cope with the demands of daily living, but having these relationships is also good for your emotional and physical health. They boost your immune system and decrease levels of stress-related hormones. Feeling connected with others also motivates you to take better care of yourself—to eat right, to rest, to get exercise, and to keep up with routine medical care. It should therefore be no surprise that people with strong social networks live longer, healthier, and happier lives.

Conversely, the research clearly indicates that women who feel that they do not have enough support from their partners, their family, or their community are more likely to suffer from depression. Having adequate support seems to be especially important for women caring for children. Without the support of others, you are more likely to feel inadequate and less confident in your abilities, and when you are faced with a stressful life event, you may have a much harder time coping. It may be especially difficult if you feel that you have been let down by others in some way and have not received the support you expected.

There are many different kinds of support, all of them valuable. Support can come in the form of having somebody to talk to or to keep you company when you are feeling low. It can be somebody who distracts you or knows how to cheer you up. It can be somebody who helps keep things in perspective and helps you to solve your problems. It can be somebody who helps you to take care of the things you need to do, like the laundry, cleaning, or cooking. But to get the support you need, you will probably have to ask for it.

Many women find it difficult to ask for help. Women are used to taking care of others and often do not make their own needs a priority. As a society we value being independent and self-reliant. However, you can't survive without the help of others, and if you are depressed, getting enough support is even more important, even though asking for help may make you feel worse about yourself. If you are depressed, you *need* the help and support of others. So how do you get the support you need and deserve?

Just ask. Admitting that you need help from others may make you feel incompetent or inadequate, or you may worry that your request for assistance will be ignored or that others will find it burdensome. Keep in mind, however, that everybody needs help from time to time. You may expect that those around you will notice that you need help. However, while they may be able to recognize that you are struggling, even those closest to you may not be totally aware of your needs. If you do not ask for help, you run the risk of not getting it.

Be specific. Even your closest friends and family members may not know *exactly* what you need and what would be the most helpful to you. You must understand that it is impossible for others to read your mind, and if you leave them guessing, there is plenty of room for misunderstanding and miscommunication. For example, your friends or family members may think you need help taking care of your children when, in fact, this is something that you really enjoy doing. Or they may think you need their advice, but what you really need is someone who can just listen. If you do not tell others what you need, they may not be able to give it to you.

Set some limits. It is important to connect with other people. But if you feel like you are the one giving all the support and getting little in return, this is not helpful. This type of interaction may make you feel even more depleted. Try to recognize who is able to give you the type of support you need. If it feels like a friend or family member is too demanding, you may need to let them know.

Create a support network. Because it is unlikely that you will find one person who can fulfill all your needs, your goal is to build a *network* for yourself. Though it is the easiest to ask for help from those who are closest to you, there may be other people who could provide assistance. Obviously, not everybody can provide the love and tenderness that a family member or close friend can, but they may be able to help you in other ways. For example, is there somebody who could help you with domestic chores or running errands? If you are having a bad day, is there somebody you know who would go for a walk with you? Think about all the people you know. Who would be able to help?

Be realistic. Asking for help can sometimes be a disappointing or frustrating experience. You may find that you do not always get what you need or want, especially when your expectations are unrealistic. For example, you may want to talk to your best friend about your frustrations with raising your children, but she is struggling with infertility problems and is not able to provide the support you need. You may count on your mother to help out with child care, but she just retired and spends much of her time traveling and is frequently out of town. Be realistic about what others can provide. What are their strengths? What are their limitations? Think about what you need and figure out who would be the best person willing and able to do the job.

Identifying Other Sources of Support

Support comes in many different forms, and there are many other things you can do to help yourself. For example, many women derive a great deal of comfort from reading and educating themselves about their problems. These days there are many books devoted to the topic of depression and many others dealing with issues related to pregnancy, childbirth, and parenting. These books are an important source of information and may help you answer many difficult questions, but they may also provide you with a sense of community. Many women who suffer from depression feel alone; it is hard to imagine that others suffer in the same way. A good book can help to combat this sense of isolation. Knowing that others suffer from the same types of problems may make you feel less ashamed about your situation. It may also make you feel more comfortable sharing your feelings and may inspire you to seek support from others.

Getting enough support may mean that you have to develop a broader social network. You may have to revitalize old friendships or make an effort to make new connections. There are many different ways to meet people, but if you are feeling depressed, it may be difficult for you to figure out what to do. You may feel less confident of yourself, and it may be difficult or uncomfortable for you to socialize. But these connections are vital, and it is important to find a way to build up your social circle.

For many women, going outside of the family for help is a foreign experience. They may feel uncomfortable talking to others—people who feel like "strangers"—about their personal problems. However, there are other types of help you may benefit from. If you have the financial resources, there are various services that may help you with child care, housecleaning, shopping, food preparation, and transportation. Seeking out some of these alternatives may help to lighten the load for those who are closest to you.

Support Groups

Many women shy away from support groups, but a good support group can be a tremendously important and enriching experience. In the appendix, you will find a list of various organizations that sponsor different types of support groups. Women who have experienced some sort of difficult loss, such as infertility or a miscarriage, often find a great deal of emotional support in making connections with women who have had similar issues. There are groups specifically for new mothers that deal with the transition to parenthood, and there are support groups that focus on how to cope with and recover from depression. If you are going through a difficult or emotionally wrenching experience, you may worry about overburdening your family or friends with your intense feelings. A support group gives you a safe place to share your problems with people who understand.

Women are also turning to Internet-based support groups. There are chat rooms and discussion boards covering almost every topic: infertility, pregnancy loss, parenting, depression, anxiety. Many women now find that they are able to build a support network via the Internet; this mode of connecting is not only more convenient but it may feel more comfortable for women who are reluctant to share their most personal feelings with others. While this type of support can be helpful, it should never feel like a substitute for face-to-face contact with other adults.

Postpartum Support Services

There are now many different services for women who have recently had a baby. Many of the services offer the same type of things that an extended family usually provides for the new mother: emotional support and reassurance, information on the basics of caring for a baby and breast-feeding, and child care. One of the advantages of using these sorts of services is that they come without the emotional baggage that family interactions often carry. The people providing these services usually receive special training and have a great deal of knowledge at their fingertips.

A doula is a woman experienced in childbirth who provides support to the mother before, during, and just after childbirth. Doulas can be a source of useful information regarding pregnancy and can help you to prepare for childbirth. They are particularly attentive to the emotional needs of a woman in labor, and some women may choose to have a doula present during labor and delivery as an extra source of support and reassurance. Doulas may also provide postpartum care to a mother after she returns to her home. Women appreciate the opportunity to be taken care of, especially when this care comes from another, more experienced woman.

Parenting Education Programs

There are also classes and groups that focus on parenting. These programs equip parents with skills that promote the healthy development of their children and improve the quality of relationships within the family. For many parents this focused approach can be extremely helpful. If you come to parenting with little experience, you will welcome the opportunity to learn about your child's development and to get a better understanding of his emotional needs. Participating in such a program will give you an opportunity to share your concerns and problems with others. It offers the chance to meet other people like you and your partner and gives you a community.

Coping with Depression As a Family

Depression is an isolating and lonely experience, yet it touches everyone close to you. Although you may be inclined to keep your problem to yourself, this is not always the best choice. If your friends and family spend any time with you, they are bound to know something is wrong. Hiding your depression from the people who are closest to you can strain your relationship with them and, most important, by not letting others know how bad you feel, you may be depriving yourself of an important source of support. Although you may worry about burdening your friends and family with your depression, you must remember that these are the people who care about you the most, and you should give them a chance to help you.

You may find it very difficult to talk about your depression with other people. This is understandable; it isn't easy to talk openly about things so personal. And what makes it worse is that many people know very little about depression, or they have negative perceptions regarding those who suffer from this illness. When you think about telling others about your depression, you may worry that they may not understand what you are experiencing or, even worse, that they will be unsympathetic or critical.

When discussing your depression with others, it is important to give an accurate picture of your situation. Do not minimize the severity of your problem; depression is not a "bad spell" or a "rough patch," it is a serious illness. If they are not familiar with depression, you may have to educate them. You also need to let them know that, because of your depression, you may not be able to do what you usually do and that you are likely to need some help. At the same time, however, you can reassure them by telling them that depression is a treatable illness. It's important to emphasize the fact that you are working to get better and with time you expect to be able to return to your normal self.

If you have children, depression can make it difficult to be the parent you want to be, and this is another reason why it is so important to involve and enlist the support of your family. Being a parent is one of the most demanding jobs you will ever have. Being depressed makes it even more demand-ing. It may be difficult to be emotionally available to your child and to pro-vide the support and patience that she needs. You may not have the energy or emotional resources to fully engage in your child's activities. However, there are steps you can take to help yourself parent more effectively and to protect your children from the negative effects of your depression.

One of the most important goals is to make sure that your child's life does not get derailed as a result of your depression. Your partner can be critical in helping you to keep up the regular routines and to make life feel as "nor-mal" as possible. This does not mean ignoring or denying your depression; it means finding a way for your family to continue moving forward *despite* your depression. Supporting your child's active and rich life outside of the home is essential and can help to make him stronger and more resilient. While you may not be able to do all the things you normally do, your part-ner can help to fill in the gaps and can help you to make sure that your chil-dren's needs are met. Other people can help as well; grandparents, other family members, and friends may be able to help you keep your family on track.

Although you will undoubtedly try very hard to keep things running smoothly, most children can pick up on relatively subtle changes in their environment and family. Even very young children can sense changes in their mother's behavior. How your child responds to you when you are de-pressed will depend on your child's age, her personality, and the nature of her relationship with you. A younger child with limited verbal skills is more likely to show his feelings through actions. Your two-year-old may express his anger by throwing temper tantrums or refusing to do what he is told. Or he may show that he is anxious by clinging and refusing to let you out of his sight. Older children have the capacity to talk about their feelings, and they may express a wide range of feelings including anger, guilt, shame, anxiety, and fear.

At some point, you will have to decide whether to tell your children about your depression. Very young children may not benefit from an expla-nation; the most important thing is that they are taken care of. With older children, however, you and your partner may decide to tell them about your depression. Sometimes you don't really have a choice: your children may see you crying and not understand why, or they may notice that you are tired and less involved in their activities. When they see these changes in your be-havior, they may ask questions about how you are feeling. Most parents want to shelter their children from their problems; however, not letting your children know what is happening to you may leave them feeling confused and insecure. They may worry that they have done something to cause your grief and feel guilty that they cannot make you better. They might fear that things will get worse and feel it is their responsibility to hold their family together. For decades, Dr. William Beardslee and his colleagues at Children's Hospital in Boston have studied how families cope when a parent is depressed. He argues very strongly that when a mother is depressed, her children, even if they are very young, must be made aware of the situation. He advocates the use of an intervention where a mental health clinician helps to educate both the depressed parent *and* family members about depression. There are family meetings where the whole family gets together on a regular basis to talk about the depression and how it affects the family. Bringing depression out of the closet can have a dramatic effect. The children who participate in this sort of intervention have a much better and more sympathetic understanding of depression and are less likely to blame themselves for the problem.

When talking to your children about your depression, it is important to remember that children of all ages often imagine the worst. They may fear that their family will fall apart, or they may worry that you are very sick and may die or may be taken away. Your children must be reassured that you are getting help and that you will eventually feel better. They need to know that they did nothing to make you feel this way, nor should they worry about trying to make you feel better. Most important, you have to emphasize that you love them and will do everything you can to take care of them.

Fighting Off Feelings of Helplessness

One of the symptoms of being depressed is feeling helpless and hopeless about your situation. Sometimes things can feel so bad that it is impossible to imagine that things will get better. Unfortunately, these negative feelings can stand in the way of your recovery. It is important to remember that while there is no quick cure for depression, people do get better. It takes hard work, persistence, patience, and a great deal of support, but there is every reason to expect that you will feel better and be able to return to your usual self.

Chapter 12

Seeking Professional Help
Treatment of Maternal Depression

Depression, once diagnosed, is highly treatable. Although women are more likely to seek help than men and are more comfortable sharing their personal issues with friends and family members, many women with depression never discuss this problem with a professional. Unfortunately, depression carries a powerful stigma, and women who become depressed are often too ashamed to ask for help and try to manage their problem on their own. This reluctance to pursue treatment is even more pronounced when depression occurs during pregnancy or after the birth of a child. When depression strikes at a time when a woman is expected to be happy, depression is often ignored or overlooked. Furthermore, if a woman is pregnant or breast-feeding, she may not seek treatment because she assumes, or has been told by others, that she cannot take any type of medication.

Many highly effective treatments for depression are available. This chapter will provide you with information on a wide array of treatments, including psychotherapy, medication, and alternative therapies, and discuss which are best for women suffering from depression during their reproductive years. It will also help you find the best care and make informed decisions regarding treatment.

When to Seek Help

Many women feel miserable, yet they tell themselves that they are not really depressed or not doing so badly that they need professional help: "I can get out of bed every day. It can't be that bad." Convinced that their problems do not merit the time or attention of a professional, they try to trudge through it on their own. But things don't have to be this way. *If you feel that it would be helpful to talk to a professional about how you are feeling, then you should do so.*

However, we are accustomed to being self-reliant and taking care of our own problems, and it is not so easy to ask for help. You may be fairly comfortable asking somebody to carry something for you when you are nine months pregnant, or you may be able to ask a friend to babysit for you, but getting help for yourself when you are depressed is probably another story. Although you may have come to the conclusion that you are depressed, there is still the challenge of finding—and asking for—the help you need. Unfortunately, there are many different reasons why you may decide not to seek out professional help, even though you are fairly certain that you need it. These include:

- I am sure that eventually things will get better.
- I should be able to take care of things on my own.
- All I need is a little more support from my husband and family.
- Why should I see a professional if I do not want to take medication?
- I can talk to my family; why do I need a therapist?
- My husband (and/or family) would never approve of me seeing a psychiatrist.
- I can't afford to see a professional.
- I don't have the time.
- I don't like the idea of talking to a stranger about personal issues.

Although it is easy to come up with reasons not to seek professional help, there are also good reasons to do so. The most important is that this is an opportunity to treat your condition, but other good, perhaps not so evident, reasons include:

- There may be a medical problem responsible for your symptoms.
- A professional may be able to direct you to sources of support and other resources you were not aware of.
- Talking to a professional may add an extra layer of support.
- It may be difficult to talk openly with your family about what is really bothering you.
- It may be comforting to know that other women feel the same way and that you are not alone.
- It may be helpful to have a professional lined up, in case things do get worse.

Furthermore, there are a number of situations where seeking the help of a professional *must* be considered. A professional should be consulted in the following situations:

- If you are not able to keep up with the basics of daily living, like eating, bathing, and getting out of bed.
- If you are not able to attend to your own or your children's medical needs, such as keeping doctor's appointments.
- If you are having difficulty caring for your children.
- If you are unable to eat or are losing a lot of weight.
- If you are drinking or using recreational drugs to make yourself feel better.
- If there is a distinct change in your personality.
- If your depression seems to be becoming more severe over time.

The following is a list of situations that are considered to be psychiatric emergencies. If you do not already have a mental health provider, you should contact your obstetrician or primary care provider so that they can help you arrange for whatever type of treatment you will need. If it is not possible to arrange for a psychiatric evaluation in a timely fashion, you should go to the nearest emergency room if:

- you are having any suicidal thoughts.
- you are having any violent thoughts directed toward your children or anyone else.
- you (or somebody else) feel that you may be at risk for harming your children.
- you are engaging in any unusual or bizarre behaviors.
- you are experiencing hallucinations (hearing voices or having visions).
- you are delusional (convinced of things that are not true or rational).

A woman who is depressed may not be fully aware or able to admit how poorly she is doing. If she is very ill, her understanding of her condition and her ability to make thoughtful decisions regarding her care may be impaired. She may be unmotivated or reluctant to pursue treatment; thus, her partner and her family must provide their support and encouragement so that she can get the care she needs.

Finding a Mental Health Professional

For many women, seeking professional help may present significant challenges. As we have discussed, it may be difficult to come to the realization that you need help. The next obstacle is finding the *right* help. There are many different kinds of mental health professionals out there, and sometimes it can be quite confusing to figure out exactly what you need. If you are pregnant or planning a pregnancy, it may be particularly difficult to find someone who is comfortable working with pregnant or postpartum women. It is essential that you find a reputable professional who is familiar with the problems you are experiencing. Landing in the office of somebody without expertise in this area may be just as bad as doing nothing at all.

Probably the best way to find a good health professional for yourself is to ask around. But while your friends and family members may be a good resource for you when you are looking for a dentist, I'd suggest that your obstetrician or primary care provider is a good place to start for this. He or she should be able to provide you with a list of mental health professionals who specialize in treating women with reproductive issues. If this approach is not fruitful, you may also try contacting Depression After Delivery or Postpartum Support International (listed in the appendix). These organizations maintain lists of professionals throughout the country who specialize in the treatment of women with depression and other psychological problems associated with pregnancy and childbirth.

Mental health providers differ in terms of their training and the services they can provide. **Psychiatrists** are physicians with a medical degree (MD) who have received the same basic four years of training in medicine as other types of physicians. In addition, they have pursued a three-year residency in psychiatry and have specialized in the diagnosis and treatment of depression and other psychiatric disorders. Some psychiatrists (also known as psychopharmacologists) choose to specialize in treatment with medication; however, many psychiatrists prescribe medication as well as provide psychotherapy. To practice medicine, a physician must have an active medical license in the state in which he or she practices.

A **clinical psychologist** has received a degree (MA, PhD, or PsyD) in clinical psychology, a field devoted to the study of all aspects of human behavior. Typically, a psychologist's training includes an average of five to seven years of graduate training during which he develops expertise in psychotherapy and diagnostic assessment. He must also complete a clinical internship. You should choose a psychologist who has graduated from an accredited program and who holds a license in the state in which he or she practices. In most states, psychologists may provide psychotherapy but cannot prescribe medication.

Social workers typically receive about two years of graduate training in mental health and a master's degree. A social worker who is a psychotherapist and is a LICSW (Licensed Clinical Social Worker) has also received specialized training in psychotherapy and has passed a licensing exam.

A **clinical nurse specialist** (sometimes called a registered nurse practitioner) is a registered nurse who has an advanced degree in psychiatric nursing. In some states, clinical nurse specialists may prescribe medication.

Psychotherapist is a generic term used to describe any one who practices psychotherapy. It may be a psychiatrist or psychologist, but this is a term used by a variety of other mental health professionals who have received some specialized training in the practice of psychotherapy. You should also be aware that in some states, anyone can call himself or herself a psychotherapist without receiving *any* specific training or a license. Before you start working with a therapist, you should ask specifically about what type of training he or she has received. In addition, you may want to verify that a therapist has a current license by contacting the state board that grants licenses to mental health professionals.

Choosing the type of professional to consult is not always so straightforward. Probably the most important thing is to choose a professional who has a good reputation and has experience in working with women with reproductive issues. Good referrals may come from your obstetrician or primary care provider. Local psychiatric societies, medical schools, and community mental health centers may be able to provide you with the names of mental health professionals in your area. Because therapy does not work well when there is not a good chemistry between you and your therapist, it is sometimes helpful to meet with a couple of therapists before beginning treatment.

An experienced clinician—whether a psychiatrist, psychologist, social worker, or clinical nurse specialist—should make a thorough diagnostic assessment and advise you regarding your options for treatment. In addition, many primary care providers and ob-gyns feel comfortable diagnosing and treating depression, although they typically refer their patients to mental health providers for psychotherapy. Only psychiatrists, other physicians, and clinical nurse specialists are medically trained to perform medical diagnostic tests and to evaluate you for other medical illnesses that may be contributing to the depression. In most states, these are the only professionals who can prescribe medications and provide detailed information regarding their use. (Although psychologists are lobbying for the right to prescribe medications, they have not been granted this professional privilege in most states.) Given these constraints, it is fairly common for a person to see one provider who can prescribe medication and another who provides psychotherapy.

Those who live in a metropolitan area may have a multitude of options, whereas those living in more remote areas may have relatively limited choices. Cost may be another factor. If you have health insurance, you may also be restricted in whom you can see. Most insurance companies cover the cost of evaluation and certain types of treatment. While medication and medication management is usually covered by insurance without restrictions, there may be limits placed on how many sessions of psychotherapy you can receive. Some people elect to pay for services out-of-pocket; social workers or clinical nurse specialists are generally more affordable than psychologists and psychiatrists. For those with limited financial resources, some clinics and mental health professionals adjust their fees on a sliding scale; ask about this option.

When you look for a mental health professional, you should choose somebody to whom you feel comfortable talking. You should feel that he or she listens closely to what you are saying and makes an effort to understand you, rather than making assumptions about how you feel. He or she should respond openly and nondefensively to your questions and concerns. If you feel that the treatment is not going well, you should point this out. When there is a healthy therapeutic relationship between you and your doctor or counselor, he or she should be able to listen to your concerns and to respond appropriately. If this is not the case, you should consider whether he or she is the right person for you.

The relationship between patient and therapist is unique. Psychotherapy can be successful only when both partners are working together to achieve a mutually agreed upon goal. Although a very special and close connection may form, the patient-therapist relationship is distinct from all others. You must be willing to reveal sometimes uncomfortable feelings and thoughts and to confront and work on your problems. And the therapist must be available to facilitate this process and to provide new insights. Essential to this relationship is mutual trust, respect, and confidentiality.

Psychotherapy

Psychotherapy, sometimes called talk therapy, is the type of treatment most commonly recommended for women with depression. With the emergence of well-tolerated and effective antidepressant medications, many women now choose to take an antidepressant medication rather than pursue therapy. Furthermore, because of the long-term nature of psychotherapy, many insurance companies limit access to it. However, for all types of depression, psychotherapy remains one of the most effective treatments. In women who are pregnant or breast-feeding, this is a particularly attractive treatment option, and several studies have demonstrated that therapy is as effective as medication for relieving the symptoms of depression. Furthermore, it seems that the most dramatic and long-lasting results are achieved when a combination of medication and therapy is used.

While medication is clearly helpful in reducing the severity of depressive symptoms, medication does not directly address environmental factors that may contribute to your depression. A key goal of therapy is to identify and work through the factors that trigger your depression. Psychotherapy may help you make significant changes in your life that may last for many years, extending way beyond the treatment itself. Acknowledging and understanding what causes depression for you may help you prevent its return. Better understanding how depression affects you may protect those who are closest to you from its negative effects. In addition, psychotherapy may provide you with techniques that help you to manage stressful stations, increase your confidence, and improve the quality of your relationships with your partner, your family, and others.

Exactly what you talk about in therapy is up to you. Most women focus on what is causing the most distress; however, among the issues that may be addressed in therapy are:

- grief following the loss of a loved one;
- stress related to child-care responsibilities, career, or financial difficulties;
- relationship issues, especially conflicts regarding parenting and child care;
- conflict with family members, friends, or coworkers;
- role transitions (getting married, becoming a mother, starting a new career);
- social isolation and loneliness.

You should not feel restricted by this list and should feel free to talk about whatever is bothering you. No problem should be considered trivial; if it is causing distress, you should talk about it.

There are several different types of individual psychotherapy to choose from. Typically, a therapist will determine what type of therapy is likely to be the most effective for you, taking into account the nature of the problem being treated, your personality, and past experiences. While some therapies are more free-flowing and open-ended, others are more structured and goal-oriented. Psychiatrists, psychologists, social workers, and other mental health professionals are all trained to provide psychotherapy. There is no evidence to suggest that one type of clinician is better than another. Some therapists rely upon a mixture of techniques, choosing those that seem to work best for an individual patient.

Interpersonal therapy (or **IPT**) is a goal-directed therapy that focuses primarily on the relationships one has with other people. It is based on the theory that depression may be triggered or exacerbated when there are problems in one's important relationships. It focuses on the conflicts and transitions that occur within relationships and works to resolve loneliness and social isolation. IPT has been demonstrated to be effective in treating depression occurring in a variety of settings and for women during pregnancy and the postpartum period.

Cognitive behavioral therapy (or **CBT**) is another form of goal-directed therapy, that focuses on the negative thought patterns and behaviors of people who suffer from depression. The goal of CBT is to eliminate beliefs or behaviors that perpetuate depression and to replace them with more positive patterns of thinking. CBT is generally short-term, lasting for about twelve to sixteen weeks. Not only is CBT effective for treating depression, there is evidence to indicate that it is helpful for people with a variety of anxiety disorders, including panic disorder, obsessive-compulsive disorder (OCD), posttraumatic stress disorder (PTSD), and social phobia.

Psychoanalysis and **psychodynamic therapy** help a person to discover and understand emotional conflicts that may be contributing to their depression. While CBT and IPT tend to be brief in duration and focus more on the present than on past experiences, these "insight-oriented" therapies tend to work with issues that have their roots in the past. The therapist helps to uncover unconscious or unresolved problems from one's childhood. Through this process, one is better able to understand how early childhood experiences influence one's feelings and behaviors and, with a greater awareness of these early conflicts, it may be possible to resolve present-day problems. This is, however, a lengthy process, typically taking several years. While psychodynamic therapy usually involves meeting once or twice per week, psychoanalysis is a more intense process, typically requiring daily sessions over a period of many years.

In addition to individual psychotherapy, there are also several other types of therapy conducted in a group setting. In **marital or couples therapy,** both partners meet with a therapist and focus on resolving conflicts within the relationship. **Family therapy** is designed to help the family work as a group to resolve problems that affect them all. The goal is to improve communication and to decrease conflict within the family. **Group therapy** consists of several unrelated people who meet with a therapist to discuss their problems together. Many different kinds of group therapy exist, and often groups are organized around a particular issue. A group may address problems related to having children, including infertility, miscarriage, and transition to parenthood. One of the major advantages of group therapy is that it gives one the opportunity to meet with and talk to others who have experienced a similar problem, and thus this may be an important source of support.

Psychotherapy may be short-term (sixteen or fewer sessions) or may be carried out over a period of months or years. This depends on the type of illness and the type of therapy selected. Generally speaking, the more severe the illness, the longer the time needed to complete therapy. Psychotherapy is effective on its own or when combined with medication. Although psychotherapy is clearly effective for treating depression and a wide range of other emotional problems, it can be prohibitively time-consuming and expensive.

Making the Decision to Use Medication

It is important to acknowledge that psychotherapy might not work for every woman. For those who do not respond to this form of treatment or for women with more severe forms of depression, there are now many effective medications available. Making the decision to take antidepressant medication is not easy for anyone. Many people suffer with depression for many years before they decide to take medication, and even after taking medication for some time, many do so only with reluctance. The pill bottle serves as a constant reminder of their problem, and some look for any opportunity to stop. Others consider medication a godsend and wish they had started using it sooner. Here are some reasons why women resist treatment.

"Taking medication is a sign of weakness." To some, an antidepressant feels like a crutch. The reality is that depression is a biological illness, and even with willpower and enormous effort on your part, you may not be able to rid yourself of its symptoms. A diabetic is not likely to consider taking insulin as a sign of moral weakness, nor should one who takes an antidepressant to treat her depression.

"A *medication won't really solve my problems.*" When it seems like the depression is the result of stressful or painful life experiences, it is hard to imagine how an antidepressant can help. If one has suffered a terrible loss, like the death of a loved one, how can a pill take that pain away? It can't. A pill will not miraculously make that loss disappear. It will not resolve your relationship problems or whisk away your financial difficulties or a stressful work situation. But an antidepressant *can* help you to deal more effectively with these situations. When you are depressed, problems may feel insurmountable, but by using an antidepressant to get your depression under better control, you may be able to approach these problems with greater confidence, clarity, and efficacy.

"A *medication may change my personality.*" Many people fear that taking an antidepressant will have a dramatic effect on their personality or that the medication will make them into a totally different person. While antidepressants may allow you to have a more positive outlook on the world or may help you to be a more cheerful and optimistic person, you are still the same person. Most people describe their antidepressant as helping them to be the person they used to be before the depression.

"*I don't want to become addicted to the medication.*" Antidepressants are not tranquilizers or narcotics, and they are not physiologically addictive. Many people will have no difficulty stopping the medication. Unfortunately, depression, like many other medical problems, tends to be recurrent, and some people experience the return of their depression after stopping an antidepressant. This does not mean that they are "addicted" to the medication; it just means that the depression has come back. It is for this reason that, while most people take an antidepressant for six months to a year, those with recurrent depression may choose to remain on an antidepressant for a longer period.

When is medication the right choice? Every situation is different, and this is a decision you should discuss with your doctor. For women who do not respond to psychotherapy or for women with more severe forms of depression, medication should be considered. Most women who are pregnant or breast-feeding believe that they cannot take any antidepressant medication, but this is not the case. Over the last ten years, we've learned a lot about the reproductive safety of many antidepressants. While information is still limited, research studies indicate that certain medications may be taken safely during pregnancy and do not increase the risk of any type of birth defect or other problems. This is an important topic we will discuss in greater detail later in the following chapter.

How Antidepressants Work

An antidepressant is not a "happy pill." If you are not depressed, an antidepressant will not have any real effect on your mood. An antidepressant will not make you high, nor will it tranquilize or numb you. However, if you are depressed, an antidepressant will, over time, improve your mood and your sense of well-being. As we discussed in chapter 2, depression occurs when there is an imbalance of certain neurotransmitter systems in your brain; in people with depression, the levels of certain neurotransmitters, including serotonin and norepinephrine, appear to be abnormally low. An antidepressant works to correct this disequilibrium and to restore the levels of these transmitters to normal. Most antidepressants increase levels of serotonin in the brain; others affect norepinephrine and dopamine levels.

Antidepressants do not work instantly. An antidepressant causes changes in the brain, but these complex biochemical changes take time, from several days to several weeks, and occur only when the medication is taken daily. This is why you may not notice any improvement for several weeks after starting an antidepressant. The time it takes to see the full effect depends on the particular medication. Your prescribing doctor will tell you what to expect.

How do I know if the medication is working? Some people notice dramatic changes in their mood, but for most people the changes become noticeable two to four weeks after starting the medication. As an antidepressant starts to work, you may notice that you are feeling a bit brighter or that you have more energy to pursue your usual activities. You may start to feel less tense or irritable and that you are better able to handle difficult situations. You may also notice that the quality of your sleep is improving and that you are feeling less fatigued and better able to focus on your activities. It is reasonable to expect that the medication will eventually help you to feel like your "normal self," the way you felt before the depression started.

How long will I have to take an antidepressant? It depends. If this is your first or second episode of depression, most experts suggest that you remain on an antidepressant for six to twelve months. Even after you feel better, you should continue taking the medication for its full course. If you stop treatment prematurely, there is a greater chance that the depression will return. It seems that the longer you stay on the medication, the better your chances for doing well after it is discontinued. However, depression in many women is recurrent. Even if you receive treatment for an adequate amount of time, there is a chance that you will have another episode at some point down the line. Thus the recommendations are a bit different if you have had three or more episodes of depression. In this situation, "maintenance" treatment is indicated. This means that you should remain on the medication for several years or even indefinitely. For some people, this may sound like a life sentence; however, the research supporting the long-term use of antidepressants is persuasive. In a recent analysis, data pooled from 4,410 patients receiving treatment with antidepressants suggested that long-term treatment with antidepressants significantly reduces the risk of relapse. Only 18 percent of those who stayed on antidepressants had another episode of depression during the follow-up period, as compared to 41 percent of those who discontinued treatment. The optimum duration of treatment remains poorly defined; however, it is apparent in some women who suffer from recurrent depression that relapse occurs whenever the medication is discontinued.

Also keep in mind that stopping certain medications abruptly may lead to uncomfortable withdrawal symptoms. Selective serotonin reuptake inhibitors (SSRIs), the most commonly prescribed antidepressants, are associated with characteristic withdrawal symptoms: dizziness or light-headedness, nausea, headaches, lethargy, anxiety, irritability, tremors, tingling, numbness, or "electric" shock–like sensations in the head or limbs. Generally, these symptoms start within a few days of stopping the medication and resolve over a period of several days. However, there are people who seem to be more sensitive to antidepressant withdrawal and experience significant symptoms for several weeks. Tapering the medication slowly over a period of several weeks can help to decrease the risk of withdrawal symptoms. If you are planning to discontinue your medication, you and your doctor should decide upon an appropriate schedule.

Types of Antidepressants
There are now a wide variety of antidepressants available in the United States. Which antidepressant you and your doctor ultimately choose will depend on your symptoms and a variety of factors. In addition, each antidepressant has certain side effects which may also influence this choice. Un-

fortunately, it is difficult to reliably predict to which medication a person will respond, and sometimes it may be necessary to try several medications before finding one that is effective. Please note: the information included in this section is not intended to be inclusive and is not a substitute for the information you will receive from the doctor who is prescribing the medication. (For more complete information regarding these medications, you may also consult the *Physicians Desk Reference*, or PDR.)

The most commonly used antidepressants are the **selective serotonin reuptake inhibitors,** or **SSRIs.** The first of these, fluoxetine (Prozac), was introduced in 1987, and since then several others have been released: setraline (Zoloft), fluvoxamine (Luvox), paroxetine (Paxil), citalopram (Celexa), and escitalopram (Lexapro). The key advantage of these medications is that they are relatively well-tolerated and free of dangerous side effects. The side effects most commonly seen with the SSRIs are stomach upset, loss of appetite, nervousness, headache, fatigue, sleep disturbance, and sexual dysfunction. Many of these side effects improve within a few days of initiating the drug and may disappear over time. Not only are the SSRIs good for depression, they are also used to treat a variety of anxiety disorders, including generalized anxiety disorder, panic disorder, obsessive-compulsive disorder, and social phobia. In contrast to most other types of antidepressants, the SSRIs are also effective for treating premenstrual mood symptoms.

Recently there has been a great deal of interest in what are called dual-action antidepressants, medications that interact with several different neurotransmitter systems. Although it was long believed that all antidepressants are equally effective, there is growing evidence to suggest that the dual-action antidepressants may act more quickly and may be more effective than other types. The **serotonin-norepeinephrine reuptake inhibitors,** or **SNRIs,** venlafaxine (Effexor) and duloxetine (Cymbalta) share many of the properties of the SSRIs combined with some of the effects on the norepinephrine system carried by an older class of antidepressants known as tricyclics. For the SNRIs, the most common side effects are stomach upset, loss of appetite, nervousness, headache, fatigue, sleep disturbance, and sexual dysfunction. At higher doses, venlafaxine may also cause increased blood pressure in some patients.

Antidepressants that are distinct from the other classes of medication and seem to have their own mechanism of action are called **atypical antidepressants.** Of this class of antidepressants, the most commonly used is bupropion (Wellbutrin). One advantage of Wellbutrin is that it does not cause the sexual side effects or weight gain frequently seen with other antidepressants. Bupropion (marketed as Zyban) also appears to be effective for smoking cessation. Although an effective antidepressant, bubropion may be less useful for treating anxiety and may exacerbate symptoms of anxiety in certain patients. The most common side effects are nervousness, nausea, loss of appetite, dry mouth, constipation, insomnia, and headache. Bupropion should not be used in patients with a history of seizure disorder or bulimia, since at higher doses it may increase the incidence of seizures.

Other atypical antidepressants mirtazapine (Remeron) and nefazodone (Serzone) are effective and may be particularly useful in patients with sleep problems. Although mirtazapine is relatively well tolerated, its use may be limited by weight gain. Nefazodone was recently pulled from the market in Canada and in Europe due to concerns that this drug may cause liver damage in some patients. Trazodone (Desyrel, a precursor of Serzone) is an antidepressant that is often used at low doses in conjunction with another antidepressant to treat insomnia. Trazodone, however, is not commonly used to treat depression because it is difficult for patients to tolerate higher doses of this medication. Especially at higher doses, trazodone may cause drowsiness, headache, dizziness, and low blood pressure.

Nowadays the older classes of antidepressants are used less frequently. The **tricyclic antidepressants,** or **TCAs,** while very effective for treating both depression and anxiety, have more significant side effects than some of the newer antidepressants, including dry mouth, constipation, sedation, blurred vision, weight gain, dizziness, and low blood pressure. In addition, people with certain cardiac problems or abnormalities of cardiac conduction may not be able to take these medications. TCAs may be useful for treating insomnia.

The **monoamine oxidase inhibitors (MAOIs),** including tranylcypromine (Parnate) and phenelzine (Nardil), were the first antidepressants developed. These medications are highly effective for depression but have very serious side effects. Patients taking MAOIs must adhere to a very strict tyramine-free diet. If they ingest any of a large number of foods containing tyramines (i.e., aged cheeses, red wine), they may experience a potentially life-threatening increase in blood pressure. The MAOIs also interact with a variety of medications, including over-the-counter cold medications, certain pain relievers, and other antidepressants. Because of these significant side effects, the MAOIs are not commonly used. However, the MAOIs remain a good choice for patients who have failed treatment with other antidepressants.

Generic Name	Trade Name	Starting Dose	Usual Dose Range
Selective Serotonin Reuptake Inhibitors (SSRIs)			
Citalopram	Celexa	20 mg	20–60 mg
Escitalopram	Lexapro	10 mg	10–20 mg
Fluoxetine	Prozac	10–20 mg	20–80 mg
Fluvoxamine	Luvox	50 mg	100–250 mg
Paroxetine	Paxil	10–20 mg	20–60 mg
Sertraline	Zoloft	50–100 mg	50–200 mg
Serotonin-Norepinephrine Reuptake Inhibitors (SNRIs)			
Duloxetine	Cymbalta	60 mg	60–120 mg
Venlafaxine	Effexor	37.5 mg	75–300 mg
Atypical Antidepressants (TCAs)			
Bupropion	Wellbutrin	100–150 mg	150–300 mg
Mirtazapine	Remeron	15 mg	15–45 mg
Nefazodone	Serzone	50 mg	300–600 mg
Trazodone	Desyrel	50 mg	200–600 mg
Tricyclic Antidepressants			
Amitriptyline	Elavil	25–50 mg	100–150 mg
Nortriptyline	Pamelor	10–25 mg	50–150 mg
Protriptyline	Vivactil	10 mg	30–60 mg
Desipramine	Norpramin	25–50 mg	100–300 mg
Imipramine	Tofranil	25–50 mg	100–300 mg
Clomipramine	Anafranil	25 mg	100–200 mg
Monoamine Oxidase Inhibitors (MAOIs)			
Phenelzine	Nardil	15 mg	15–90 mg
Tranylcypromine	Parnate	10 mg	30–60 mg

While it was long believed that all antidepressants were equally effective, current research suggests that some antidepressants may be better for treating certain symptoms of depression. For example, SSRIs may be better than other agents for treating the obsessional and intrusive thoughts that sometimes come along with depression. Bupropion may be helpful for treating symptoms of attention deficit disorder. There is also research to indicate that certain antidepressants, including the dual-acting agents venlafaxine and duloxetine, may be more effective than other antidepressants.

Dr. Susan Kornstein and her colleagues from the Medical College of

Virginia hypothesize that one's gender may also influence the effectiveness of an antidepressant, such that certain antidepressants may be better for women than for men, and vice versa. A recent study demonstrated that pre-menopausal women responded slightly better to SSRIs than to the older tri-cyclic agents. Although not all studies indicate that gender affects treatment response, other studies have demonstrated that women with hormonally mediated mood disorders, including premenstrual dysphoric disorder and postpartum depression, may respond better to SSRIs (or other antidepres-sants that affect the serotonin neurotransmitter system) than to other antide-pressants.

Coping with Side Effects

There is no such thing as a perfect antidepressant. All medications have side effects; some are relatively benign and easy to tolerate, while others are more serious and may prompt the discontinuation of the medication. Fortu-nately, most of the newer antidepressants are relatively well tolerated and free of life-threatening side effects. In the table below, you will find the side effects most commonly seen in patients taking antidepressants, as well as other side effects that occur less often but are medically serious. The follow-ing list is not intended to be complete. For a more extensive list of side effects, you should consult the package insert or the *Physicians Desk Refer-ence* (available online at pdr.net). Furthermore, your doctor will discuss the side effects of every medication prescribed to you and will take into consid-eration interactions with other medications you may be taking.

Though many people experience side effects while taking an antidepres-sant, this is not always a reason to abandon treatment. Being patient is the key here; side effects often resolve within a few days or weeks of initiating treatment. However, if you are worried about the side effects or if they per-sist over time, it is important to discuss this problem with your doctor. There are many things that can be done to alleviate or eliminate these trouble-some problems. Sometimes changing the amount or frequency of the dosage, changing how it is delivered (time release, extended release), or switching to a different medication is the solution. You should not, however, make *any* changes in your treatment without first discussing them with your physician.

Nausea and stomach upset are side effects seen with most of the antide-pressants; when severe, weight loss may occur. The antidepressant least likely to cause stomach upset is mirtazapine (Remeron). Although these side effects tend to disappear within a few days of initiating treatment or rais-

Antidepressant	Side Effect
Selective Serotonin Reuptake inhibitors (SSRIs) *and* Serotonin-Norepinephrine Reuptake Inhibitors (SNRIs)	Jitteriness, anxiety Heartburn, loss of appetite Diarrhea Headache Fatigue Excessive sweating Sleep disruption Sexual dysfunction High blood pressure (venlafaxine)
Tricyclic Antidepressants (TCAs)	Sedation Dry mouth Constipation Blurred vision Weight gain Sexual dysfunction Dizziness, low blood pressure Irregular heart rhythm
Bupropion	Jitteriness or anxiety Insomnia Constipation Dry mouth Hand tremor Sedation Increased risk of seizure in some patients
Nefazodone *and* Trazodone	Headache Sedation Fatigue Dizziness, low blood pressure Liver function abnormalities (nefazodone)
Mirtazapine	Weight gain Sedation
Monoamine Oxidase Inhibitors (MAOIs)	Severe high blood pressure Serotonin syndrome Insomnia Sexual dysfunction Dizziness and low blood pressure

ing the dosage, you should talk to your doctor if the problem persists. You may consider some of the following options:

- Divide the antidepressant into several smaller doses to be taken over the course of the day.
- Take the medication with or immediately after meals.
- Consider using antacids.
- Ask your doctor if it may be helpful to use medications that reduce acid production by the stomach, such as famotidine (Pepcid), ranitidine (Zantac), omeprazole (Prilosec), or pantoprazole (Protonix).
- Ask your doctor if it may be possible to lower the dose of medication or to switch to another medication less likely to cause stomach upset.

Constipation occurs most commonly with the tricyclic antidepressants but may also be seen with other antidepressants. Generally, this is not a significant problem but is more of a nuisance. To reduce constipation, you may:

- increase the amount of fiber in your diet;
- increase your intake of fluids;
- consider adding fiber supplements (Metamucil, FiberChoice);
- consider using a stool softener, such as Colace (docusate sodium 50–200 mg daily) or Peri-Colace (docusate sodium plus a laxative casanthranol 1–2 tablets daily).

Drowsiness and fatigue are problems common to many of the antidepressants. The tricyclic antidepressants (especially imipramine and amitryptyline), nefazodone (Serzone), and mirtazapine (Remeron) are the most sedating, and this side effect can be an advantage when treating a patient who has difficulty sleeping. In contrast, bupropion (Wellbutrin) and the SSRIs tend to be a bit more activating, although some women do experience fatigue while taking the SSRIs. Over time, you may be able to adjust to this side effect, but if it persists, you should discuss these options with your physician:

- Take the medication in the evening or at bedtime.
- If your fatigue during the daytime is a result of insomnia at night or restless sleep, ask your doctor about using a sleep medication to improve the quality of your sleep at night.
- Ask your doctor about switching to a less sedating antidepressant (such as Wellbutrin).

- If you are on an antidepressant other than an MAOI, ask your doctor about adding a medication to increase wakefulness during the daytime.
  - Modafenil (Provigil) 100–200 mg
  - Bupropion (Wellbutrin) 75–150 mg
  - Methylphenidate (Ritalin) 10–20 mg twice daily

Sleep disruption is a common problem in those suffering from depression. Insomnia, when it is a symptom of the depression itself, tends to improve with the resolution of the depression. However, certain antidepressants, including bupropion (Wellbutrin) and the SSRIs, may exacerbate sleep problems and may make it more difficult to fall asleep or may cause restless sleep.

- Take your medication in the morning or earlier in the day.
- Avoid caffeinated beverages late in the day.
- Avoid taking naps during the day. If you must take a nap, try to make it less than half an hour.
- Ask your doctor about using a medication for sleep. Trazodone (Desyrel) and mirtazapine (Remeron) are sedating antidepressants that are sometimes used to promote sleep. Benzodiazepines (lorazepam, clonazepam, temazepam) may also be useful and are especially indicated when it seems that anxiety is making it difficult to sleep. Other sleep-promoting agents, including zolpidem (Ambien) and zaleplon (Sonata), may also be helpful for short-term use.
- Ask your doctor about switching to a more sedating antidepressant (such as mirtazapine [Remeron], nefazodone [Serzone], or the tricyclic antidepressants).

Weight gain is another common problem reported by patients taking antidepressant medications. It is most common with mirtazapine (Remeron) and the tricyclic antidepressants, and it is less often seen in patients taking the SSRIs and the SNRIs. The only antidepressant that seems to be free of this side effect is bupropion (Wellbutrin).

- Evaluate your eating behaviors and try to eliminate calorie-rich items from your diet.
- Consult with a nutritionist.
- Establish a routine exercise plan. This will help you burn calories and it may also improve your mood.

- Ask your doctor about switching to a medication less likely to cause weight gain (for example, bupropion, or Wellbutrin).
- Ask your doctor about adding topiramate (Topamax) to your regimen. Topiramate (25–200 mg daily) may decrease appetite and cause weight loss.

Sexual dysfunction is a problem seen with most antidepressants, but it appears to be particularly common with the SSRIs, affecting about half of patients. The degree of sexual dysfunction varies. Loss of libido is common. Women may also have difficulty attaining orgasm or may complain of decreased or altered sensation. Men often describe delayed time to orgasm but may occasionally experience impotence. While many other side effects may be tolerable, this is one that many are unable to live with, and it is estimated that 15 percent to 20 percent of patients discontinue antidepressant treatment because of sexual side effects. While mirtazapine (Remeron) and nefazodone (Serzone) are less commonly associated with sexual side effects, the only antidepressant free of this problem is bupropion, or Wellbutrin. There are a variety of strategies that can be used to manage the sexual side effects caused by antidepressants.

- Consult with your doctor to determine if there may be any medical causes for the sexual problems.
- Consult with your doctor to determine if it is possible to lower your dose of medication. Lowering the dose, however, may increase your chances of having the depression recur.
- Ask your doctor for an antidote. Bupropion (Wellbutrin) may be used at a dose of 75 to 150 mg one hour before anticipated sexual intercourse, or if this does not work, it may be prescribed at a dose of 150 to 300 daily in combination with your antidepressant.
- Other antidotes for sexual side effects include:
  - Stimulants (including methylphenidate [Ritalin] up to 20 to 30 mg per day)
  - Yohimbine (5.4 to 10.8 mg per day or as needed)
  - Buspirone (BuSpar) (5 to 20 mg three times per day)
- Ask your doctor about using sildenafil (Viagra). At this point its use in women is experimental. This treatment is not recommended for those with a history of coronary artery disease and should not be used in pregnant or lactating women.
- Ask your doctor about switching to another medication with fewer sexual side effects (such as bupropion [Wellbutrin] or mirtazapine [Rem-

eron]). Sometimes sexual side effects resolve after switching to another antidepressant in the same class.

Dizziness occurs most commonly with the tricyclic antidepressants, MAOIs, nefazodone (Serzone), and trazodone (Desyrel). Usually dizziness is a symptom associated with low blood pressure on rising from a reclining or seated position (a problem physicians call orthostatic hypotension).

- Maintain adequate hydration.
- Rise slowly and carefully after you have been sitting or lying down.
- Consider switching to a medication that is less likely to lower blood pressure, such as an SSRI, venlafaxine (Effexor), or bupropion (Wellbutrin).

Other Medications Used to Treat Depression and Anxiety

While many women with depression can be treated effectively with one medication, some require several medications to treat their symptoms. In some cases, a second medication is added to augment the action of an antidepressant or to treat its side effects. In other situations, a medication may be added to treat coexisting symptoms. For example, a woman with major depression *and* an anxiety disorder may require treatment with an antidepressant combined with another medication specifically for anxiety. Sometimes the treatment can become quite complicated. In this section, you will find some basic information regarding other medications that may be used to treat symptoms of depression and anxiety.

Anxiolytic Agents

Anxiolytic agents are medications used specifically to treat anxiety. While many of the antidepressants, including the SSRIs, TCAs, and SNRIs, may be effective for alleviating anxiety symptoms, these agents are often combined with antianxiety medications. The most commonly used anxiolytic agents are the benzodiazepines. This is a class of medications related to diazepam (Valium). Although the benzodiazepines are highly effective, one negative aspect is their potential for physical dependence and abuse. In general, the benzodiazepines are well-tolerated. Common side effects include drowsiness, lethargy, and decreased mental sharpness. When the dose is too high, slurring of speech, impaired coordination, or unsteadiness of gait may occur. Benzodiazepines can also intensify the effects of alcohol;

thus, you should drink very little alcohol and should refrain from drinking if you plan to drive a car within a few hours.

In addition, the benzodiazepines should never be discontinued abruptly because serious withdrawal symptoms may occur: anxiety, poor concentration, disruption of sleep, headache, shakiness, sweating, muscle cramping or twitching, and, in severe cases, seizure. The benzodiazepines most commonly associated with withdrawal are those with short half-lives, such as alprazolam (Xanax). Withdrawal symptoms are more likely to occur in those who have taken high doses of benzodiazepines over a long period of time. Agents with longer half-lives, such as clonazepam (Klonopin), are generally preferred because they have less abuse potential and are less likely to elicit withdrawal symptoms when discontinued.

A structurally unrelated anxiolytic agent with low potential for abuse is buspirone (BuSpar). Compared to the benzodiazepines, BuSpar is less sedating and less likely to cause significant problems with cognitive and motor functioning. However, unlike benzodiazepines, which have a more immediate effect, BuSpar takes two to four weeks to be fully effective. Furthermore, BuSpar may be less effective for more severe anxiety symptoms and panic disorder. Commonly seen side effects include nausea, dizziness, and light-headedness.

Mood Stabilizers
This is a group of medications that are used to stabilize mood in patients with bipolar disorder. Not only do these medications protect one from depression, they reduce the risk of manic or hypomanic episodes. Although these medications are used primarily in patients with bipolar disorder, they may also be useful in certain patients with unipolar depression and may augment the action of a conventional antidepressant. Lithium was the first mood stabilizer. Lithium is a naturally occurring salt that has both antimanic and antidepressant properties. Side effects include fatigue, nausea, stomach upset, diarrhea, thirst, and hand tremor: often these symptoms resolve over time. Over time, treatment may be associated with other problems, including weight gain and acne. Long-term use is also associated with more serious problems, specifically hypothyroidism and impaired kidney function. When lithium levels are too high, nausea and/or vomiting, diarrhea, abnormal muscle movement, impaired coordination, slurred speech, blurred vision, dizziness, and confusion may occur. Frequent blood monitoring is required to assess lithium levels and to monitor thyroid and kidney functioning.

More recently, there has been a greater interest in using antiseizure, or anticonvulsant, medications. Valproic acid (Depakene) and carbamazepine (Tegretol) have been demonstrated to be effective for preventing relapse in patients with bipolar disorder. Side effects of these agents include nausea, sedation, decreased mental acuity, dizziness, tremor, hair loss (valproic acid), and weight gain. More serious but less common side effects include blood cell and liver function abnormalities. Signs of toxicity are nausea and/or vomiting, poor coordination, slurred speech, blurred vision, and confusion. Blood monitoring is required to assess drug levels and to monitor liver function and blood cell counts.

Newer anticonvulsants—including gabapentin (Neurontin), levetiracetam (Keppra), oxcarbazepine (Trileptal), tiagabine (Gabitril), topiramate (Topamax), and zomisamide (Zonegran)—are currently being investigated for use as mood stabilizers. Lamotrigine (Lamictal) shows great promise in treating depression in patients with bipolar disorder. It is better tolerated than other anticonvulsants; the most common side effects are headache, nausea, tremor, and sleepiness. The main concern with lamotrigine is that it may cause a severe rash and a potentially life-threatening condition called Stevens Johnson syndrome. This complication is rare, occurring in less than 0.1 percent of patients, and can be prevented by increasing the dose of medication very slowly.

Antipsychotic (Neuroleptic) Agents

These medications are specifically used to treat psychotic symptoms. They are used primarily in patients with psychotic disorders, such as schizophrenia, but many other patients may benefit from these medications. The newer, or atypical, antipsychotic agents—for example olanzapine (Zyprexa) and quetiapine (Seroquel)—are much more tolerable and have fewer serious side effects than the older antipsychotic agents and are being used very widely. Patients with bipolar disorder may benefit from the mood-stabilizing activities of these medications. There is also evidence to suggest that they may be effective in patients with refractory, or treatment-resistant, anxiety or depression.

While long-term use of the older antipsychotic agents has been associated with abnormal involuntary movements of the face and other parts of the body (the worst of these being tardive dyskinesia), the risk of this type of side effect appears to be very low in patients treated with the newer agents. Common side effects include sedation, weight gain, sexual dysfunction, blurred vision, and low white blood cell count (clozapine; Clozaril). More recently researchers have been concerned about the potential of these medications to affect glucose metabolism and to increase the risk of diabetes in certain individuals.

Sedative-Hypnotic Agents

These agents, including zolpidem (Ambien), zaleplon (Sonata), and eszopiclone (Lunesta), are medications specifically used to induce or maintain sleep. Typically, these medications are used for a short period, as they may lose their effectiveness over time. A better option for treating sleep disruption may be a sedating antidepressant, such as trazodone or mirtazapine.

Stimulants

These are drugs, such as methylphenidate (Ritalin), that have a stimulating effect. Typically, these medications are used to treat attention deficit disorder, but they are now used to treat certain medication side effects, such as sedation, apathy, or inattentiveness. Like the benzodiazepines, there is the potential for abuse with these medications, and they are, for this reason, used relatively sparingly. Other side effects include sleep disturbance, decreased appetite and weight loss, anxiety, restlessness, agitation, and increased blood pressure.

Bright Light Therapy

Exposure to bright light for one to two hours each day may have an antidepressant effect. Light therapy is most commonly used for people who have seasonal affective disorder (SAD). Those with SAD become more depressed during the autumn and winter months when the daylight hours are shorter. Light therapy works best if given early in the morning, and the brighter the light, the greater the benefit. It is typically administered using a light box consisting of high-intensity fluorescent bulbs, filtered to remove harmful UV (ultraviolet) light. The amount of light needed varies widely from individual to individual; typically 10,000 lux is the recommended brightness. While light therapy seems to work best in patients with seasonal depression, there is evidence to suggest that this treatment may be effective in patients with other forms of depression as well. One of the real advantages of light therapy is the low incidence of side effects. Some patients experience headaches, eye irritation, and slight nausea. These side effects are generally the most severe at the beginning of treatment and disappear altogether after several exposures. In patients with bipolar disorder, however, light therapy may induce hypomania or mania, so it should be used with caution.

Class	Generic Name	Trade Name
Antianxiety Agents (Benzodiazepines)	Alprazolam	Xanax
	Chlordiazepoxide	Librium
	Clonazepam	Klonopin
	Diazepam	Valium
	Lorazepam	Ativan
	Temazepam	Restoril
Antianxiety Agents (Nonbenzodiazepine)	Buspirone	BuSpar
Mood Stabilizers	Lithium	Eskalith, Lithobid
	Carbamazepine	Tegretol
	Divalproex sodium	Depakote
	Gabapentin	Neurontin
	Lamotrigine	Lamictal
	Levetiracetam	Keppra
	Oxcarbazepine	Trileptal
	Tiagabine	Gabitril
	Topiramate	Topamax
	Valproic acid	Depakene
	Zomisamide	Zonegran
Antipsychotic Agents (Typical or Conventional)	Chlorpromazine	Thorazine
	Haloperidol	Haldol
	Perphenazine	Trilafon
	Trifluoperazine	Stelazine
Antipsychotic Agents (Atypical)	Aripiprazole	Abilify
	Clozapine	Clozaril
	Olanzapine	Zyprexa
	Quetiapine	Seroquel
	Risperidone	Risperdal
	Ziprasidone	Geodon
Sedative-Hypnotics	Zaleplon	Sonata
	Zolpidem	Ambien
	Eszopiclone	Lunesta
Stimulants	Dextroamphetamine	Dexedrine
	Methylphenidate	Ritalin, Concerta
	Modafinil	Provigil

Electroconvulsive Therapy

Electroconvulsive, or electroshock, therapy (also known as ECT) was one of the first treatments available for depression. In the 1930s and 1940s, doctors first discovered that after having a seizure some patients with psychiatric illness experienced a complete resolution of their symptoms. ECT is now carried out using a general anesthetic and a muscle relaxant. An electric stimulus is applied briefly to produce a generalized seizure lasting for about one minute. Because of the muscle relaxants and anesthesia, the patient does not experience any muscle spasms and feels no pain. Treatments are usually given three times a week, with a full course of ECT consisting of six to twelve treatments. Side effects from ECT include headache, muscle aches, nausea, and confusion; usually these symptoms resolve within a few hours. Over the course of ECT, patients may experience memory problems, although this side effect typically resolves over the days and weeks following completion of ECT. Some patients describe more long-term memory loss.

While ECT is one of our most effective treatments for depression, many people continue to fear ECT and are reluctant to pursue this option. When they think of ECT, they recall the terrifying image of Jack Nicholson in *One Flew Over the Cuckoo's Nest*. While this is not an accurate portrayal of ECT as performed today, it is difficult to erase the fears many people have regarding ECT. Even though celebrities like pianist Vladimir Horowitz and TV personality Dick Cavett have spoken openly about their very positive experiences with ECT, this treatment is generally used only for severely depressed patients for whom psychotherapy and medication have proven to be ineffective or for those who are at imminent risk of suicide.

Complementary and Alternative Treatments

Alternative medicine is defined as any form of treatment that lies outside the realm of conventional modern medicine, and it encompasses a broad range of healing philosophies and therapies. These are not practices that are commonly taught in traditional medical schools, and often they are provided by practitioners with no traditional medical training. Examples of alternative treatment include acupuncture, herbal medicines, dietary supplements, aromatherapy, and massage therapy. If a therapy is used alone or instead of conventional treatment, it is called *alternative medicine*. If this treatment is received in combination with a conventional medical treatment, it is referred to as *complementary medicine*. For example, many hospitals are now using acupuncture to manage pain and nausea in certain populations, such as those undergoing cancer chemotherapy or surgery.

In the United States, alternative treatments have been used much more widely over the last decade. Recent studies indicate that about half of all Americans have used alternative therapies to treat a wide range of medical ailments and emotional problems, including depression and anxiety. In many instances, the alternative treatments are combined with conventional strategies in the hope of obtaining a more successful outcome. Although alternative and complementary strategies seem very attractive and are often touted as "natural" remedies, it is important to recognize that they are not risk-free. If you are pregnant or nursing, bear in mind that there is no regulatory body overseeing the safety of these alternative treatments. They may have serious side effects. Furthermore, many of these treatments have not been systematically studied and have not been proven to be effective. Using a treatment without proven efficacy can delay or replace an effective conventional treatment. Given the wide availability of these treatments, many people are diagnosing and treating themselves; without the input of an experienced health professional, serious conditions may be missed or mismanaged. Finally, alternative strategies are not covered by most insurance companies and may thus end up being more costly than conventional treatments.

Acupuncture

Acupuncture is a procedure in which fine needles are inserted into very specific acupuncture points throughout the body. Traditional Chinese medicine has relied upon acupuncture for thousands of years to treat a wide array of medical conditions. While there are various theories to explain how acupuncture works, its mechanism of action remains poorly understood. Over the last decades there has been increased interest in using acupuncture to treat certain conditions, including intractable pain. Although one small double-blind study found that acupuncture may also be helpful in treating patients who suffer from depression, further study is clearly warranted.

Herbal Medicines

Herbal remedies have long been used in other cultures to treat a wide variety of ailments. A 1997 survey estimated that 12.1 percent of U.S. adults had used an herbal medicine in the previous year, and the popularity of herbal remedies continues to grow. Most herbal products in the United States are considered dietary supplements and thus are not regulated as medicines and therefore are not required to meet the standards for drugs specified in the Federal Food, Drug, and Cosmetic Act. Unlike conventional medications, herbal medicines are not evaluated by the Food and Drug Administration (FDA) and may be marketed without solid proof of their efficacy and/or safety. A particular concern for women of childbearing age is that herbal medicines have been found to contain high concentrations of lead, mercury, and other heavy metals. Both lead and mercury are potent neurotoxins and can lead to a number of psychiatric problems, including anxiety, irritability, sleep disturbance, seizure, and dementia. In addition, exposure to lead and mercury in pregnant women has been associated with miscarriage and intrauterine growth retardation. Children are particularly vulnerable to lead exposure, and there is evidence that exposure to even relatively low lead levels either *in utero* or after birth may result in developmental delays, cognitive problems, attentional deficits, and mental retardation. Unfortunately, the problem of heavy metal contaminants has not received adequate attention, and the public is largely unaware of the serious side effects of some herbal preparations.

Although there is a tendency to think of herbal remedies as being safer or more benign than conventional medications, the truth is that herbal remedies can pose serious health risks. Like conventional medications, they do have side effects and may interact with other prescribed medications. While there is some data to support the use of certain herbal medicines in patients who suffer from depression, the use of these herbal treatments in pregnancy is clearly a more complicated issue. While an herbal medicine may be considered a "natural" remedy, it would be a mistake to automatically assume that it is safe for use during pregnancy. Herbal medications are not compounds that are normally found in the body or in one's diet, and the effects of these agents on the developing fetus have not been adequately studied. The manufacturers of herbal remedies are not required to collect information on the safety of these compounds during pregnancy.

St. John's Wort. Many different herbal remedies have been touted as being effective for the treatment of depression, including ginkgo biloba, ginseng, kava kava, black hellebore, and borage. There are, however, no rigorous studies to support the use of these agents in patients with depression. Of all the herbal remedies used to treat depression, St. John's wort (also known as *Hypericum perforatum*) is probably the one with the most evidence to support its effectiveness. Although the active ingredient has not been identified, this preparation contains a mixture of compounds that inhibit the uptake of several neurotransmitters, including serotonin and dopamine.

It appears that St. John's wort (usually used at doses of 900 mg per day) is more effective than placebo for the treatment of depression. However, most of these studies have included only patients with mild to moderate depression. In several recent studies evaluating patients with more severe depression, St. John's wort did not appear to be much more effective than placebo. Furthermore, there is little information on the long-term use of this preparation. Given these results, St. John's wort is recommended only for the short-term treatment of patients with mild depression who are not and do not plan to become pregnant and are not breast-feeding.

It is important to note that St. John's wort may have significant side effects. Reported side effects include gastrointestinal symptoms, dizziness, confusion, fatigue, dry mouth, restlessness, headache, allergic skin reactions, sexual dysfunction, frequent urination, and swelling. St. John's wort, particularly at higher doses, may also cause photosensitivity, and severe skin reactions after exposure to sunlight have been reported. Although some women may choose to use natural remedies while pregnant or breast-feeding, there is not sufficient data regarding the safety of St. John's wort in pregnant or breast-feeding women. At this point the literature includes limited data on the use of St. John's wort during pregnancy. With regard to breast-feeding, there is a report suggesting some adverse events, including drowsiness and colic, in nursing infants exposed to St. John's wort in the breast milk.

Phytoestrogens. Over the last decade, there has been an increasing interest in herbal remedies with estrogenic activity for the treatment of a variety of disorders in women. Given the recent concerns regarding the long-term use of estrogen replacement therapy, the search for natural alternatives to estrogen has intensified. The phytoestrogens are a family of naturally occurring plant compounds with estrogen-like activity. Various classes of phytoestrogens exist, including isoflavones, lignans, coumestans, resorcylic acid lactones, and mycotoxins. Of all of these, it is probably only the isoflavones and lignans that have biological activity in humans. Soybeans and soy products, including tofu, tempeh, soy flour, and soy milk, are rich in isoflavones. Other food sources include alfalfa, apples, green tea, sesame, and wheat. Lignans are found in flaxseed (linseed), rye, red clover, berries, fruits, vegetables, and whole grains.

Recent research has focused on the capacity of these compounds to reduce menopausal symptoms. Others have raised the possibility that the phytoestrogens may reduce the risk of certain types of cancer or cardiovascular disease. Given the estrogenic activity of these compounds, it has also been postulated that this group of compounds may be effective antidepressants in women; whether or not they have an effect on mood and psychological well-being is a question that remains unanswered.

While supplementing one's diet with soy products and other natural sources of phytoestrogens is probably a benign intervention, no such presumption of safety can be made when using preparations of isolated, often high-dose, isoflavone and lignan phytoestrogens that are currently sold over the counter. In fact, there has been some concern that exposure to high doses of the estrogenic phytoestrogens may carry some of the same types of risk as seen with estrogen. Until more information is available regarding the safety of these compounds, it is recommended that women do not consume excessive amounts of phytoestrogens, especially if they are pregnant or breast-feeding.

Evening Primrose Oil. Evening primrose oil is another natural remedy that has been promoted for the treatment of mood symptoms in women, especially those suffering from premenstrual syndrome, or PMS. Evening primrose oil is a rich source of omega-6 essential fatty acids, primarily gamma-linolenic acid (GLA) and linoleic acid, both essential components of cell membranes in the brain. While the manufacturers of evening primrose oil preparations promote this agent as improving mood and decreasing anxiety, the most rigorously conducted studies show that evening primrose oil is no more effective than placebo in women who suffer from PMS. In addition, evening primrose oil may increase the risk of seizure and should not be used in those individuals with a history of seizure or in combination with drugs that lower seizure threshold (e.g., tricyclic antidepressants, bupropion). There is very little information on the safety of this compound taken during pregnancy, and there is one report that suggests that evening primrose oil may actually increase the risk of certain complications, including prolonged labor. Its use is not recommended in pregnant or breast-feeding women.

Dietary Supplements

Although supplementing the diet with the recommended doses of vitamins and minerals is a sound practice, the risks associated with taking high doses of nutritional supplements are not well understood. Furthermore, there is evidence that even natural compounds, including vitamins that are required by the body, may carry some risk when taken at higher than recommended doses. For example, there is some evidence that excessive doses of vitamin A taken during pregnancy may be associated with an increased risk of certain types of birth defects.

S-adenosyl-L-methionine (SAMe). S-adenosyl-L-methionine (SAMe) is an amino acid derivative that is important for the synthesis of several different neurotransmitters in the brain, including serotonin and norepinephrine. Although the antidepressant effects of SAMe were first discovered in Europe in 1974, SAMe was not used in the United States until 1999, after the development of a stable oral preparation. Approximately 1,400 patients have participated in clinical trials using SAMe, and the accumulated data have shown that SAMe (in doses of 200 to 1600 mg per day) is superior to placebo and may be as effective as tricyclic antidepressants for the treatment of depression. Furthermore, SAMe may be better tolerated and may have a more rapid onset of action than conventional antidepressants; the only significant side effect was gastrointestinal distress (including nausea and diarrhea), particularly in patients taking higher doses. SAMe also appears to be free of serious drug-drug interactions, although it is not recommended that this agent be combined with an MAO inhibitor. This preliminary data on SAMe are promising; however, there are little data to support the use of this compound in pregnancy. SAMe is not recommended for use during pregnancy or while nursing infants.

Omega-3 Fatty Acids. Fish oil has received a great deal of interest lately. Fish oil is rich in omega-3 fatty acids, and it is hypothesized that the omega-3 fatty acids found in our diet are essential for normal brain development and function. What has excited a great deal of interest in fish oil are the studies that have reported lower rates of depressive illness in countries with high rates of fish or fish oil consumption. In addition, there is some preliminary evidence to suggest that the omega-3 fatty acids contained in fish and fish oil, including eicosapentaenoic acid (EPA) and docosahexaenoic acid (DHA), have a positive effect in patients with unipolar depression and bipolar disorder. Another study indicated that EPA may enhance the effects of a conventional antidepressant. However, the data are preliminary, and it should be noted that not all studies have shown a beneficial effect.

The best way to get omega-3 fatty acids is by increasing the amount of fish in your diet; fishes especially rich in omega-3 fatty acids include mackerel, salmon, trout, herring, pilchards, anchovies, and sardines. Fish oil also comes in capsules. Although some of the studies used up to 10 grams of fish oil daily, most people use 3 to 4 grams per day. Fish oils are generally well tolerated. Side effects may include gas (belching, flatulence), bloating, abdominal discomfort, and diarrhea. Fish oil prepared from the liver of the fish (such as cod liver oil) is generally not recommended, especially during pregnancy, because this preparation of fish oil contains high levels of vitamin A that may be harmful. Whether or not other preparations of omega-3 fatty acids are safe in pregnant or breast-feeding women is not known, nor have the effects of very high doses of these fatty acids on the developing fetus been studied systematically. In addition, women of childbearing age have been urged to limit their intake of certain kinds of fish, which may contain high levels of mercury. For now, eating a balanced diet is the safest approach.

Many Effective Treatments Are Available

Depression is not something you have to battle on your own. It is a treatable illness and there are many different treatments available. One of the most important aspects of your care is finding a mental health professional whom you can trust and rely upon. The person you choose should be able to give you a good sense of what options are available to you and should help to select the treatment that is most likely to work. Ideally, this should feel like a collaborative experience, where you feel comfortable to ask questions and to express your concerns regarding your treatment. And keep in mind that, while the first treatment you try may not be successful, there are many different options and you are likely to find one that works for you.

Chapter 13

Understanding Your Options
Treating Depression During Pregnancy and the Postpartum Period

While there are many effective treatments available for depression, for women who are pregnant or nursing, selecting the most appropriate treatment is more complicated. The primary concern is that, if a woman takes any kind of medication to treat her symptoms, her child may be exposed to this medication passed through the placenta or into the breast milk. Because our understanding of how these medications may affect the child is limited, many women are understandably reluctant to use medication while they are pregnant or breast-feeding and doctors typically advise their pregnant and nursing patients to avoid treatment with antidepressants and other medications.

While this approach appears to be the safest option, withholding or withdrawing treatment for depression can have disastrous results. We now know that a significant proportion of women suffer from depression or anxiety during pregnancy. And the risk of illness is particularly high in those women who have been treated with medication but discontinue this treatment near the time of conception. What options are available to women who suffer from depression during pregnancy or after the birth of a child? While non-pharmacologic interventions, including psychotherapy, may be helpful in alleviating the symptoms of depression and anxiety, they are not always effective. Further, many women require ongoing treatment with a medication to maintain their emotional well-being. Without medication, the symptoms may be so severe that they compromise a woman's ability to function and may place her and her family at risk.

Historically, only those women with the most debilitating symptoms have been advised to take medication if they are pregnant or breast-feeding. Over the last decade, we have witnessed a shift in attitudes regarding the treatment of childbearing women. With more information on the reproductive safety of certain medications, both physicians and patients are now more willing to consider the use of certain medications during pregnancy and the postpartum period when it is indicated. Also contributing to this shift in attitude is our understanding that if a mother suffers from depression, whether it is mild or relatively severe, it is *not* a benign event when it occurs during pregnancy or in the early years of a child's life. To recap, when a pregnant mother is depressed, certain physiologic changes may occur that negatively affect the unborn child and place the pregnancy at risk. Depression during pregnancy is a strong risk factor for depression after delivery. Postpartum depression affects a woman's ability to parent and may place her child at risk for developmental delay, behavioral problems, and ongoing interpersonal difficulties. Fortunately, new research indicates that childbearing women who suffer from depression may safely pursue certain types of treatment that will allow them to remain emotionally healthy, and these interventions can help to protect both the mother and her family from the negative repercussions of this illness.

In the previous chapter, we reviewed the wide array of treatments available; here we will focus on those that are the most appropriate and effective for women who experience depression or anxiety during pregnancy or the postpartum period. Under no circumstances should this information be considered a substitute for consultation with a well-trained professional. Each woman's situation is different, and while this chapter will attempt to address a broad range of scenarios, it is *essential* that you discuss your particular situation with your own physician. The information provided in this chapter will help you, in collaboration with your doctor, to choose the safest and most appropriate options for your treatment.

How Is Depression During Pregnancy Treated?

Making Decisions Before Your Pregnancy. If you have a history of depression or anxiety, you may be wondering how pregnancy and having a child will affect you. Unfortunately, there is a good chance that you may experience some recurrent symptoms during pregnancy or after childbirth. Although it may be your nature to just delve into your pregnancy and to see how things go, you should do some advance planning. You should meet with a health care professional to discuss your options should your symptoms recur during pregnancy. There may be things you have not considered, and there may even be things that you can do to minimize your risk of illness during pregnancy.

When Joelle discovered she was pregnant, she called her obstetrician right away. Although she and her husband were planning to start a family in the near future, the pregnancy had happened sooner than she expected. She was worried because she had been taking Celexa for a depression that

started about a year before. Her obstetrician recommended that she immediately stop her medication.

Although she was excited about her pregnancy, Joelle was also worried.
She knew that her baby had been exposed to the medication for several
weeks and was concerned that she might have hurt her baby. She wondered if she should terminate the pregnancy. She also had other concerns:
she had had several episodes of depression in the past, and the last was her
worst. How would she do after she stopped the medication? If the depression came back, what would she do? Her obstetrician told her that she
should not take any type of antidepressant during pregnancy. Did that
mean she would have to suffer with the depression until the baby was born?

Joelle's first trimester was difficult. The morning sickness made her feel
horrible, and she felt drained of energy. It was hard to get up in the morning, and nothing interested or excited her. Her obstetrician was very supportive and tried to reassure her that things would get better in the second
trimester. Joelle very much wanted to believe her doctor, but she had experienced these symptoms before and feared that it was the depression creep-
ing back into her life.

By the second trimester, things were even worse. Joelle felt better physically, but she felt depressed and was having difficulty functioning at work.
Her obstetrician did not feel comfortable prescribing an antidepressant but
referred her to a psychiatrist with expertise in this area. Ultimately Joelle
decided to restart the Celexa. She and her husband weighed the information regarding the reproductive safety of Celexa and decided that the risks
were small compared to the risks associated with her depression. Although
Joelle felt guilty about her decision and was reluctant to tell her friends or
family that she was taking the medication, she felt she had made the right
decision. Within a few weeks, her depression started to subside. Her pregnancy went very well, her baby was healthy, and she felt incredibly fortunate.

With the advent of effective and well-tolerated antidepressants, the number of women taking psychotropic medications during their reproductive
years has grown tremendously. Unfortunately, women who take antidepressants regularly face a difficult decision when they plan to conceive or inadvertently become pregnant. Should they stop their medication and risk that
the depression may return? Or should they continue their medication during their pregnancy? For many medications, including antidepressants,
there is limited information regarding reproductive safety, and most doctors

advise their patients to avoid taking *any* medication during pregnancy whenever possible. But is this the appropriate approach for everyone?

Although a woman with a potentially serious medical illness, like high blood pressure or a seizure disorder, would never be advised by her physician to discontinue or to avoid treatment with a medication, depression is often considered to be a more "benign" condition, the treatment of which is "optional." In many cases, this decision to discontinue an antidepressant is made reflexively, without full consideration of the impact that withdrawal of treatment may have on the mother's well-being. Of course, it is important that you understand the risks of taking medication during pregnancy, but you also need to appreciate and take into consideration the risks of discontinuing treatment. Many women assume that discontinuing medication is the safest option, but this is not always the case. Research from Dr. Lee Cohen and his colleagues at the Center for Women's Mental Health indicates that about 68 percent of women who make the decision to stop antidepressant medication during pregnancy experience recurrent symptoms during pregnancy.

Given the fact that depression tends to be a recurrent illness and that pregnancy does not appear to protect a woman from depression, many women who have histories of depression and who have done well on medication may prefer to remain on their medication during pregnancy, rather than risk becoming ill. Depression hinders a woman's ability to care for herself during pregnancy, and women with severe depression are at risk for suicidal and other self-injurious behaviors. For many women, getting depressed takes such a tremendous toll that they are unwilling to accept this risk, if there is something that can be done to prevent it.

If you are taking a medication for depression or anxiety and are planning to become pregnant, you will have to decide whether or not to continue your medication during your pregnancy. This is by no means an easy decision, and there is no single correct choice. You should take the time to consider your options carefully in collaboration with your partner and your doctor. If you and your doctor feel that your risk for recurrent depression is low, you may want to try to stop the medication during your pregnancy. But even if all your medications are discontinued, close monitoring during pregnancy is essential. If you have stopped your medication, you are at risk for relapse during pregnancy, and early recognition and prompt treatment of recurrent illness may help to keep your depression from having a negative effect on you and your family.

Women who are at higher risk for developing depression during pregnancy must consider remaining on medication during pregnancy. For example, if you have had multiple episodes of depression, or if your symptoms have been particularly severe in the past, you may decide that it is safest to maintain treatment with an antidepressant throughout your pregnancy rather than risk becoming ill again. If you answer yes to any of the following questions, you may be at higher risk for illness during pregnancy, and you should discuss the possibility of continuing your medication during pregnancy with your doctor.

- Are you currently depressed?
- Have you been depressed within the past year?
- If you have ever tried to discontinue or lower the dose of your medication, did your symptoms return within a few weeks or months?
- Have you had three or more episodes of depression during your lifetime?
- Have you ever been diagnosed with bipolar disorder?
- Have you suffered from depression during a prior pregnancy?
- Have you ever had postpartum depression or postpartum psychosis?
- Have you ever required hospitalization for your depression?
- Have you ever been suicidal or made a suicide attempt?
- Have you ever had psychotic symptoms?
- Are you experiencing marital difficulties?
- Are you dealing with any other stressful life situations?

In making recommendations regarding your treatment, your doctor will take into consideration many different factors, including the severity of your symptoms in the past and your response to treatment. Your doctor should discuss with you which treatments can be used safely during pregnancy. In addition, you should have a sense of what can be done if your depression reappears or worsens during your pregnancy. Ideally, you should have this discussion with your physician *before* you are pregnant. This gives you ample time to discuss your options for treatment and, if you decide to use a medication, gives you the opportunity to choose the antidepressant that is the safest and the most effective for you.

If you had an episode of mild to moderate depression one or more years ago and have remained well without medication since that time, you most likely will decide to pursue a pregnancy without taking a medication, although your risk of depression during pregnancy is higher than that of a woman with no history of depression. But even if you are not taking a medication, psychotherapy may provide an additional layer of support and may be help-ful in reducing your levels of stress and protecting you from depression. Meeting with a mental health professional on a regular basis throughout your pregnancy may also help you to identify the symptoms of depression should they reemerge.

If you have had one to two episodes of mild to moderate depression and have been doing well on medication for the past one or more years, you may consider discontinuing your treatment during pregnancy. If you decide to stop your medication, it should be done slowly over a period of a month or so. If you are not already in therapy, you may consider meeting with a thera-pist regularly as a means of reducing your risk of recurrent depression. Should symptoms recur either during or after discontinuation, you may need to resume treatment with a medication.

If you have had three or more episodes of depression or if your depressive episodes have been very severe, your chances of having another episode of de-pression are fairly high if you discontinue your medication, even if you have been doing relatively well over the past few years. In this situation, many women make the decision to maintain their medication throughout their pregnancy. Similarly, if you have tried on one or more occasions to stop the medication and have experienced recurrent symptoms, it is likely that you will experience recurrent symptoms during pregnancy if you stop your med-ication.

If you have recently been depressed or are currently depressed, you are at higher risk for suffering from depression during pregnancy. As we discussed in chapter 6, pregnancy is not necessarily a mood-elevating experience and women who have been depressed within the past year or who are depressed at the time of conception are more likely to experience depression during pregnancy. In this situation, you should meet with a mental health profes-sional. If you are already taking medication, some changes in your regimen may help you to stabilize your condition. If you are not receiving any type of treatment, you may want to consider getting treatment *before* you conceive. Individual psychotherapy may be very helpful for relieving the symptoms of depression, but if your symptoms do not seem to improve or if you feel that your depression is worsening, you should consider taking an antidepressant medication. Ideally, you should have your symptoms well under control be-fore attempting to conceive. The longer you remain on medication and feel well, the more likely you are to *stay* well. Just how long you should wait be-fore you try to get pregnant is not entirely clear. A full course of antidepres-sant treatment is about six to twelve months, and we know that the risk of becoming ill is very high in women who discontinue treatment early. However, if you have had recurrent illness (three or more episodes of depression), you will probably be advised to maintain antidepressant treatment for a longer period of time. You may ultimately make the decision that you want to remain on your medication throughout your pregnancy.

Pregnant and Depressed: What Are Your Options?

Most women approach pregnancy with a certain degree of optimism, and we tend to view pregnancy as a time of emotional well-being. The unfortunate reality is that 10 percent to 15 percent of women suffer from depression during pregnancy, and rates of depression are even higher among women who discontinue maintenance treatment with an antidepressant prior to conception. Depression is an unexpected, often extremely unsettling experience. Women suffering depression during pregnancy may be forced to make some very difficult decisions. They are often very worried that the medication might pose a risk to their unborn child, yet they know they need treatment for their depression.

You may try psychotherapy, and this is often a good option. But what if it doesn't help? You don't necessarily have to tough it out. There are other options. Although no antidepressant has yet been approved by the Food and Drug Administration (FDA) as being safe for use during pregnancy, research accumulated over the last thirty years suggests that some medications may be used safely.

Finding the Help You Need. What often makes decisions regarding treatment so difficult to make is not being able to find accurate and up-to-date information on the treatment of depression during pregnancy. Your obstetrician may be able to provide information on the reproductive safety of various medications but may not have a good sense of your psychiatric history and may not feel comfortable prescribing psychotropic medications. Your psychiatrist can manage your illness but may not be sure whether or not certain medications are safe when used during pregnancy. To make matters worse, many women get conflicting opinions. Their psychiatrist recommends one thing; their obstetrician suggests another.

Far too often, women are not able to locate any clinician who has any expertise in this area. Over the last decade, a number of programs specializing in perinatal psychiatry have been set up throughout the United States and Canada. These provide information and counseling so that women and their doctors may make intelligent and careful decisions regarding the use of medication during pregnancy. (These resources are listed in a separate section at the end of the book.) However, if you do not have access to one of these centers, it is essential that you find a well-trained psychiatrist whom you trust and who can help you to make well-informed decisions regarding your treatment. But keep in mind that even with the best of information, the decision to take—or to avoid—medication during pregnancy is never easy.

Psychotherapy Remains One of the Safest Options

When a woman is depressed, what treatment she ultimately chooses will depend on the severity of her depression. Many women with mild to moderate depression may benefit from some type of psychotherapy and may not require medication. In the previous chapter, we discussed the various kinds of therapy that may be helpful for treating women with depression. In a recent study, Dr. Margaret Spinelli at the College of Physicians and Surgeons of Columbia University demonstrated that interpersonal psychotherapy (IPT) was not only successful in resolving the symptoms of depression during pregnancy, it seemed to protect women from postpartum depression later on. Other types of individual psychotherapy, although not specifically studied in this population, may also be effective, and psychotherapy remains an important treatment option.

The clear advantage of psychotherapy is that it does not involve the use of medication and therefore poses no risk to the unborn child. However, not all women respond fully to this treatment, and it is important to evaluate its effectiveness on an ongoing basis. If you feel that psychotherapy is not working or if you continue to experience lingering symptoms of depression, therapy alone may not be enough. In addition, if the depression is so severe that it is compromising your health or your ability to function, it is important to talk to your doctor about other treatment options, including the use of medication. Many women, especially those with more severe or recurrent illness, do best with a combination of medication *and* therapy. Whatever option you choose, it should be effective; adhering to a treatment that is ineffective means that you are losing precious time.

Understanding the Risks. When it comes to treating depression during pregnancy, the goal is to alleviate the symptoms of depression in the mother while at the same time minimizing risk to the unborn child. It is also important to remember that maintaining mood stability during the pregnancy reduces the risk of postpartum depression. We now have research to support the use of certain antidepressants during pregnancy. However, our information remains incomplete. Even with the best research, it is impossible to prove beyond doubt the safety of a given medication taken during pregnancy. It is your doctor's responsibility to provide accurate and up-to-date information on the reproductive safety of various medications so that you, working in collaboration with your doctor, may select the most appropriate treatment strategy. When medication is taken during pregnancy, there are several different types of risk we must take into consideration:

- Does the medication increase the risk of miscarriage or pregnancy loss?
- Is there any risk of organ malformation or birth defect?
- Are there any side effects or withdrawal symptoms observed in the infant after delivery?
- Does exposure to this medication *in utero* have any long-term effects on the child?

It is important for you to understand these risks. Keep in mind that this is a rapidly changing field, and new research studies come out nearly every week. It is also important to note that there are many controversies in the practice of perinatal psychiatry, and you may discover that different doctors offer very different suggestions. This chapter will help you to better understand the various treatment options. However, the information provided here is by no means a substitute for a discussion with your own doctor, and he or she should supplement the information provided in this book with the most current research in this area so that you can make well-informed decisions regarding your care.

So what is the *safest* antidepressant? To help medical professionals make decisions regarding the use of medications during pregnancy, the Food and Drug Administration (FDA), the governmental agency that oversees the safety of drugs, established a system that classifies the reproductive safety of medications using five risk categories (A, B, C, D, and X) based on data derived from human and animal studies (Appendix B). Long before a drug is released in the market, it is tested in animals to determine its safety. If it is deemed sufficiently safe, the drug is then tested in humans. Most drugs, however, are never tested in pregnant women or children, and information regarding reproductive safety is usually gathered after the medication is on the market. Some of this information comes from patients who report pregnancy outcomes directly to the manufacturer or the FDA. Sometimes the manufacturer collects this information in a more systematic fashion. Another important source of information is the research carried out by various independent investigators. While this system of classification is often considered to be the gold standard for judging a medication's safety, it is far from perfect.

Category A medications are those designated as safe for use during pregnancy. This category includes drugs such as folic acid, vitamin B_6, and thyroid hormone. While we consider many medications to be relatively safe for use during pregnancy, the FDA has not included any psychiatric medications in this safest category. Most psychotropic medications are classified as category C, agents that may carry some risk. Although this may indicate that animal studies may have suggested a problem, what it more commonly means is that there have been no well-controlled studies in humans and there is not enough information to draw definitive conclusions regarding safety. At this point, it is reassuring to note that no psychiatric medications have been listed in category X; these drugs, such as thalidomide and isotretinoin (Accutane), are *never* used during pregnancy because they are known to cause harm to the developing fetus that outweighs any benefit to the patient.

Although these guidelines have been established to provide guidance to physicians and patients seeking information on the reproductive safety of various prescription medications, this system of classification has been criticized because it is frequently ambiguous and sometimes misleading. For example, certain tricyclic antidepressants have been labeled as category D, indicating "positive evidence of risk," although the published data do not support this assertion. In fact, these drugs are frequently used during pregnancy. Furthermore, one cannot assume that all medications within a given category are equally safe. For example, both fluoxetine (Prozac) and mirtazapine (Remeron) are category C drugs; however, the use of Prozac during pregnancy has been very well studied whereas there is no data yet collected regarding the use of the newer antidepressant Remeron. Since 1997, the FDA has been working to develop a more reliable pregnancy labeling system. In the meantime, we must rely on other sources of information.

Do Antidepressants Cause Miscarriage or Pregnancy Loss?

One of the most common questions is whether antidepressants can cause miscarriages. While most reports do not indicate that antidepressants increase the risk of miscarriage, there is some controversy. A handful of studies suggests a small increase in the risk of miscarriage among women treated with serotonin reuptake inhibitor antidepressants and venlafaxine (Effexor) during the first trimester of pregnancy.

While it is important to take note of this information, there is no need for alarm. Reassuringly, the rates of miscarriage in antidepressant-exposed women are low, ranging from 10 percent to 15 percent, and within the range of what we would normally expect in women with no known drug exposure. While this small increase in risk may be attributed to exposure to an antidepressant, there are other ways to interpret the finding. One alternative explanation for the finding is that the depression itself—not the medication—may increase the risk of miscarriage. Some authors also suggest that the number of miscarriages may have been overestimated in these studies because some women may choose to report a miscarriage, when in fact they had decided to terminate their pregnancy. Is this possibly minimally higher risk of miscarriage a reason to avoid taking an antidepressant during pregnancy? For most women, it is not. And most experts in the field feel that untreated depression is more of a risk than the risk of miscarriage.

Do Antidepressants Cause Birth Defects?

Most of the research on the reproductive safety of medications has focused on the capacity of these medications to cause serious malformations in the developing child. To better understand this type of risk, it helps to know a little bit about how the fetus develops. At conception, the sperm fertilizes the egg to make a zygote. The zygote then divides over and over again until there is a rapidly dividing ball of cells. This ball of cells floats around the uterus for a couple of weeks and then implants itself into the wall of the uterus. After implantation, the placenta forms, connecting the fetus to the mother's circulatory system providing the developing fetus with nutrients. The next ten to twelve weeks are the most critical time for fetal development; during this period called *organogenesis*, all the baby's major organs will develop and, by the end of the first trimester, there is a fully formed human being. If anything disrupts this process of organogenesis, a malformation or birth defect can occur. Or if the problem is very severe, there may be a miscarriage.

Many different things can disrupt this very complicated process of development. A *teratogen* is an agent or a substance—a virus, drug, chemical, or environmental agent—that affects fetal development and causes a physical defect. Some examples of teratogens are thalidomide, which causes limb malformations, and the rubella virus, which may cause eye defects, hearing loss, and heart defects. Although these and other teratogens may increase the risk of having a birth defect, they do not necessarily cause problems in *all* cases of exposure. This is in part because a child's vulnerability to birth defects is also determined by genetic factors. And the timing of exposure is also very important. Insults that occur during the first two weeks after conception typically result in loss of the pregnancy and are unlikely to cause a birth defect, whereas events that occur later in organogenesis may result in an organ malformation or birth defect. There is a critical development period for each organ or organ system. During that time that organ or organ system may be susceptible to the effects of a teratogen. For example, the neural tube forms and transforms itself into the brain and spinal cord within the first four weeks after conception. Formation of the heart and the major blood vessels takes place from three to eight weeks after conception. Formation of the lip and palate is typically complete by week ten. If an insult occurs during any of these critical periods, a congenital malformation, or birth defect, may occur.* However, there would be no risk of malformation of a particular organ system if the exposure occurs either before or after this critical period.

In the United States the overall incidence of major congenital malformations in newborns is somewhere between 2 percent and 3 percent. In about two-thirds of birth defects, the cause is unknown. Abnormalities in a single gene or in the number of chromosomes may cause birth defects. Birth defects may also occur as a result of exposure to certain environmental factors, viral infections, chemicals, and maternal drug or alcohol abuse. Less commonly, exposure to certain prescription medications may cause fetal malformations.

Of all the antidepressants, fluoxetine (Prozac) has the most information to support its reproductive safety. The data collected from over 1,500 cases indicate that fluoxetine does not appear to increase the risk of major congenital malformations in exposed infants, as compared to nonexposed children. Given the weight of this data, fluoxetine is the antidepressant we use most commonly during pregnancy. Some women, however, do not respond to Prozac or are unable to tolerate its side effects; thus, we often must use other

---

* There is always some confusion as to when a pregnancy actually starts. Your obstetrician will start counting at the day of your LMP (the first day of your last menstrual period); however, teratologists, those who specialize in the study of fetal development and birth defects, start the clock at the time of conception, which typically occurs about two weeks *after* your LMP.

antidepressants. Information regarding the reproductive safety of other anti-depressants is more limited but has been accumulating over time and has been quite reassuring.

There have been several studies assessing the reproductive safety of the selective serotonin reuptake inhibitors (SSRIs) including sertraline (Zoloft), paroxetine (Paxil), fluvoxamine (Luvox), and citalopram (Celexa). Thus far, the largest of these studies is one including 969 infants exposed to SSRIs during the first trimester—most commonly citalopram (375 infants). This study did not demonstrate an increased risk of major malformation in children exposed to SSRIs. The remaining studies were smaller yet their findings suggest that pregnancy outcomes did not differ significantly be-tween the exposed and nonexposed groups in terms of risk for congenital malformation. While these initial reports regarding other SSRIs indicate no increase in the risk of major malformation, studies involving larger numbers of exposed children are required to establish the reproductive safety of a par-ticular medication. Experts believe that you need to examine at least 400 to 600 children exposed to a given medication to be able to detect a significant increase in risk for a particular malformation over what is observed in the general population.

Unfortunately, this area is not without its controversies. A preliminary study sponsored by GlaxoSmithKline, the manufacturer of Paxil, looked at pregnancy outcomes in more than 4,000 women who took antidepressants during pregnancy. It was observed that infants exposed to Paxil during the first trimester, as compared to infants exposed to other antidepressants, had a twofold increase in the overall frequency of birth defects and risk of heart malformations. The prevalence of birth defects among Paxil-exposed in-fants was about 4 percent, or 43.6 per 1,000 births. (Keep in mind that the rate of malformations in the general population is somewhere between 2 percent and 3 percent.) Of the heart-related defects observed, the majority were ventricular septal defects (a hole in the muscular wall that separates the right and left ventricles of the heart). This is the most common type of heart defect; most cases are mild and resolve spontaneously over time.

These reports are complemented by a recent meta-analysis conducted by researchers at the Motherisk Program in Toronto; combining the results of seven prospective studies including a total of 1,774 infants exposed to anti-depressants (mostly SSRIs) *in utero*, it appears that antidepressants do not increase the risk of major malformations over what is observed in the gen-eral population. Another recent report analyzing data from the Swedish Medical Birth Registry assessed outcomes in 4,291 infants born to mothers taking SSRIs in early pregnancy. The overall prevalence of major malformations was 2.9%, which did not differ significantly from the rate observed in unexposed infants.

This new study is somewhat difficult to interpret. At this point, we do not know if Paxil causes birth defects; however, researchers have urged caution regarding the use of Paxil during the first trimester of pregnancy until more data are collected. It is nonetheless reassuring to note that, in this study, the vast majority of babies born to women taking Paxil and other antidepressants were born healthy.

Tricyclic antidepressants, an older class of medication, are not used very commonly today; however, they may be a good option for women during pregnancy. Although early case reports suggested a possible association between first-trimester exposure to tricyclic antidepressants and limb malformation, a more recent analysis from Dr. Lori Altshuler at the UCLA Mood Disorders Research Program examined more than 400 cases of first-trimester exposure to the tricyclic antidepressants—nortriptyline (Pamelor), amitriptyline (Elavil), imipramine (Tofranil), desipramine (Norpramin), and clomipramine (Anafranil)—and found no significant association between fetal exposure to tricyclic antidepressants and risk for any major malformation. This information is made even more reassuring by the fact that tricyclic antidepressants have been in use since the 1950s and were the primary antidepressants used during pregnancy before the release of Prozac in 1987. Among this class of medications, desipramine (Norpramin) and nortriptyline (Pamelor) are preferred since they are less likely to cause side effects, such as constipation and low blood pressure. In addition to the SSRIs, the tricyclic antidepressants are frequently used during pregnancy and are effective for a wide range of symptoms, including depression, anxiety, and sleep disturbance.

Among the newer antidepressants, a recent study of 150 women exposed to venlafaxine (Effexor) during the first trimester indicated no increase in risk of major malformation as compared to nonexposed infants. Another study of 58 women exposed to trazodone (Desyrel) and 89 women exposed to nefazodone (Serzone) similarly showed no negative effects. Although these studies were relatively small, the results are encouraging. To date, the medical literature does not include data on the use of mirtazapine (Remeron) and duloxetine (Cymbalta). Similarly, there is little information available regarding the safety of monoamine oxidase inhibitors (MAOIs) during pregnancy; the MAOIs have typically been avoided due to concerns that they may have serious complications. In a preliminary report, the manufacturer of bupropion (Wellbutrin) demonstrated no increase in risk of malformations in over 1,200 women exposed to this drug during the first trimester of pregnancy; these results have not yet been published in a peer-reviewed journal.

Do Babies Exposed to Antidepressants Experience Other Problems After Delivery?

While over the last five to ten years, studies have indicated that antidepressant use during pregnancy does not appear to cause harm to the developing fetus, several more recent studies have raised concerns that infants born to women taking SSRIs while pregnant may experience some problems *after* delivery. A recent study published by Dr. Kari Laine from Turku University in Finland suggested that infants exposed to SSRIs were four times as likely to have symptoms of restlessness and jitteriness as compared to infants with no drug exposure. Other studies show similar results; the most commonly reported symptoms in the newborns exposed to SSRIs include tremors, restlessness, irritability, increased crying, poor feeding, and sleep disruption. There have also been scattered reports of babies with respiratory distress (usually rapid breathing) or neurologic symptoms (such as increased muscle tone). In 2004, these studies prompted the FDA to issue a stronger warning regarding the use of certain antidepressants during pregnancy.

These studies have created anxiety among women taking or planning to take antidepressants during pregnancy. Obviously, no woman wants to do anything that may harm her child. While these recent reports should not be ignored, it is important to keep this information in perspective. All of the studies have reported symptoms that are relatively mild. (In fact, many larger studies have demonstrated *no* serious problems in antidepressant-exposed children.) Moreover, the symptoms appear to be short-lived and resolve within a few days without any specific intervention; there appear to be no long-lasting effects. Dr. Laine and his colleagues observed no differences between the children with SSRI symptoms and those without at two weeks or at two months. Another study followed these children for eight months and also observed no differences between the two groups.

It is not entirely clear what causes these transient symptoms of distress in the newborn. Several researchers have urged caution regarding the interpretation of these results and have questioned whether these neonatal symptoms may be attributed to other factors. There have been several reports suggesting that the children born to depressed, *unmedicated* mothers tend to be more jittery and irritable. In fact, a recent study from Dr. Shaila Misri and her colleagues at the University of British Columbia demonstrated that higher levels of depression and anxiety were reported among the mothers of children who experienced neonatal distress than in the mothers of children who did not have these symptoms after birth. Like their depressed mothers, the infants are exposed to higher levels of stress hormones, including cortisol, and this may affect their behavior. Thus, it may be the underlying depression—not the medication—that affects the infant's well-being after delivery. If this is the case, withholding medication may actually increase the risk of problems in the newborn.

Other researchers have hypothesized that these symptoms—jitteriness, sleep disruption, and appetite changes—are a sign of toxicity, a signal that there is too much serotonin. Adults taking SSRI antidepressants experience similar symptoms, so it is not surprising that infants exposed to these agents may also have side effects. There has also been speculation that these symptoms may constitute some sort of antidepressant withdrawal syndrome. Adults who abruptly stop antidepressants may experience some withdrawal symptoms, the most common of which are fatigue, dizziness, nausea, headache, tremor, irritability, insomnia, and loss of appetite. It is possible that after delivery infants may experience an abrupt decrease in the amount of antidepressant and thus may be at risk for withdrawal symptoms. Several reports suggest that infants exposed to tricyclic antidepressants *in utero* have characteristic withdrawal symptoms of jitteriness and irritability. Withdrawal symptoms (irritability, excessive crying, feeding problems, sleep disruption and, less commonly, respiratory distress) have also been reported in infants exposed to paroxetine (Paxil) *in utero*, although several studies of Paxil-exposed children did not report any concerning symptoms after delivery. In all reported cases of adverse events, these symptoms resolved completely within hours or a few days without any specific intervention.

Because of these reports of problems in infants born to mothers treated with antidepressants, some physicians have recommended lowering the dose or discontinuing antidepressant medication several days or weeks prior to delivery in order to minimize risk to the infant. It is not yet clear if this type of intervention eliminates the risk of problems in the infant. What is clear, however, is that withdrawing treatment shortly before a woman is about to enter into the postpartum period—a time when she is at very high risk for depression—places the mother at significant risk for recurrent illness. The women who make the decision to take antidepressants during pregnancy are usually those with the most severe illness, and they are extremely vulnerable to depression during the postpartum period. Withdrawing treatment before delivery just doesn't make sense given that postpartum depression may have such a profound impact on the child's well-being. Although the recent data suggests that some infants may experience symptoms related to antidepressant exposure, it is important to recognize that the overall incidence of serious problems is very low and that an infant's ability to adjust to life outside of the womb is also dependent upon the mother's emotional well-being. If a mother is not doing well because she is depressed, her child may suffer.

What Are the Long-Term Risks?

Most of the studies looking at the reproductive safety of medications have focused on the short-term risks. We know much less about whether or not exposure to these medications *in utero* has any long-term effects on the child's health and well-being. In particular, many women wonder if these antidepressants may affect the developing brain and if they may alter or interrupt their child's cognitive or emotional development. Unfortunately, our understanding of the long-term consequences of exposure to psychotropic medications remains incomplete.

The structures of the brain form during the first few weeks of the first trimester, but the brain continues to grow in size and complexity throughout pregnancy and the early years of a child's life. The question is whether or not these psychotropic medications, which interact with structures within the brain, affect this complicated process of development. To date, we have limited information regarding the impact of antidepressants taken by the mother on the developing fetal brain. While it may be relatively easy to detect a birth defect, more subtle developmental problems that may arise as a result of exposure to a particular medication are much harder to detect. There are many questions. For example, are children exposed to antidepressants *in utero* at risk for developmental delays or similar problems? Are they more likely to have behavioral problems later? Are they at higher—or lower—risk for depression as a result of this early exposure to antidepressants?

This is clearly a very important area of research yet very difficult to pursue, given the multiple and often uncontrollable variables that may affect a child's development. However, several studies suggest that antidepressants taken during pregnancy do *not* have a negative effect on a child's subsequent development. In a landmark study published in 1997, Dr. Irena Nulman and her colleagues at the Motherisk Program in Toronto followed a group of children exposed to either tricyclic antidepressants or fluoxetine (Prozac) during pregnancy. A total of 135 exposed children and 84 children with no exposure to these drugs were followed up to seven years of age. The two groups of children did not differ in terms of IQ or cognitive development. Nor were any other differences observed between the two groups across a number of different domains, including temperament, behavior, emotional reactivity, mood, distractibility, and activity level. A more recent report from the same research group followed another group of 87 children exposed to fluoxetine (Prozac) or tricyclic antidepressants for the *entire duration of the pregnancy.* (The previous study included some children who were exposed for briefer periods of time during pregnancy, including children who were exposed only during the first trimester of pregnancy.) Again they found no differences between the exposed and nonexposed children. These findings are very reassuring and suggest that fluoxetine and the tricyclic antidepressants do not have a negative effect on brain development. However, these studies were relatively small, and we still need more research in order to better assess the long-term effects of prenatal exposure to antidepressants and other psychotropic medications.

How to Make the Best Decisions Regarding Your Treatment

Each woman is unique and will base her choices on her history and her personal preferences. In making the decision to use medication during pregnancy, many women want to be assured there is absolutely no risk associated with a particular medication. Unfortunately, there are no guarantees, and there may be risks that we do not yet know about. We do know, however, that even in its milder forms, depression can have a negative effect on a mother's well-being and may put the pregnancy at risk. Depression during pregnancy is also a potent risk factor for postpartum depression. In order to make well-informed decisions, you need the best and most current information on hand. This book can serve as a foundation. The reference section lists many medically oriented articles on the use of medication during pregnancy. However, this is a rapidly changing field, and you and your doctor should consult other sources of information, too. Your doctor will have access to the most current medical literature. You may also access this literature using PubMed, an Internet-based service of the National Library of Medicine that indexes biomedical articles dating back to the 1950s. In addition, the Web site of the Center of Women's Health at womensmental health.org includes the most current information on the use of medication during pregnancy.

Consider nonpharmacologic options first. Although much of this chapter focuses on the use of medication, this does not imply that medication is always the best option. Psychotherapy may help to relieve the symptoms of depression and anxiety and may also protect you from depression by giving you skills that help you to better manage stressful life situations. Women with panic disorder, obsessive-compulsive disorder, or other types of anxiety disorder may benefit from cognitive-behavioral therapy. Women with chronic sleep problems may find relief using certain relaxation strategies and other behavioral interventions. If these strategies are effective for you, you may be able to avoid taking medications during pregnancy.

Try to select a medication with the best reproductive safety profile. There is a great deal of data regarding reproductive safety for some antidepressants; other medications, especially some of the newer agents, have not been well studied. Generally, we like to use the antidepressants that have been studied the most extensively. Fluoxetine (Prozac), with the most extensive literature supporting its use during pregnancy, is a first-line choice. There is also a growing literature to suggest the reproductive safety of the newer SSRIs; of these, citalopram (Celexa) is an attractive alternative. The tricyclic antidepressants should also be considered as first-line agents.

At this point, there is more limited information regarding the use of the other antidepressants during pregnancy, including sertraline (Zoloft), paroxetine (Paxil), fluvoxamine (Luvox), venlafaxine (Effexor), duloxetine (Cymbalta), bupropion (Wellbutrin), nefazodone (Serzone), trazodone (Desyrel) and mirtazapine (Remeron). If you are pregnant or planning to conceive and you are already taking one of these antidepressants, you will have to decide whether you should continue with this medication or switch to another agent which is better characterized. For example, if you are taking Remeron, you may decide to switch to an agent such as fluoxetine (Prozac) or a tricyclic antidepressant. On the other hand, you and your doctor may decide that switching is *not* a good option, if, for example, you do not respond to Prozac or the tricyclic antidepressants or cannot tolerate their side effects. If you have very severe or difficult-to-treat depression, changing your medication may put you at risk for recurrent illness and you may be unwilling to take this sort of risk. In these situations, we are often forced to use medications for which the information on reproductive safety is limited.

Use a medication that is effective. If you have made the decision to take a medication during pregnancy, it is important that you use one that is effective for you. Some women, in an effort to choose the "safest" option, end up taking a medication that is not particularly effective for them. It makes no sense to take a medication during pregnancy if it is not working for you.

Use an adequate dosage. If you are taking a medication, you should take a dosage that is high enough to achieve the desired effect. Frequently, the dosage of an antidepressant is reduced during pregnancy in an attempt to limit risk to the child; however, this may place the woman at greater risk for recurrent illness. You should also be aware that, as the pregnancy progresses, your fluid volume increases, as does your ability to metabolize and clear medications from your system. This means that drug levels tend to decline gradually as a pregnancy proceeds. Toward the middle or end of the second trimester, women often experience a more significant drop in their drug levels. When this happens, the concentration of drug in the blood may decline to a level that is no longer effective for treating your symptoms. If you find yourself experiencing recurrent symptoms of depression, you should talk to your doctor about increasing the dosage of your medication.

Try to simplify your treatment regimen. As discussed in chapter 12, polypharmacy, the use of multiple medications, is a relatively common practice. This is a reasonable approach for a woman who is not pregnant, but during pregnancy you want to make sure that you are taking as few medications as possible. For example, if you have anxiety symptoms and are taking an antidepressant *and* an antianxiety medication like lorazepam (Ativan) or clonazepam (Klonopin), it may be possible to gradually taper the antianxiety medication and use an SSRI or a tricyclic antidepressant to treat both depression and your anxiety. Or if your depression comes with severe insomnia, rather than taking an antidepressant plus a sleep medication, you may benefit from treatment with a more sedating antidepressant, like a tricyclic antidepressant.

What About Other Medications?

Many women who suffer from depression are treated with other types of medications in addition to antidepressants. Anxiety is a common complication of depression, and many women take antianxiety medications; other medications may be used to treat sleep problems. Women with bipolar disorder often receive a complicated mixture of medications, including mood stabilizers, antidepressants, and antianxiety medications. Although this chapter has focused mainly on the antidepressants, the safety of these other medications must also be considered.

Antianxiety Medications

Although certain antidepressants, including the SSRIs and the tricyclic antidepressants, may help to relieve anxiety, many women treat their anxiety symptoms with benzodiazepines, including diazepam (Valium), clonazepam (Klonopin), lorazepam (Ativan), and alprazolam (Xanax). The information on the reproductive safety of these medications has been somewhat controversial. Although initial reports suggested that there may be an increased risk of cleft lip and cleft palate associated with first-trimester use of these drugs, more recent reports have found no association between exposure to benzodiazepines and risk for cleft lip or cleft palate. Experts now believe that, if there is any risk, it is very small and is estimated to be less than 0.6 percent. Given this controversy, some women are uncomfortable taking benzodiazepines during the first trimester. For women with milder anxiety symptoms, it may be possible to avoid using the benzodiazepines during the first trimester. If an antianxiety agent is required, it may also be possible to switch to an SSRI or a tricyclic antidepressant. Many women with more severe anxiety symptoms, especially those with panic disorder, must use benzodiazepines during their pregnancy in order to control their symptoms.

Infants exposed to these drugs *in utero*, especially when used at higher doses, may experience some side effects after delivery, including drowsiness and respiratory depression, although serious events appear to occur infrequently. In addition, there have been reports of benzodiazepine withdrawal symptoms in children exposed to these drugs *in utero*. Signs of withdrawal include jitteriness, tremulousness, respiratory distress, poor temperature regulation, and, less commonly, seizure. Exactly how often these symptoms occur is unclear, but they appear to be relatively uncommon and are probably more likely to occur in those women treated with shorter-acting agents like alprazolam (Xanax). Agents with longer half-lives, like clonazepam (Klonopin) and diazepam (Valium), seem to carry less of a risk. In a recent study from the Center of Women's Mental Health, Dr. Lisa Weinstock followed 38 pregnant women treated with 0.5 to 3.5 mg of clonazepam (Klonopin) during pregnancy and found no evidence of neonatal toxicity or withdrawal syndromes in the newborns.

Although there have been some concerns about the use of benzodiazepines, these drugs are used commonly during pregnancy. In many cases, the risks of untreated illness in the mother outweigh the risks associated with medication exposure. Untreated anxiety during pregnancy may place the pregnancy at risk, and several studies indicate that anxiety in the mother can increase the likelihood of preterm labor and other complications, including preeclampsia, at the time of delivery. Infants born to mothers with higher levels of stress and anxiety may also have lower Apgar Scores and signs of neonatal distress.

Mood Stabilizers

Women with bipolar disorder face a significant dilemma when considering treatment during pregnancy. Dr. Adele Viguera from the Center for Women's Mental Health recently reported that about 75 percent of women with bipolar disorder experience recurrent illness during pregnancy if they discontinue their treatment. However, the mood stabilizers most commonly used to treat bipolar disorder, including lithium and valproate (Depakote or Depakene), may cause congenital malformations when used during pregnancy. For women who need a mood stabilizer during pregnancy, lithium is one of the safest options, though when used during the first trimester, it carries a 0.05 percent to 0.1 percent risk of a serious cardiac malformation called Ebstein's anomaly. Although lithium may cause heart defects, we often prescribe lithium during pregnancy to women suffering from bipolar disorder. The risk of Ebstein's anomaly is relatively small—it occurs in fewer than 1 in 1,000 children exposed to lithium. One way of eliminating this risk may be to briefly discontinue the lithium during the first trimester, when formation of the heart takes place. This may not, however, be the best option for a woman with more severe bipolar illness; even a brief disruption of treatment may put her at risk for recurrent illness. Women who take lithium during the first trimester should have a high-resolution ultrasound and fetal echocardiogram at sixteen to eighteen weeks to detect any cardiovascular defects.

There have been several reports of hypothyroidism in infants exposed to lithium; however, this appears to be relatively rare. There have also been several reports of polyhydramnios (excessive amniotic fluid); if this complication occurs, lithium levels should be lowered to decrease the risk of preterm labor. Other complications have also been observed, including lower Apgar Scores, poor muscle tone, lethargy, and respiratory distress; these complications are more common in infants with high levels of lithium. To reduce the risk of complications, lithium treatment may be suspended 24 hours before a scheduled caesarean section or induction or at the onset of labor in the event of spontaneous delivery. Lithium treatment should be reinitiated after delivery.

Antiseizure medications or anticonvulsants are also used to treat bipolar disorder. Unfortunately, some of the anticonvulsants commonly used pose a much greater risk to the developing fetus than lithium. Carbamazepine (Tegretol) carries a 1 percent risk of neural tube defect, a malformation of the structures of the brain and spinal cord. Valproate (Depakote or Depakene) is associated with a 3 percent to 6 percent risk of neural tube defect, as well as an increased risk of other malformations affecting the heart, limbs, and genitals. There is also evidence that exposure to valproate *in utero* may result in developmental delays or other neurobehavioral problems. Folic acid supplements given during pregnancy decrease the risk of neural tube defects in the general population. While it is not clear if folic acid reduces the risk of neural tube defects in women taking anticonvulsants, it is recommended that all women of child-bearing age who are prescribed anticonvulsants take 4 mg of folic acid per day. Women taking these anticonvulsants often switch to lithium or to a safer anticonvulsant, such as lamotrigine (Lamictal).

There is less information on the reproductive safety of the newer anticonvulsants used to treat bipolar disorder, specifically gabapentin (Neurontin), oxcarbazepine (Trileptal), topiramate (Topamax), tiagabine (Gabitril), levetiracetam (Keppra), and zonisamide (Zonegran). However, there is a growing body of information on the reproductive safety of lamotrigine (Lamictal), and the preliminary data suggest that lamotrigine may be a useful alternative for some women with bipolar disorder. The manufacturer of Lamictal maintains a pregnancy registry for lamotrigine and has presented data regarding the outcomes of children exposed to lamotrigine *in utero*. (A copy of this report may be obtained from GlaxoSmithKline at 800-336-2176.) The registry identified 1,082 pregnant women taking lamotrigine during pregnancy. Of the 707 children exposed to lamotrigine alone, 2.8 percent had a major malformation, which is within the range of 2 percent to 3 percent observed in women with no known exposure to a teratogen. However, when lamotrigine was used in combination with another anticonvulsant, particularly valproic acid, the risk of malformation was higher than expected. This preliminary data is very encouraging regarding the safety of lamotrigine, and many women taking mood stabilizers that pose a significant risk to the fetus, or that lack data regarding their reproductive safety, may consider switching to lamotrigine.

Antipsychotic Medications

Although this class of medications is used primarily for patients with psychotic disorders like schizophrenia, the antipsychotic agents, particularly the newer drugs, are used to treat a wide spectrum of illnesses, including bipolar disorder, obsessive-compulsive disorder, posttraumatic stress disorder, and depression. Most of our data comes from several large studies in which certain antipsychotic medications were used to control nausea and vomiting during pregnancy; these studies indicate no increased risk of malformation among children exposed to these agents. A study pooling the data from multiple sources has suggested that while there appears to be no increased risk of congenital malformation associated with exposure to the higher-potency drugs, including perphenazine (Trilafon) and trifluoperazine (Stelazine), lower-potency agents, including chlorpromazine (Thorazine) may increase the risk of malformation. One very small study assessed the use of haloperidol (Haldol) and demonstrated no increase in risk of malformation.

These data support the use of some of the older, or "typical," antipsychotic agents during pregnancy. At this point, however, it is the newer or "atypical" antipsychotic agents that are used more commonly. In one preliminary report of 34 infants exposed to olanzapine (Zyprexa), there appeared to be no increase in the risk of malformation; however, studies including larger numbers of women are needed to establish reproductive safety. Even more limited is the information regarding the reproductive safety of other atypical agents: clozapine (Clozaril), risperidone (Risperdal), quetiapine (Seroquel), ziprasidone (Geodon), and aripiprazole (Abilify). Given the lack of adequate information, women treated with these newer antipsychotic agents are typically advised to discontinue the medication or to switch to one of the older antipsychotic medications during pregnancy, like perphanazine (Trilafon) or trifluoperazine (Stelazine). Many women, however, do not respond as well to these agents or may develop intolerable side effects. Under these circumstances, a woman may elect to continue treatment with an atypical agent, even though it has not been as well studied as the older drugs.

Stimulants

Stimulants are typically taken by patients with attention deficit disorder but may be also used to treat a variety of other symptoms including fatigue, cognitive problems, and antidepressant-induced sexual dysfunction. Stimulants may also be used to enhance the action of an antidepressant. There are many different preparations on the market; the most commonly used agent is methylphenidate, the key ingredient of Ritalin and Concerta. To date, the information regarding the use of stimulants during pregnancy is very limited. There are no data to suggest that the stimulants cause any type of major malformation. However, the stimulants, particularly when used at higher doses, may cause other problems, including intrauterine growth retardation, low birth weight, and preterm labor and delivery.

Because the stimulants are generally used to treat relatively benign symptoms, such as fatigue or attentional problems, it is generally recommended that they be discontinued during pregnancy. Especially when there is so little known about these medications, it seems difficult to justify the use of the medications during pregnancy. There may be some other alternatives. For example, a woman with attention deficit disorder may be able to switch over to a tricyclic antidepressant, such as desipramine. The reproductive safety of atomoxetine (Strattera)—another drug used to treat ADHD—has not been studied and this drug is generally not used during pregnancy. However, there may be some women who are unable to function without a stimulant. They have severe attention problems or the stimulant is being used in conjunction with an antidepressant to improve its effectiveness. If there are no other options, a woman may elect to continue treatment with a stimulant with careful monitoring.

Sleep Medications

Although many different psychotropic medications may be used to improve sleep, there are currently only three drugs on the market specifically designed for promoting sleep: zolpidem (Ambien), zaleplon (Sonata), and eszopiclone (Lunesta). Unfortunately, there are no data regarding the reproductive safety of these agents, so they are typically not used during pregnancy, especially during the first trimester. If you do need a sleep medication, other options include using a sedating tricyclic antidepressant like amitriptyline or a benzodiazepine such as lorazepam (Ativan) or clonazepam (Klonopin).

Electroconvulsive Therapy

As discussed more fully in chapter 12, electroconvulsive therapy remains one of the most effective treatments for depression. Several recent studies have demonstrated that ECT is safe for use during pregnancy and does not pose a significant risk to the fetus, although ECT may be avoided in the later stages of pregnancy, as it may increase the risk of premature labor. ECT has several advantages over conventional pharmacologic treatment. With ECT, the fetus is exposed to fewer drugs. And a positive response to ECT can occur very quickly, with some women showing improvement one to two weeks after initiating treatment. Furthermore, in cases of severe depression that has responded poorly to treatment with conventional antidepressants, ECT is more likely to be effective than medication.

Bright Light Therapy for Depression During Pregnancy

Several preliminary studies have suggested that bright light therapy may be useful for the treatment of depression during pregnancy. In a recent pilot study from Dr. Neill Epperson and her colleagues at the Yale School of Medicine, 10 women who developed depression during pregnancy were treated with light therapy. After ten weeks of treatment, bright light therapy demonstrated a beneficial effect. Although none of the women had SAD, many of the women in this study had seasonal worsening of their depression and received treatment during the winter months. These results are encouraging, but it is not yet clear if bright light therapy would work for all women who experience depression during pregnancy. If your depressions occur in the winter months or if you have had success with bright light therapy in the past, you may want to discuss this option with your doctor. For more information, see chapter 12.

What About Alternative or Complementary Treatments?

Taking a conventional medication during pregnancy understandably raises concerns, and for some women, alternative therapies may feel safer or more "natural." While an herbal medicine or dietary supplement may be considered a "natural" remedy, it would be a mistake to assume that it is safe for use during pregnancy. In most cases, these are compounds not normally found in one's diet, and their effects on the developing fetus have not been studied. Unfortunately, the manufacturers of herbal remedies and dietary supplements are not required to collect information on the safety of these compounds during pregnancy.

Depression is a serious illness, and it is essential that you select a treatment that is both safe and effective. One of the major disadvantages to using these alternative treatments is that many of them have not been systematically studied and may not be as effective as conventional therapies. Although some interventions—for example, exercise, dietary modification, acupuncture, and yoga—may have a positive benefit on mood and are likely to pose little threat to the pregnancy, there is little evidence to support the effectiveness of these alternative strategies in women suffering from moderate to severe depression. Although alternative and complementary treatments may seem more attractive to some, it is important to stick with what is proven to be effective. While certain alternative or complementary therapies may not pose a direct threat to the pregnancy, using a treatment that is ineffective *is* harmful in that it stands in the way of your getting effective treatment for your illness.

How Is Postpartum Depression Treated?

Making the Decision to Get Professional Help. Women with postpartum depression often avoid treatment because they are breast-feeding and are worried about the effects medication may have on their baby. This is an understandable concern; however, there are many different types of treatment available for women who suffer from postpartum depression. Psychotherapy can be a highly effective intervention and poses no risk whatsoever to the baby. But even if you are breast-feeding, you may consider taking an antidepressant medication. While there has been a tendency to avoid using medications in nursing women, recent research supports the safety of several different antidepressants in breast-feeding women.

What postpartum depression looks like varies widely, with some women having relatively mild symptoms while others experience a more disabling form of this illness. What type of treatment you receive will depend on the severity and type of symptoms you experience. However, before initiating any type of psychiatric treatment, you should have a thorough medical evaluation to make sure there is not a medical cause for your mood disturbance, such as hypothyroidism or anemia. This initial evaluation can be performed by your primary care provider or your obstetrician and should include a thorough history, physical examination, and routine laboratory tests.

Whether your depression is mild or severe, the first thing you must do is come to the realization that postpartum depression is a "real" illness. It does not indicate that you are incompetent or unprepared to be a mother. It is not a symptom of sleep deprivation. It is a biologically driven illness that represents a crisis for you and your family. Under no circumstances should it be ignored. And to recover from depression, you will need extra help. This support may come in many different shapes and forms—from your partner, family, friends, or trained professionals. Having this additional support may help to alleviate the symptoms of depression; however, if you continue to struggle, it is important to seek the help of a professional. Not only is this important for your emotional well-being, you are doing something that benefits your entire family.

Psychotherapy Is Effective for Postpartum Depression

For women with mild to moderate depression, individual psychotherapy or counseling can be very helpful. Psychotherapy may also be helpful for women with more severe forms of depression; however, in this situation, psychotherapy is often combined with a medication. In chapter 12, we discussed the various types of psychotherapy and how they work. While there are many different types of psychotherapy available, only a handful of studies have explored the effectiveness of these treatments in women suffering from postpartum depression.

In one small study, Dr. Louis Appleby and his colleagues at the University of Manchester treated women with postpartum depression using either fluoxetine (Prozac) or short-term cognitive behavioral therapy (CBT), a type of therapy that focuses on the negative patterns of thinking that often accompany depression. These women started to show improvement after one session of counseling, and it was demonstrated that six sessions of counseling were as effective in decreasing depressive symptoms as treatment with Prozac. It should be noted, however, that most of the women participating in this study suffered from mild to moderate depression.

Several studies from Drs. Michael O'Hara and Scott Stuart at the University of Iowa have explored the use of interpersonal therapy (IPT) in women with mild to moderate postpartum depression. IPT primarily focuses on how problems within close relationships in your life may contribute to your depression and, in turn, how depression may affect these important social connections. IPT may be particularly useful for treating postpartum depression as it focuses on many of the issues that are important to new mothers, including managing the stress associated with taking on a new role, maintaining healthy and satisfying relationships, and coping with social isolation. Not only is IPT effective for treating the symptoms of depression, women who receive IPT also experience significant improvements in the quality of their interpersonal relationships.

Although there are many different types of therapy, most therapists use a combination of techniques. Whatever type of therapy you choose, women with postpartum depression may find it helpful to address the following issues in therapy:

Role Transition	What are your feelings regarding your new role as a mother? What about other roles you play both in and outside of the home? How have they been affected by having a child? How has your image of yourself changed?
Feelings of Loss	Are there activities that you are no longer able to pursue? Has having a baby had a negative effect on your

	relationships with your friends or family? Your partner? Your career?
Feelings of Inadequacy or Incompetence	Do you feel satisfied with your ability to care for your child? Do you find yourself comparing yourself to others? Are your expectations of yourself realistic? Do you feel pressure from other people to behave in a certain way?
Support	Do you feel that you have enough support? Do others understand what you are experiencing? Do they know how they can be helpful to you?
Conflict with Your Partner	Do you have disagreements with your partner regarding how your child should be cared for? Is your partner supportive and appreciative of you? How has your relationship changed after having a child? Is there anything you miss?
Social Isolation	Are you spending enough time with others? With your partner? If you are feeling lonely or isolated, what can you do to solve the problem?
Disappointment	Is being a mother what you expected? Did childbirth go as you had planned? Is your baby what you had hoped for?

Therapy can give you a place to talk about issues that are uncomfortable to bring up with friends or family members. Having an impartial observer may also help you to better understand your problems and to look at them from a different vantage point. Therapy can also give you new strategies for dealing with difficult situations. However, the most important thing is that the therapy is effective for treating your depression. Although therapy may have many positive effects, it is not always effective for eliminating the symptoms of depression. If you feel that your depression is not getting any better—or if it is getting worse—then you should discuss this with your therapist and you may need to consider other types of treatment.

Medications Are Highly Effective

If your symptoms do not seem to get better with therapy or if you have very severe symptoms, you may consider treatment with an antidepressant medication. There are many different antidepressants on the market, all of which are highly effective for the treatment of women with depression. (More specific information about these drugs can be found in chapter 12.) One of the advantages of antidepressants is that they can bring about improvement relatively quickly, usually within two to four weeks. Although they can have side effects, antidepressants are generally very well-tolerated. For many women with postpartum depression, antidepressants may be required to fully treat the depression; however, antidepressants are most effective when they are combined with therapy.

To date, only a few small studies have systematically tested the effectiveness of conventional antidepressants in the treatment of postpartum depression. The antidepressants thus far studied include fluoxetine (Prozac), sertraline (Zoloft), fluvoxamine (Luvox), paroxetine (Paxil), venlafaxine (Effexor), and bupropion (Wellbutrin). Although the information is somewhat limited, it seems that postpartum depression responds well to antidepressants and is no more difficult to treat than other type of depression. Whether the depression is mild or more severe, the symptoms improve relatively quickly using standard dosages of the conventional antidepressants. These studies indicate that, when treated with these antidepressants, about 80 percent of the women with postpartum depression experience a significant reduction in their symptoms.

What antidepressant you and your doctor ultimately choose will be influenced by several factors and you should not feel that you are restricted to using only the medications listed above. If you have had a good response to a particular antidepressant in the past, it makes sense to use that medication again if you have postpartum depression. The choice of an antidepressant will also be guided by a given medication's side effect profile. Specific serotonin reuptake inhibitors (SSRIs) and serotonin-norepinephrine reuptake inhibitors (SNRIs) are ideal first-line agents. They are nonsedating, have few side effects, and are helpful for treating the anxiety symptoms that often mingle with postpartum depression. These drugs also have anti-obsessional activity and are effective for women who suffer from obsessive thoughts or full-blown obsessive-compulsive disorder. The tricyclic antidepressants (TCAs) are frequently used and, because they tend to be more sedating, the TCAs may be a good choice for women who present with prominent sleep disturbance. However, there is some suggestion that the tricyclic antidepressants and bupropion (Wellbutrin) may be slightly less effective for treating postpartum depression and anxiety than the SSRIs or SNRIs.

Given the prevalence of anxiety symptoms among women with postpartum depression, using a medication specifically for the treatment of anxiety may be helpful. The SSRIs, SNRIs, tricyclic antidepressants, and some other antidepressants (including nefazodone and mirtazapine) are effective for relieving anxiety, but it may take several weeks for the effects of these medications to kick in. Women who are having severe anxiety, panic attacks, or significant sleep disturbance may benefit from the addition of an antianxiety medication. In this situation, benzodiazepines (members of the Valium family) are commonly used. The shorter-acting agents, such as lorazepam (Ativan), may be helpful both for initiating sleep and for the rapid treatment of anxiety symptoms. Clonazepam (Klonopin) is a potent, longer-acting agent useful for the treatment of panic attacks and generalized anxiety.

Bipolar Disorder and Postpartum Depression

Although most women with postpartum depression suffer from the most common sort of depression, unipolar depression, some women may have bipolar disorder (also known as manic depression). Women with bipolar disorder are very vulnerable to depression after the birth of a child, and, as we discussed in chapter 9, these woman are also at risk for postpartum psychosis. If you have a history of bipolar disorder and become depressed after pregnancy, antidepressants are generally not the first choice for treatment and may actually make your symptoms worse. If you are taking an antidepressant and you feel that it is making you feel more anxious, agitated, irritable, or if you feel energized and euphoric, you should discuss this with your doctor; these may be symptoms of bipolar disorder. The treatment for bipolar disorder is much more complicated than for unipolar depression. If bipolar disorder is suspected, a mood stabilizer is indicated. This is a medication that treats the depression while protecting you from having hypomanic or manic episodes. The mood stabilizers most commonly used to treat depression in this setting are lithium and lamotrigine (Lamictal); other mood stabilizers, like valproate (Depakote or Depakene), may work for controlling manic symptoms but may be less effective for depression.

Are Hormonal Treatments Effective?

While individual psychotherapy and antidepressants remain the most commonly prescribed treatments for postpartum depression, many experts have questioned the use of hormonal therapies for women with this disorder. Progesterone was once a very popular treatment for postpartum depression and continues to be used outside of the United States. However, there is evidence to suggest that synthetic progesterone compounds do not help to alleviate the symptoms of postpartum depression. In fact, these progesterone-like drugs may actually make depression worse. More recently, a natural form of progesterone has been developed and marketed. In the body, natural progesterone is metabolized into allopregnanolone, a steroid that enhances the activity of specific neurotransmitter systems in the brain and may thus reduce anxiety. Natural progesterone has not yet been evaluated for the treatment of postpartum depression.

Several studies suggest that estrogen may be helpful for the treatment of postpartum depression. In one study from Dr. Alain Gregoire, women receiving treatment with an estrogen patch showed improvement within four weeks. What makes this study somewhat difficult to interpret is that about half of the women were also taking an antidepressant, so it is not clear if the estrogen acted on its own or if it merely enhanced the activity of the antidepressant. In another study, Dr. Antti Ahokas from the University of Helsinki in Finland treated a group of women with postpartum depression with sublingual estrogen. Within two weeks 19 of the 23 women experienced a complete remission of their symptoms.

Although estrogen may be an intriguing alternative, its use for this purpose is still under investigation. Estrogen is associated with several risks, including endometrial overgrowth (hyperplasia) and blood clots (thromboembolism). Especially during the postpartum period, estrogen may increase the risk of blood clots and may put women at increased risk for complications, including deep vein thrombosis and stroke. It may also diminish the production of breast milk in nursing mothers. Given these concerns, antidepressants remain at this time the safest and the most effective treatment for women with postpartum depression.

Antidepressants and Breast-feeding

If your doctor suggests that you take an antidepressant medication and you are breast-feeding, you will be forced to make a very difficult decision. You may not feel comfortable breast-feeding while taking a medication and exposing your child to medication in your milk. However, you may feel that breast-feeding is too important to give up and you may opt to postpone treatment. On the other hand, your symptoms may not allow you to defer treatment and you may be encouraged (or feel obliged) to discontinue breast-feeding before starting a medication. Having to give up breast-feeding may give rise to feelings of sadness and loss; for many women, breast-feeding is an essential and deeply gratifying aspect of being a mother.

Having to wean before you are ready may leave you with the sense that you have somehow failed as a mother.

But taking medication does not necessarily mean that you have to stop nursing. Although there has been a tendency to avoid using medication in breast-feeding women, information collected over the last decade suggests that certain antidepressants may be safe in this setting. It is true that all medications taken by the mother, including antidepressants, are secreted into the breast milk and thus may be transferred to the nursing infant; however, it is reassuring to note that the current research suggests that, under most circumstances, the nursing infant is exposed only to very small doses of medication. Furthermore, the risk of problems in the nursing infant appears to be relatively low.

What remains unanswered at this point is the question of whether exposure to trace amounts of antidepressant in the breast milk poses any long-term neurodevelopmental risks. A child's brain continues to develop during the first two decades of his life, and we do not yet know how the small amounts of antidepressant passed into the breast milk might affect development. Several small studies have looked at the cognitive development of children exposed to antidepressants while nursing; the exposed children (some of them followed up to five years of age) did not demonstrate any differences in cognitive abilities as compared to unexposed children. However, it should be noted that these few studies, while reassuring, are very preliminary, and more extensive study is clearly needed to better understand the long-term effects of this exposure.

So far, we have the most breast-feeding data for the tricyclic antidepressants, fluoxetine (Prozac), sertraline (Zoloft), and paroxetine (Paxil). Our information regarding the use of these newer medications is accumulating, and there are reports on smaller numbers of women breast-feeding on some of the newer antidepressants, including fluvoxamine (Luvox), citalopram (Celexa), venlafaxine (Effexor), and bupropion (Wellbutrin). The studies thus far have been encouraging. Although medication can be detected in the breast milk, the studies that have measured the levels of these medications in the infants' blood demonstrate that the levels of drug are either very low or undetectable. This means two things. First, it means that the amount of drug that the baby absorbs from the breast milk is very small. It also means that the drug does not accumulate in the baby; full-term babies are able to metabolize and get rid of these drugs so the drug levels do not reach toxic levels.

If you look at the data as a whole, it looks as if breast-feeding while taking most antidepressants does not pose a significant risk to the child. Nonetheless, one cannot ignore the handful of reports in the literature that suggest the occurrence of side effects in a very small number of nursing infants exposed to antidepressants in breast milk. There have been rare reports of a variety of symptoms in these infants, including jitteriness, irritability, sleepiness, feeding difficulties, and sleep disruption. For the most part, no serious or life-threatening problems have been reported, although there was one report of a seizure that may have been related to exposure to bupropion (Wellbutrin). (In this report, it could not be demonstrated that the bupropion actually *caused* the seizure. Neonatal seizures are relatively common, and children are more vulnerable to seizures during the first ten days of life than at any other time.) While raising some concerns, these reports are somewhat difficult to interpret, since it's impossible to determine if a particular adverse event is the direct result of antidepressant exposure or an unrelated problem that occurred simultaneously. Many of the reported side effects are rather nonspecific (e.g., sleep disruption, feeding problems) and frequently occur in healthy infants who are not exposed to any type of medication. On the other hand, it makes sense that infants exposed to these medications, like adults, may experience certain side effects. The important thing to remember is that the symptoms reported are, in general, relatively benign, short-lived, and do not pose any significant threat to the baby.

When selecting a medication for a breast-feeding woman, we try to choose those medications that have been the best studied. At this point, the preferred medications are nortriptyline, sertraline, and paroxetine (Paxil); serum levels of these drugs in the nursing infant are generally very low or undetectable and these drugs appear to carry the lowest risk of adverse events in nursing infants. Several reports have suggested that fluoxetine (Prozac) may be found at higher levels in the nursing infant; however, the data regarding fluoxetine and the other antidepressants suggest a relatively low incidence of serious problems among nursing infants exposed to these drugs. Because there has been concern that Prozac may be passed into the breast milk at higher levels, many women taking Prozac during pregnancy question whether they should change to Paxil or Zoloft after delivery. In general, this is not recommended. It does not make sense to make this switch after delivery because making this change may increase a woman's risk for relapse during the postpartum period.

Although we have sufficient data on only a few antidepressants, these are not the only antidepressant drugs we use in nursing women. There may be times when we decide to use a medication that is not on this short list—for example, when a woman has not responded to or cannot tolerate any of these well-characterized medications. A similar choice may also be made when a women has been taking one medication throughout her pregnancy. Should she switch to a different one for breast-feeding? Usually the antidepressant used throughout her pregnancy is continued during the postpartum period, as making a switch may increase a woman's likelihood of becoming ill after delivery.

The total amount of medication to which an infant is exposed depends on several factors, including the dosage of the medication. In situations where the mother is taking a higher dose of the medication, more medication will be passed into the breast milk and the baby will be exposed to higher levels of the drug. The extent of exposure is also influenced by the frequency and timing of the infant's feedings. A baby who is breast-feeding exclusively around the clock will be exposed to more medication than an older infant who is also taking formula or solid food. The amount of medication in the breast milk also depends on when the medication is taken. Dr. Zachary Stowe and his colleagues at Emory University have focused on the complicated issue of medication passage into the breast milk and have determined that drug levels in the breast milk seem to peak six to eight hours after the mother takes an antidepressant drug. Given this relatively predictable pattern, some experts have advocated a "pump and dump" technique to reduce exposure to the drug in the nursing infant. With this technique women are instructed to pump six to eight hours after taking medication and to discard this breast milk that contains higher levels of the antidepressant. Dr. Stowe's studies indicate that this approach decreases the baby's exposure by about 25 percent. From a theoretical standpoint this technique may seem quite attractive as a means of decreasing exposure; however, it is a very cumbersome proposition, especially for women breast-feeding young infants who feed every two to three hours around the clock. It is difficult to imagine trying to take care of a hungry baby on an on-demand feeding schedule while at the same time pumping and throwing away precious breast milk. On the other hand, if you have an older baby who nurses less frequently, you may be able to adjust the timing of feedings so that your baby nurses only at times when drug concentrations are at their lowest in the breast milk. (For example, you may take your medication at bedtime and nurse your baby shortly before taking the medication and then wait to nurse the baby again in the morning, ten to twelve hours after that dosage.)

The general consensus is that the benefits of the breast-feeding outweigh the risks of exposure to most antidepressant medications. There are only a few situations where you may be advised not to breast-feed if you are taking a medication. If your baby is premature or has signs of jaundice, your baby's liver may not be fully mature and may not have the capacity to metabolize drugs carried in the breast milk. Thus, your baby may be exposed to higher levels of the drug and may be more likely to experience negative effects related to this exposure. In addition, if your baby has a serious medical problem, your pediatrician may have some concerns about exposure to medication. If you make the decision to use a medication while breast-feeding, it is essential that you inform your pediatrician so that your baby can be evaluated appropriately. Your baby does not necessarily require monitoring that is any more rigorous than the average baby, but if you notice any changes in your baby's behavior or habits after you start taking a medication, you should discuss them with your pediatrician. Your doctor can help you to evaluate what is normal and what is more concerning.

Breast-feeding in Women with Bipolar Disorder. For women with bipolar disorder, breast-feeding may be more problematic. First, there is concern that on-demand breast-feeding may significantly disrupt the mother's sleep and thus may increase her vulnerability to illness during the acute postpartum period. Second, while there is relative comfort in using antidepressants in nursing women, there have been reports of toxicity in nursing infants exposed to various mood stabilizers—including lithium, valproate (Depakote or Depakene) and carbamazepine (Tegretol)—in the breast milk. Lithium is secreted at relatively high levels into the mother's milk, and consequently infant lithium levels may be high, about one-quarter of the mother's serum levels, increasing the risk of toxicity in the infant. Also of concern is the fact that exposure to carbamazepine and valproate in the breast milk may cause liver damage in the nursing infant. Information regarding the use of the newer anticonvulsant mood stabilizers and antipsychotic medications is still quite limited. Given these risks and inadequate data on certain drugs, many women with bipolar disorder choose not to breast-feed.

Are Complementary or Alternative Treatments Useful?
Despite the growing interest in nontraditional remedies for depression and other medical illnesses, none has been adequately studied and for most there is no evidence to show that these forms of treatment are effective for the treatment of depression. The list of complementary or alternative treatments is long and includes herbal remedies, dietary supplements, acupuncture, homeopathy, hypnosis, meditation, yoga, and massage therapy. (In

chapter 12, you will find a discussion of some of these treatments in greater detail.)

At this time, there is little data to support the use of herbal remedies for the treatment of postpartum depression. Herbalists have recommended various herbs for PPD including evening primrose oil, licorice root, skullcap, and motherwort. St. John's wort has been used commonly to treat mild to moderate depression; however, there is no data to support its use or the use of other herbal remedies for the treatment of postpartum depression. Further, the data on the use of herbal remedies in breast-feeding women is very limited, with one recent report suggesting some side effects, such as irritability and drowsiness, in nursing infants exposed to St. John's wort in the breast milk.

There is some preliminary evidence to suggest that the omega-3 fatty acids contained in fish and fish oil, including eicosapentanoic acid (EPA) and docosahexanoic acid (DHA), have an antidepressant effect. Mothers selectively transfer DHA to their baby during pregnancy and through the breast milk to support neurological development. Thus, childbearing women may become depleted of DHA, and it has been hypothesized that DHA deficiency may make mothers more vulnerable to depression during the postpartum period. One study suggested that eating more fish during pregnancy may reduce your risk of postpartum depression; in contrast, mothers with lower seafood consumption and lower DHA concentrations in breast milk were more likely to develop postpartum depression. Whether or not omega-3 fatty acids are a cure for postpartum depression is far from clear; it appears that supplementing the mother's diet with the omega-3 fatty acid, docosahexaenoic acid (DHA), after delivery does not decrease the risk for depression.

Postpartum Depression Can Be Prevented

It is difficult to reliably predict exactly who will experience postpartum illness. It is possible, however, to identify women who are at high risk for this illness. Current research also indicates that if you are at high risk, there are steps you can take during pregnancy or near the time of delivery to decrease your risk of illness after delivery. The following questionnaire is based on the work of Cheryl Tatano Beck, a prominent researcher in the field of postpartum depression, who has developed several questionnaires—including the Postpartum Depression Predictors Inventory—that can be used to assess a woman's risk for postpartum depression. By answering the questions listed next, you can determine your own risk for depression after delivery.

WHAT IS YOUR RISK FOR POSTPARTUM DEPRESSION?		
Have you ever suffered from depression?	Yes	No
Have you ever suffered from postpartum depression or psychosis?	Yes	No
Are you married or living with your partner?	Yes	No
Are you experiencing any marital difficulties?	Yes	No
Have you recently experienced any stressful life events—for example, the death of a loved one, medical illness, unemployment, financial difficulties?	Yes	No
Was this an unplanned or unwanted pregnancy?	Yes	No
Do you have adequate support from your partner, family members, and friends?	Yes	No
Do you struggle with feelings of inadequacy or low self-esteem?	Yes	No
Did you experience any episodes of depression during pregnancy?	Yes	No
Did you experience significant anxiety during pregnancy?	Yes	No
Does your baby have a difficult temperament? Is your baby colicky, irritable, or difficult to soothe?	Yes	No
Do you have any stress related to child-care issues?	Yes	No

One of the most important things you can do to minimize your risk of postpartum depression is to bolster your support network *before* your baby arrives. Women who receive more support after the birth of a child appear to be less vulnerable to depression. Chapter 11 talks more specifically about how to get the support you need and deserve, but here are a few important things that you can do to prepare for the new baby:

- Discuss with your partner his availability during the first few months after the baby is born. Will your partner be able to take time off from work? What will his hours be like? Will he have to do any out-of-town traveling?
- Make arrangements with friends and family members to help you out during the first few months.
- Consider hiring someone to help you to care for the baby or your older children.
- Arrange for help around the house and with cooking.
- Find out about new mothers' groups and other similar resources in your community.

Making sure that you are your partner are working together as a team is also important. To prepare you for the arrival of your baby, it may be helpful for the two of you to attend a Preparation for Parenthood class. Not only will this type of class give you practical information that will help you to better take care of your child, it will give you and your partner the opportunity to talk about your expectations and your anxieties surrounding the arrival of your child. If you find that you and your partner are having difficulties communicating or making decisions, you may consider meeting with a couples therapist so that you can address some of the more pressing issues *before* your baby is born.

After answering the above questionnaire, if you are concerned that you are at risk for postpartum depression, meet with a mental health professional before the baby arrives. This will allow you to get a better sense of your situation and will provide you with information on what interventions may be available to you. Having a professional lined up may also help to give you an added sense of security. If your risk for postpartum depression is low, you may not need to do anything other than to make sure you have enough support. The following table can help you to decide which strategies are the most appropriate for your situation.

RISK LEVEL	DESCRIPTION	INTERVENTION
Low	No history of mood disorder	Routine monitoring
	Remote history of depression	Routine monitoring Increase supports
Moderate	Recent history of depression	Increase supports Individual psychotherapy Consider antidepressant
	Marital problems	Couples therapy Increase supports Individual psychotherapy
	Inadequate support	Increase supports Individual psychotherapy
High	History of recurrent depression *or* Postpartum depression	Close monitoring Increase supports Individual psychotherapy Antidepressant prophylaxis
	History of bipolar disorder *or* Postpartum psychosis	Close monitoring Increase Supports Individual psychotherapy Lithium prophylaxis

There is evidence that certain types of psychotherapy received during pregnancy may reduce the risk of illness in women at high risk for postpartum depression. Interpersonal therapy (IPT) is a technique that helps women develop new ways of understanding and dealing with interpersonal conflicts and lapses in communication. This type of therapy also aims to help women deal with the various role transitions that occur after childbirth and to adjust to becoming a mother. In a study from Dr. Caron Zlotnick and her colleagues at Brown University School of Medicine, a group of women at high risk for postpartum depression received a brief course of IPT during pregnancy. None of these women became depressed after giving birth, whereas one-third of the women who did not receive this intervention developed postpartum depression.

If you have a history of a mood or anxiety disorder, you should also discuss with your doctor what types of pharmacologic interventions may help to reduce your risk of postpartum depression. Women with histories of postpartum depression have a 50 percent risk of having another episode following a subsequent pregnancy. Although these are fairly grim statistics, there are several studies that indicate that treatment with an antidepressant initiated around the time of delivery may significantly reduce this risk. In a recent study from Dr. Katherine Wisner and her colleagues at the University of Pittsburgh School of Medicine, women with histories of postpartum depression received either Zoloft or placebo immediately after delivery. Half of the women in the placebo group developed postpartum depression, in contrast to only 1 in 14 (about 7 percent) of the women treated with Zoloft. It is interesting to note that although antidepressants typically take two to four weeks to start working, in this study the antidepressant did not have to be introduced prior to delivery to have a beneficial effect.

Although it has not been well studied, it is believed that antidepressants may also help to protect other groups of women at high risk, specifically those women with histories of depression prior to pregnancy. Women with histories of severe or recurrent depression are counseled to maintain treatment with an antidepressant during the postpartum period to minimize their risk of depression after delivery. However, if you have a history of depression and have remained well off medications during your pregnancy, you may prefer to take a wait-and-see approach.

Another group at high risk for postpartum depression are women with bipolar disorder. Several studies have demonstrated that women with histories of bipolar disorder benefit from preventative treatment with lithium initiated either prior to delivery (at 36 weeks gestation) or no later than the first forty-eight hours postpartum. Not only does lithium significantly reduce the risk of postpartum illness, it appears to decrease the severity of symptoms if they do occur. Although many other mood stabilizers may be used to treat bipolar disorder, only lithium has been studied as a preventative treatment in postpartum women with bipolar disorder.

Depression Is a Treatable Illness

There are many misconceptions regarding depression and its treatment that may discourage a woman from seeking treatment. Furthermore, while there are many effective strategies available for the treatment of depression, the situation is much more complicated in pregnant and postpartum women. However, you should not assume there is no treatment available to you. As we discussed in this chapter, there are many types of interventions — including psychotherapy — that do not pose any risk to your child. And over the last ten years, investigations have yielded important information regarding the reproductive safety of many antidepressant medications. While this information is still limited, research studies indicate that certain medications may be taken safely during pregnancy and while nursing and do not appear to pose a significant risk to the child. The most important thing is that you get the information you need so that you can make the best and the safest decisions regarding your care.

Chapter 14

For Families and Friends
How You Can Help

I f somebody close to you is depressed, you want to help. However, it is difficult to know exactly what to do. Depression is often so pervasive, affecting every aspect of a person's life, that it may seem impossible to eradicate this problem and to make things better. Because depression colors how one views the world, it may also be difficult to know when you are being helpful or when progress is being made. To make things worse, depression can change one's personality and behavior and, in this way, can totally transform—or in the worst cases, destroy—even the strongest relationships. You may end up feeling that you are losing the person you love and respect. You may feel that your efforts are not appreciated or go nowhere. Although you might be tempted to ignore the problem and just walk away, you can't. While caring for or living with somebody who is depressed can be a stressful, frustrating, and exhausting business, taking care of somebody who needs your help can also be immensely rewarding. And if your partner is depressed, your support is vital to hold your family together.

Understanding Depression
The first step in helping somebody with depression is understanding the nature of the problem. While depression is a biologically driven illness, just like diabetes or high blood pressure, many people have a hard time appreciating how depression can alter one's personality and behavior. If your friend or family member appears angry or irritable, you may worry that you have done something wrong. If she pulls away from you, you may assume the she no longer cares for you. You may try to help her but feel that your efforts are either ignored or rejected; she may tell you that nobody can help her. While these are the typical symptoms of depression, it is hard not to take things personally. Helping someone who is depressed can be a challenging and frustrating experience; however, here are some things to keep in mind that can make it easier to care for a friend or family member who is depressed:

Depression is a real illness. It is not a sign of laziness or weakness or lack of willpower. Under no circumstances should depression be ignored or tolerated. Although you may expect her to "snap out of it," getting better isn't simply a matter of taking a more positive outlook on life.

Depression is treatable. With treatment, your friend or family member will recover. However, you may need to help her to recognize that there is a problem and to encourage her and help her to get the professional help she needs. Also keep in mind that it may take time for the depression to resolve completely, and you need to be patient, optimistic, and reassuring while you are waiting for the treatment to take effect.

Depression has many negative consequences. Depression affects one's ability to function and derive pleasure from life. It also can make it very difficult to connect with and maintain relationships with others. It hinders a woman's ability to care for and nurture her children. Reminding her of these consequences may make her more willing to pursue treatment.

Your support is essential. Although you may feel that your efforts to help are not appreciated or are rejected, when a friend or family member is depressed, she needs your help. You can support her by being a person to talk to and to share her feelings with, and you can help her by taking on some of the responsibilities she may be struggling with. You can also help her to get the treatment she needs.

When Your Partner Is Depressed

Depression can entirely change the nature of your relationship with your partner, and even the most supportive and caring relationship may be threatened when depression intervenes. Depression, and caring for someone who is depressed, may be so consuming that you feel cut off from and unable to enjoy many other facets of your life. Author Anne Sheffield coined the term "depression fallout" to describe the painful and complicated feelings that emerge when you are living with and caring for a person who is depressed. At first you feel confused; you may not be able to understand why your partner is behaving so differently. She used to be loving and affectionate, now she is cool and distant. Now she is angry or hostile and seems to treat others with more kindness and consideration than she treats you. You may wonder what happened to the woman you fell in love with. Does she still love you? Does she believe in your relationship? How do you explain what is happening?

You may blame yourself for what is going on, and you may work hard to make things better. However, when nothing you do seems to improve the situation, you may end up feeling hopeless. Without the love and affection of your partner, you may feel unwanted, unloved, and very lonely. It is hard to retain a positive and healthy outlook on life when someone so close to you is depressed, and you may end up feeling humiliated or demoralized. Unfortunately, these feelings may extend beyond the boundaries of your relationship, affecting your sense of self-esteem, your effectiveness at work, and your relationships with others.

If your efforts to be supportive and caring are ineffective or are rejected over and over again, you will eventually start to become resentful. You may feel angry and frustrated that you have had to suffer with your partner's depression for so long. When you feel hurt or angry, it is hard to be empathic and understanding. You may find yourself pulling away from your partner in an effort to protect yourself, or you may find yourself fighting back, making negative or critical remarks. If things persist in this way long enough, you will eventually start to think about how to escape this painful and unpleasant situation. You may think about separation or divorce, or you may find a way to emotionally distance yourself from the relationship in order to protect yourself.

But you shouldn't let things go this far. If you and your partner are experiencing problems, you should look for professional help. The earlier, the better.

What You Can Do to Help

As a family member or friend, you want to help the person you love, but it may be difficult to know exactly what to do. Depression is often an alienating and isolating experience, and those who suffer from depression often retreat and are reluctant to seek or accept the help of others. Under these circumstances, offering help may feel a bit like trying to break through a bolted and barricaded door. If you are rebuffed over and over again, it may be hard to accept that she wants or needs your help. In addition, she may not appear to appreciate the help she receives. She may criticize or reject your efforts, and you may end up feeling helpless and demoralized. You may feel so hurt that you just want to want to walk away and leave her alone. However, it is important to remember that this rejecting attitude is a symptom of the depression and not a reflection of her true feelings for you. If someone you love is depressed, they do need your help. Here are some things that you can do.

Show you care. When a woman is depressed, she may feel isolated and lonely, convinced that nobody loves her or is available to help her. Let her know that you care for her and are willing to help. You may also need to remind her that there are many other people who care about her.

Listen to what she is saying. It may be difficult to bear the intensity of her feelings, or her depression may make you feel helpless and hopeless. Do not dismiss or try to avoid the painful issues she may be struggling with, and resist the temptation to "fix" all of her problems; just try your best to understand what she is experiencing.

Ask how you can help. Rather than assuming that you know what she wants or needs, ask her how you can be helpful. There are many different ways to help. Does she need you to listen to her problems? Does she need a shoulder to cry on? Or does she just need a hand doing the housework?

Help her to recognize when she needs help. Many women who suffer from depression feel helpless yet are reluctant to ask for assistance. You can help your friend or family member to identify situations in which she may need help. While she may not know what type of assistance she needs, you are in a position to help her figure this out.

Help her to identify other sources of support. When a woman is depressed, she may not be able to see that there are other people who are willing to help and to provide support. The hopeless feelings that come along with depression can prevent her from thinking constructively about what can be done to solve a particular problem. What you can do is help to identify and pursue other resources.

Getting Professional Help

There are many things you can do to help a depressed person; however, one of the most important things is helping her to get professional help. Although your support is vital, it is not a substitute for professional care, and you should not feel that you have to shoulder the burden of another person's depression on your own. While you should make yourself available to provide assistance, you should not feel that you are taking on the role of a therapist. This is not your job. Your job is to get your friend or family member the professional help she needs. However, getting her to pursue and to accept this help is not always easy, and you should be prepared to work hard to overcome the resistance you may encounter.

First of all, help her to acknowledge that there is a problem. Often, a woman suffering from depression does not seek help because she is not aware or willing to admit that there is a problem. She may not see herself as being depressed or she may blame how bad she feels on her circumstances. You may have to convince her that what she is experiencing is depression and that she needs professional help.

Help her to understand how the depression affects her life. She may be better able to appreciate the importance of getting professional help if you try to make her more aware of how the depression is affecting her and the people around her. Is she able to do the things that she used to do? Is she enjoying herself? Has she experienced any changes in her relationships with friends or family members? When she is more aware of the toll that depression takes on her life and on those around her, she may be more motivated to seek help.

Educate yourself about depression and its treatment. A woman may be reluctant to pursue treatment because she doesn't know what she needs or where to go for help. Make it clear to her that depression is a treatable medical condition, not a sign of weakness. Assure her that those suffering from depression do feel better if they get help. This book can help you to better appreciate what she is struggling with, and by learning more about depression, you may be able to help your friend or family member to come to a better understanding of her illness and find the type of treatment that is most appropriate for her.

Help her to find a mental health professional. Finding a compassionate and caring professional is not always easy, and, if one is depressed, the task may seem overwhelming. It may be helpful for you to take the lead here. First of all, you will have to help her find a reputable professional; chapter 12 discusses how to go about finding one. In addition, you may need to help her make the first appointment, and your encouragement and support may be necessary to get her to the first visit.

Enlist the support of other family members, friends, and medical professionals. If you feel that you are not making any headway or you need extra help, it may be useful to enlist the aid of others. Hearing the same message from several different people may have a greater impact. Other people may also be able to help you to find and obtain the treatment she needs.

Help to monitor the effectiveness of her treatment. When one is depressed, everything looks bleak, and it may be difficult to assess whether or not things are getting any better. As an outside observer, you can provide useful information on how the treatment is working. It is often helpful for a family member to come along to some appointments. This is an opportunity for you to better understand the depression and its treatment, but you can be very helpful in providing additional information regarding the progress of the treatment.

Seek immediate help in case of emergency. On page 230, you will find a list of situations that warrant immediate attention. If at any point, you are concerned that your depressed friend or family may be a danger to herself or to others, or if she talks about death or suicide, this is an emergency. Contact her doctor, go to your local emergency room, or call 911.

Keeping Your Family Healthy

Depression affects the entire family. If you have children, it is essential to help them to understand what is happening. Not wanting to burden their children, most parents usually try to hide their depression. However, when their mother is depressed, even very young children are aware that something is amiss. It is essential for everyone in the family to understand what is going on and to give them an opportunity to share their feelings and concerns. In chapter 3, you will find more information about how depression affects your family and how you can help children better understand this illness. By allowing every family member to discuss this important issue, you can identify problematic areas.

It may feel as if your partner's depression is derailing your family's life. Especially if you have children, it is important to try to keep things as consistent and normal as possible. Nor can you allow yourself to be cut off from your family, your friends, or other activities that are important to you. As the depression starts to resolve, it may be helpful to gently encourage—not push—your partner to pursue activities or hobbies, sports, and games that have given her pleasure in the past. However, there may be times when your partner may not be able to keep up with her routine activities and you may need to step in. You may need to take more of a role in child care, or you may need to recruit help from family members or friends. Although this may seem like a great deal of effort, remember that you and your family will do better when at least some of the usual routines can be maintained. Eventually your partner will be able to return to her usual activities and responsibilities.

Depression can cause a great deal of friction. You may be tempted to try to ride things out, figuring that the problems will go away as the depression resolves. However, depression may place a great deal of strain on certain relationships, and it may be helpful to see a couples or family therapist to help negotiate these issues. This may also provide you with a safe place to discuss how much of a strain the depression has placed on the family.

Protecting Yourself

Being a caregiver is hard work. It is difficult to see somebody you love suffering and to feel that you can do little to eliminate this pain. Many caregivers fail to recognize their own needs or fail to do anything about them, and if somebody close to you is depressed, you may feel you have lost one of *your* most important sources of support. Especially when depression becomes a more chronic or recurrent problem, taking care of somebody who is depressed can lead to a host of problems for you, including anxiety, depression, insomnia, irritability, and exhaustion. But there are some things you can do to protect yourself.

Have realistic expectations. If someone is depressed, she may not have the emotional resources or energy to do what she usually does. No matter how much you encourage her, she may not be able to do what she used to do. Furthermore, it is important to recognize that recovery is a slow process and you must be patient.

Attend to your own feelings and emotions. You may feel angry, frustrated, depressed, disappointed, or despairing. It is important not to ignore these feelings. If you feel that it is difficult to handle these feelings or if you feel that they are interfering with your ability to live your own life, it may be helpful to speak with a therapist.

Take care of yourself. Dealing with somebody who is depressed may feel like a full-time job. You still need to find the time to take care of yourself. If you are not tending to your own needs, it will be more difficult to help another person. Taking care of yourself means eating well, getting enough rest and exercise, and keeping up with your usual activities. But it also means finding somebody to talk to about *your* feelings and *your* experiences as a caregiver.

Set limits. Taking care of someone who is depressed is extremely diffi-cult work, and it is easy to feel overwhelmed and overburdened. If you are feeling burned out, you may need to give yourself a little distance from the situation and to get more support for yourself. If you feel that you are being poorly treated or unappreciated for your efforts, say something. If you do not protect yourself, nobody else will.

Light at the End of the Tunnel

Remember that things do get better. Depression is a treatable illness and, with appropriate treatment, most people recover completely. Depression makes it difficult to ask for and to get help, so the most important thing you can do is to help her to get the treatment she needs. Although you may feel hopeless at times, your support can make a huge difference. Getting better may take some time and effort, but your love, patience, and encouragement can make the process of recovery much easier.

Author's Note

Whe n I started writing this book and began to meet with various publishers, the first one I met did not seem particularly interested in the book. "Depression is a real downer," he told me. "The world is a really negative place these days; nobody wants to read about depression." It is true, depression can be depressing. Obviously, this is a problem. But it is a topic we all need to know about. We can't simply sweep it under the rug and hope that it goes away. Over the last few years, when I told friends and acquaintances about this project, I was impressed by the number of them who confided that they had suffered from depression either during pregnancy or after the birth of a child. Many more told me about a friend or a family member who had experienced depression under the same circumstances.

If you suffer from depression, understanding what you are experiencing—and why—is one of the most important steps to feeling better. Many women who suffer from depression know that something is wrong but never have a name for it. Their families know something is wrong, but they don't know how to fix it. Although learning to accept this illness as a part of your life is certainly not easy, acknowledging that depression is a problem may bring a sense of relief. By addressing the problem head on, you can begin to get the help you need and you and your loved ones can take the first steps toward helping you to feel better.

Even though depression can be a debilitating illness, there is certainly room for optimism, and I want to leave all who read this book with a sense of hopefulness. Depression is not something to live with or suffer through. Depression is not a terminal disease. Depression is a treatable illness, and there are many highly effective treatments available today. Depression is, like other problems, something you can manage, and, most important, you can learn how to protect yourself and your family from its negative effects.

One of our most powerful tools for combating depression in women during the childbearing years is teaching women, their families, and the physicians who care for them how to identify the problem. The central message of this book is that depression is highly treatable. When women recognize depression and seek appropriate treatment, its damaging effects can be minimized, if not eliminated.

My ultimate goal in writing this book is to convey hope. Books about medical conditions can be hard to digest. After all, depression is, by definition, a "downer," just like that first publisher said. However, I find my work incredibly uplifting. There is immense satisfaction in helping women to successfully negotiate a potentially life-ravaging illness through a stressful time. Mothers benefit, the children benefit, marriages benefit, and society benefits. It's not all that common in the practice of medicine that education, recognition, and treatment can have such profound and lasting effects, and I consider myself lucky to have stumbled into this field. Perhaps most important, I feel privileged to be able to help the women I take care of, and look forward to continuing my work for a long, long time.

Appendix A
Edinburgh Postnatal Depression Scale (EPDS)

Circle the answer which comes closest to how you have felt IN THE PAST 7 DAYS, not just how you feel today. The first item in the scale is an example, already completed.

	I have felt happy.	Yes, all the time
		<u>Yes, most of the time</u>
		No, not very often
		No, not at all
1	I have been able to laugh and see the funny side of things.	As much as I always could (0)
		Not quite so much now (1)
		Definitely not so much now (2)
		Not at all (3)
2	I have looked forward with enjoyment to things.	As much as I ever did (0)
		Rather less than I used to (1)
		Definitely less than I used to (2)
		Hardly at all (3)
3	I have blamed myself unnecessarily when things went wrong.	Yes, most of the time (3)
		Yes, some of the time (2)
		Not very often (1)
		No, never (0)
4	I have been anxious or worried for no good reason.	No, not at all (0)
		Hardly ever (1)
		Yes, sometimes (2)
		Yes, very often (3)

EPDS is reproduced from J. L. Cox, J. M. Holden, and R. Sagovsky (1987), "Detection of Postnatal Depression: Development of the 10-item Edinburgh Postnatal Depression Scale," *British Journal of Psychiatry*, 150:782–86.

5	I have felt scared or panicky for not very good reasons.	Yes, quite a lot (3) Yes, sometimes (2) No, not much (1) No, not at all (0)
6	Things have been getting on top of me.	Yes, most of the time I haven't been able to cope at all (3) Yes, sometimes I haven't been coping as well as usual (2) No, most of the time I have coped quite well (1) No, I have been coping as well as ever (0)
7	I have been so unhappy that I have had difficulty sleeping.	Yes, most of the time (3) Yes, sometimes (2) Not very often (1) No, not at all (0)
8	I have felt sad or miserable.	Yes, most of the time (3) Yes, quite often (2) Not very often (1) No, not at all (0)
9	I have been so unhappy that I have been crying.	Yes, most of the time (3) Yes, quite often (2) Only occasionally (1) No, never (0)
10	The thought of harming myself has occurred to me.	Yes, quite often (3) Sometimes (2) Hardly ever (1) Never (0)

If you score a 12 or higher, there is a good chance you have postpartum depression, and you should contact your obstetrician, your primary care provider, or a mental health professional for a more thorough evaluation. If your answer is yes to question 10, indicating that you are having suicidal thoughts, you should contact your doctor as soon as possible for a more thorough evaluation. Although this questionnaire may be a useful tool for you, it is important to remember that this is not a substitute for a good evaluation from a trained professional. If you—or somebody who knows you well— think that you may be suffering from postpartum depression, you should discuss this with your doctor.

Appendix B
FDA Pregnancy Categories

The FDA requires that all prescription drugs be classified according to one of five pregnancy categories (A, B, C, D, X) based on studies carried out in animals and humans. The identifying letter signifies the level of risk to the fetus (with A being the safest category) and is to appear in the precautions section of the package insert. The categories described by the FDA are as follows:

CATEGORY	DESCRIPTION
A	Adequate, well-controlled studies in pregnant women have not shown an increased risk of fetal abnormalities.
B	Animal studies have revealed no evidence of harm to the fetus, however, there are no adequate and well-controlled studies in pregnant women. OR Animal studies have shown an adverse effect, but adequate and well-controlled studies in pregnant women have failed to demonstrate a risk to the fetus.
C	Animal studies have shown an adverse effect and there are no adequate and well-controlled studies in pregnant women. OR No animal studies have been conducted and there are no adequate and well-controlled studies in pregnant women.
D	Studies, adequate well-controlled or observational, in pregnant women have demonstrated a risk to the fetus. However, the benefits of therapy may outweigh the potential risk.
X	Studies, adequate well-controlled or observational, in animals or pregnant women have demonstrated positive evidence of fetal abnormalities. The use of the product is contraindicated in women who are or may become pregnant.

Appendix C
Women's Mental Health Programs

This is a list of programs specializing in the treatment of women during pregnancy and the postpartum period. Most of these programs are affiliated with universities or medical centers and offer a combination of clinical care and research. This is by no means a complete list of mental health professionals with expertise in this area; there are many psychiatrists and therapists in the community who treat women during pregnancy and the postpartum period. Your obstetrician or primary care provider may be able to help you to locate well-trained professionals in your area.

Arizona
Women's Mental Health Program
Director: Marlene Freeman, MD
University of Arizona
Department of Psychiatry
1501 N. Campbell Ave.
PO Box 245002
Tucson, AZ 85724-5002
Telephone: 520-626-3273

California
Behavioral Neuroendocrinology
   Program
Director: Natalie Rasgon, MD
Department of Psychiatry and
   Behavioral Sciences
Stanford University School of
   Medicine
401 Quarry Road
Stanford, CA 94305

UCLA Pregnancy and Postpartum
   Mood Disorders Program
Director: Lori Altshuler, MD
300 UCLA Medical Plaza,
   Suite 1544
Los Angeles, CA 90095-7057

Women's Life Center
Director: Vivien K. Burt, MD, PhD
UCLA Neuropsychiatric Institute
Telephone: 310-206-5135
www.npi.ucla.edu/wlc/

Women's Mood Disorders Clinic
Director: Barbara Parry, MD
University of California at San Diego
   Medical Center
9500 Gilman Drive
La Jolla, CA 92037
Telephone: 619-543-7393

Women's Wellness Program
Director: Regina Casper, MD
Department of Psychiatry and
   Behavioral Sciences

Stanford University School of
  Medicine
401 Quarry Road
Stanford, CA 94305
Telephone: 650-725-1353

Connecticut
Yale Behavioral Gynecology Program
Director: Cynthia Neill Epperson, MD
Department of Psychiatry
Yale University School of Medicine
University Towers
100 York Street, Suite 2H
New Haven, CT 06511

Georgia
Emory University Women's Mental
  Health Program
Director: Zachary Stowe, MD
Emory University School of
  Medicine
Emory Clinic Building B
1365 Clifton Road NE, Suite 6100
Atlanta, GA 30322
Telephone: 404-778-2524
www.emorywomensprogram.org

Illinois
Women's Mental Health Program
Director: Laura J. Miller, MD
University of Illinois at Chicago
912 S. Wood St., M/C 913
Chicago, IL 60612
Telephone: 312-355-1223
www.psych.uic.edu/clinical/women
  .htm

Maryland
Women's Mood Disorders Center
Directors: Jennifer L. Payne, MD,
  and Karen L. Swartz, MD
The Johns Hopkins Hospital

Meyer Building, Room 3-181
600 North Wolfe Street
Baltimore, MD 21287
www.hopkinsmedicine.org/Psychiatry
  /Moods/womensmood.html

Massachusetts
MGH Center for Women's Mental
  Health
Director: Lee Cohen, MD
Massachusetts General Hospital
Simches Research Building
185 Cambridge Street
Boston, MA 02114
Telephone: 617-724-2933
www.womensmentalhealth.org

Michigan
Women's Mental Health Program
Director: Sheila Marcus, MD
2101 Commonwealth
Ann Arbor, MI 48105
Telephone: 800-525-5185
www.med.umich.edu/depression

Minnesota
Hennepin Women's Mental Health
  Program
Director: Helen Kim, MD
Hennepin County Medical Center
Hennepin Faculty Associates
914 South 8th Street, Suite D-110
Minneapolis, MN 55404
Telephone: 612-347-3996
www.hcmc.org/depts/psych/mental
  health.htm

New York
Perinatal Psychiatric Consultation
  Clinic
Director: Linda Chaudron, MD
Strong Memorial Hospital

University of Rochester School of
   Medicine
Rochester, NY 14642
Telephone: 585-275-3750

Maternal Mental Health Program
Director: Margaret Spinelli, MD
New York State Psychiatric Institute
722 West 168th Street, Room 1105
New York, NY 10032

Payne Whitney Women's Program
Director: Catherine Birndorf, MD
Payne Whitney Manhattan
525 East 68th Street
New York, NY 10021
Telephone: 212-821-0779

Pennsylvania
Women's Behavioral HealthCARE
Director: Katherine Wisner, MD
Western Psychiatric Institute and
   Clinic
3811 O'Hara Street
Pittsburgh, PA 15213
Telephone: 800-436-2461
www.womensbehavioralhealth.org

Virginia
Virginia Commonwealth University
   Institute for Women's Health
Director: Susan Kornstein, MD
9000 Stony Point Parkway
Richmond, VA 23235
Telephone: 804-560-8950 or 866-
   829-6626
www.womenshealth.vcu.edu/index
   .html

Washington, DC
Women's Mood Program
Director: Wendy Hookman, MD
Georgetown University Hospital
3800 Reservoir Road, NW
Washington, DC 20007
Telephone: 202-687-8609

Canada
The British Columbia Reproductive
   Mental Health Program
Director: Shaila Misri, MD
BC Women's Health Centre
H214-4500 Oak Street
Vancouver, BC V6H 3N1
Telephone: 604-875-3060 or
   604-875-2025
www.bcrmh.com

Motherisk
Director: Gideon Koren, MD
Hospital for Sick Children
555 University Avenue
Toronto, ON M5G 1X8
Telephone: 416-813-6780
www.motherisk.org

Women's Health Concerns Clinic
Director: Claudio Soares, MD
McMaster University
Hamilton, Ontario
Telephone: 905-522-1155
www.stjosham.on.ca/whcc/home
   .htm

Resources

Pregnancy

American College of Obstetricians
and Gynecologists (ACOG)
409 12th Street, Southwest
P.O. Box 96920
Washington, DC 20090-6920
Telephone: 800-673-8444 or
202-638-5577
www.acog.org

American Pregnancy Association
1425 Greenway Drive, Suite 440
Irving, TX 75038
Telephone: 800-672-2296
www.americanpregnancy.org

Baby Center
163 Freelon Street
San Francisco, CA 94107
www.babycenter.com

March of Dimes
1275 Mamaroneck Avenue
White Plains, NY 10605
www.marchofdimes.com

Motherisk
Hospital for Sick Children
555 University Avenue
Toronto, ON M5G 1X8
Telephone: 416-813-6780
www.motherisk.org

National Women's Health
Information Center
8270 Willow Oaks Corporate Drive
Fairfax, VA 22031
Telephone: 800-994-WOMAN
(800-994-9662)
www.4woman.gov

Organization of Teratology
Information Specialists (OTIS)
Telephone: 866-626-OTIS or
866-626-6847
www.otispregnancy.org

Mental Health (General)

American Psychiatric Association
1000 Wilson Boulevard, Suite 1825
Arlington, VA 22209-3901
Telephone: 703-907-7300
www.psych.org

American Psychological Association
750 First Street, NE
Washington, DC 20002-4242
Telephone: 800-374-2721 or
202-336-5500
www.apa.org

Anxiety Disorders Association of
America (ADAA)
8730 Georgia Avenue, Suite 600
Silver Spring, MD 20910
Telephone: 240-485-1001
www.adaa.org

Depression and Bipolar Support
  Alliance (DBSA)
730 N. Franklin Street, Suite 501
Chicago, IL 60610-7224
Telephone: 800-826-3632 or
  312-642-0049
www.DBSAlliance.org

Families for Depression Awareness
300 Fifth Avenue
Waltham, MA 02451
Telephone: 781-890-0220
www.familyaware.org

HealthyPlace.com
www.healthyplace.com

Madison Institute of Medicine
7617 Mineral Point Road
Suite 300
Madison, WI 53717
Telephone: 608-827-2470
www.miminc.org

National Alliance for the
  Mentally Ill
Colonial Place Three
2107 Wilson Blvd., Suite 300
Arlington, VA 22201-3042
Telephone: 703-524-7600
www.nami.org

National Institute of Mental Health
6001 Executive Boulevard
Room 8184, MSC 9663
Bethesda, MD 20892-9663
Telephone: 866-615-6464 or
  301-443-4513
www.nimh.nih.gov

National Mental Health Association
2001 N. Beauregard St., 12th Floor
Alexandria, VA 22311
Telephone: 703-684-7722
www.nmha.org

Psychiatric Illness During Pregnancy

The British Columbia Reproductive
  Mental Health Program
BC Women's Health Centre
H214-4500 Oak Street
Vancouver, BC V6H 3N1
Telephone: 604-875-3060 or
  604-875-2025
www.bcrmh.com

Emory University Women's Mental
  Health Program
Emory University School of
  Medicine
Emory Clinic Building B
1365 Clifton Road NE, Suite 6100
Atlanta, GA 30322
Telephone: 404-778-2524
www.emorywomensprogram.org

MGH Center for Women's Mental
  Health
Massachusetts General Hospital
Simches Research Building
185 Cambridge Street
Boston, MA 02114
Telephone: 617-724-2933
www.womensmentalhealth.org

Postpartum Depression

(See also resources listed under *Psychiatric Illness During Pregnancy*)

Depression After Delivery, Inc.
www.depressionafterdelivery.com

Postpartum Support International
927 N. Kellogg Avenue
Santa Barbara, CA 93111
Telephone: 805-967-7636
www.postpartum.net

Pacific Post Partum Support Society
1416 Commercial Drive,
   Suite 104
Vancouver, BC, V5L 3X9
Telephone: 604-255-7999
www.postpartum.org

The Postpartum Stress Center
1062 Lancaster Avenue
Rosemont Plaza, Suite 2
Rosemont, PA 19010
Telephone: 610-525-7527
www.postpartumstress.com

Pregnancy Loss
The Miss Foundation
PO Box 5333
Peoria, AZ 85385-5333
Telephone: 623-979-1000
www.missfoundation.org

Share: Pregnancy and Infant Loss
   Support, Inc.
St. Joseph Health Center
300 First Capitol Drive
St. Charles, MO 63301-2893
Telephone: 800-821-6819 or
   636-947-6164
www.nationalshareoffice.com

Infertility
American Fertility Association
666 Fifth Avenue, Suite 278
New York, NY 10103
Telephone: 888-917-3777
www.theafa.org

International Council on Infertility
   Information Dissemination, Inc.
PO Box 6836
Arlington, VA 22206
Telephone: 703-379-9178
www.inciid.org

RESOLVE
7910 Woodmont Avenue, suite 1350
Bethesda, MD 20814
301-652-8585
888-623-0744
www.resolve.org

Recommended Reading

Depression and Other Mood Disorders

Burns, David D. *Feeling Good: The New Mood Therapy.* New York: Avon, 1999.
———. *The Feeling Good Handbook.* New York: Plume, 1999.
Miklowitz, David J. *The Bipolar Disorder Survival Guide: What You and Your Family Need to Know.* New York: Guilford, 2002.
O'Connor, Richard. *Undoing Depression.* New York: Little, Brown, 1997.
Solomon, Andrew. *The Noonday Demon: An Atlas of Depression.* New York: Scribner, 2001.
Thase, Michael E., and Susan S. Lang. *Beating the Blues: New Approaches to Overcoming Dysthymia and Chronic Mild Depression.* Oxford University Press, 2004.

Depression and Other Mood Disorders: Personal Experiences

Jamison, Kay Redfield. *An Unquiet Mind: A Memoir of Moods and Madness.* New York: Vintage, 1997. (Bipolar Disorder)
Resnick, Suan Kushner. *Sleepless Days: One Woman's Journey Through Postpartum Depression.* New York: St. Martin's Press, 2001.
Shields, Brooke. *Down Came the Rain: My Journey Through Postpartum Depression.* New York: Hyperion, 2005.
Styron, William. *Darkness Visible: A Memoir of Madness.* New York: Vintage, 1992.
Thompson, Tracy. *The Beast: A Journey Through Depression.* New York: Plume, 1996.

Psychological Issues in Pregnancy and the Postpartum Period

Barrett, Nina. *I Wish Someone Had Told Me: A Realistic Guide to Early Motherhood.* Chicago: Academy Chicago Publishers, 1997.
Cohen, Lee S., and Ruta Nonacs. *Mood and Anxiety Disorders During Pregnancy and Postpartum.* Arlington, VA: American Psychiatric Publishing, 2005.
Kleiman, Karen, and Valerie Raskin. *This Isn't What I Expected: Overcoming Postpartum Depression.* New York: Bantam, 1994.
Placksin, Sally. *Mothering the New Mother: Women's Feelings and Needs After*

Childbirth, a Support and Resource Guide. New York: Newmarket Press, 2000.

Depression and Its Impact on the Family

Goodman, Sherryl H., and Ian H. Gotlib. *Children of Depressed Parents: Mechanisms of Risk and Implications for Treatment.* Washington, DC: American Psychological Association, 2001.

Murray, Lynne, and Peter J. Cooper, eds. *Postpartum Depression and Child Development.* New York: Guilford, 1997.

Sheffield, Anne. *Sorrow's Web: Hope, Help, and Understanding for Depressed Mothers and Their Children.* New York: Free Press, 2001.

——. *Depression Fallout: The Impact of Depression on Couples and What You Can Do to Preserve the Bond.* New York: Harper Paperbacks, 2003.

Infertility

Domar, Alice D., and Alice Lesch Kelly. *Conquering Infertility: Dr. Alice Domar's Mind/Body Guide to Enhancing Fertility and Coping with Infertility.* New York: Viking, 2002.

Falker, Elizabeth Swire. *The Infertility Survival Handbook: Everything You Never Thought You'd Need to Know.* New York: Riverhead, 2004.

Wisot, Arthur L., and David R. Meldrum. *Conceptions & Misconceptions: The Informed Consumer's Guide Through the Maze of In Vitro Fertilization & Assisted Reproduction Techniques.* Point Roberts, WA: Hartley and Marks, 1997.

Pregnancy Loss

Douglas, Ann, and John R. Sussman. *Trying Again: A Guide to Pregnancy After Miscarriage, Stillbirth, and Infant Loss.* Dallas: Taylor Publishing, 2000.

Cirulli Lanham, Carol. *Pregnancy After a Loss: A Guide to Pregnancy After a Miscarriage, Stillbirth or Infant Death.* New York: Berkley Books, 1999.

Kohn, Ingrid, Perry-Lynn Moffitt, and Isabelle A. Wilkins. *A Silent Sorrow: Pregnancy Loss—Guidance and Support for You and Your Family.* New York: Brunner-Routledge, 2000.

Lerner, Henry M. *Miscarriage: Why It Happens and How Best to Reduce Your Risks—A Doctor's Guide to the Facts.* New York: Perseus, 2003.

Parenting and the Transition to Parenthood

Belsky, Jay, and John Kelly. *The Transition to Parenthood: How a First Child Changes a Marriage: Why Some Couples Grow Closer and Others Apart.* New York: Delacorte Press, 1994.

Cowan, Carolyn Pepe, and Philip Cowan. *When Partners Become Parents: The Big Life Change for Couples.* New York: Basic Books, 1992.

Gottman, John. *Why Marriages Succeed or Fail and How You Can Make Yours Last.* New York: Simon & Schuster, 1995.

Gottman, John, and Nan Silver. *The Seven Principles for Making Marriage Work: A Practical Guide from the Country's Foremost Relationship Expert.* New York: Crown, 1999.

Jordan, Pamela L., Scott M. Stanley, and Howard J. Markman. *Becoming Parents: How to Strengthen Your Marriage as Your Family Grows.* New York: Jossey-Bass Publishers, 1999.

Karen, Robert. *Becoming Attached: First Relationships and How They Shape Our Capacity to Love.* New York: Oxford University Press, 1998.

Siegel, Daniel J., and Mary Hartzell. *Parenting from the Inside Out: How a Deeper Self-Understanding Can Help You Raise Children Who Thrive.* New York: Jeremy P. Tarcher, 2003.

References

1. A Neglected Problem: Depression During the Childbearing Years

Cohen LS, Nonacs RM, Bailey JW, Viguera AC, Reminick AM, Altshuler LL, Stowe ZN, Faraone SV: Relapse of depression during pregnancy following antidepressant discontinuation: A preliminary prospective study. *Archives of Women's Mental Health* 2004; 7(4):217–21.

Evans J, Heron J, Francomb H, Oke S, Golding J: Cohort study of depressed mood during pregnancy and after childbirth. *British Medical Journal* 2001; 323(7307):257–60.

Evins GG, Theofrastous JP, Galvin SL: Postpartum depression: A comparison of screening and routine clinical evaluation. *American Journal of Obstetrics and Gynecology* 2000; 182(5):1080–82.

Gilman, CP: The yellow wallpaper. *New England Magazine* 1892; 5:647–56.

Goodman SH, Gotlib IH, eds.: *Children of depressed parents: Mechanisms of risk and implications for treatment.* Washington, DC: American Psychological Association, 2001.

Kessler RC, McGonagle KA, Swartz M, Blazer DG, Nelson CB: Sex and depression in the National Comorbidity Survey I: Lifetime prevalence, chronicity and recurrence. *Journal of Affective Disorders* 1993; 29:85–96.

Marcus SM, Flynn HA, Blow FC, Barry KL: Depressive symptoms among pregnant women screened in obstetrics settings. *Journal of Women's Health* 2003; 12(4):373–80.

Murray C, Lopez A, eds.: *The global burden of disease and injury series, volume 1: A comprehensive assessment of mortality and disability from diseases, injuries, and risk factors in 1990 and projected to 2020.* Cambridge, MA: Harvard University Press, 1996.

Murray L: Postpartum depression and child development. *Psychological Medicine* 1997; 27:253–60.

National Institute of Mental Health. *Depression research at the National Institute of Mental Health.* Washington, DC: National Institute of Mental Health, 1999.

National Institute of Mental Health. *The numbers count: Mental disorders in America.* Washington, DC: National Institute of Mental Health, 2001.

Regier DA, Narrow WE, Rae DS, Manderscheid RW, Locke BZ, Goodwin FK: The de facto U.S. mental and addictive disorders service system. Epidemiologic catchment area prospective 1-year prevalence rates of disorders and services. *Archives of General Psychiatry* 1993; 50(2):85–94.

Resnick SK: *Sleepless nights: one woman's journey through postpartum depression.* New York: St. Martin's Press, 2000.

2. Hormones and Mood: Understanding What Causes Depression in Women

Diagnostic and statistical manual of mental disorders, DSM-IV-TR. Arlington, VA: American Psychiatric Publishing, 2000.

Amin Z, Canli T, Epperson CN: Effect of estrogen-serotonin interactions on mood and cognition. *Behavioral & Cognitive Neuroscience Reviews* 2005; 4(1):43–58.

Barnett RC: Women and multiple roles: Myths and reality. *Harvard Review of Psychiatry* 2004; 12(3):158–64.

Barnett RC, Marshall NL: Worker and mother roles, spillover effects, and psychological distress. *Women & Health* 1992; 18(2):9–40.

Barnett RC, Marshall NL, Singer JD: Job experiences over time, multiple roles, and women's mental health: A longitudinal study. *Journal of Personality & Social Psychology* 1992; 62(4):634–44.

Barrett AE, Raskin White H: Trajectories of gender role orientations in adolescence and early adulthood: A prospective study of the mental health effects of masculinity and femininity. *Journal of Health & Social Behavior* 2002; 43(4):451–68.

Barrett LF, Lane RD, Sechrest L, Schwartz GE: Sex differences in emotional awareness. *Personality and Social Psychology Bulletin* 2000; 26(9):1027–35.

Briere J, Runtz M: Childhood sexual abuse: Long-term sequelae and implications for psychological assessment. *Journal of Interpersonal Violence* 1993; 8(3):312–30.

Brown GW, Harris TO: *Social origins of depression: A study of psychiatric disorder in women.* Cambridge: Cambridge University Press, 1978.

Brown GW, Bifulco A, Harris TO: Life events, vulnerability and onset of depression: Some refinements. *British Journal of Psychiatry* 1987; 150:30–42.

Brown GW, Harris TO, Hepworth C: Loss, humiliation and entrapment among women developing depression: A patient and non-patient comparison. *Psychological Medicine* 1995; 25(1):7–21.

Brown GW, Moran PM: Single mothers, poverty and depression. *Psychological Medicine* 1997; 27(1):21–33.

Checkley S: The neuroendocrinology of depression and chronic stress. *British Medical Bulletin* 1996; 52(3):597–617.

Costello EJ: Married with children: Predictors of mental and physical health in middle-aged women. *Psychiatry* 1991; 54(3):292–305.

Cyranowski JM, Frank E, Young E, Shear MK: Adolescent onset of the gender difference in lifetime rates of major depression: A theoretical model. *Archives of General Psychiatry* 2000; 57(1):21–27.

Harris TO, Borsanyi S, Messari S, Stanford K, Cleary SE, Shiers HM, Brown GW, Herbert J: Morning cortisol as a risk factor for subsequent major depressive disorder in adult women. *British Journal of Psychiatry* 2000; 177:505–10.

Helgeson VS: Relation of agency and communion to well-being: Evidence and potential explanations. *Psychological Bulletin* 1994; 116(3):412–28.

Joffe H, Cohen L: Estrogen, serotonin, and mood disturbance: Where is the therapeutic bridge? *Biological Psychiatry* 1998; 44:798–811.

Jorm AF: Sex and age differences in depression: A quantitative synthesis of published research. *Australian & New Zealand Journal of Psychiatry* 1987; 21(1):46–53.

Kapusta MA, Frank S: The book of Job and the modern view of depression. *Annals of Internal Medicine* 1977; 86(5):667–72.

Kessler R, McLeod J: Sex differences in vulnerability to undesirable life events. *American Sociological Review* 1984; 49:620–31.

Kessler RC, McGonagle KA, Swartz M, Blazer DG, Nelson CB: Sex and depression in the national comorbidity survey I: Lifetime prevalence, chronicity and recurrence. *Journal of Affective Disorders* 1993; 29:85–96.

Levine S: Influence of psychological variables on the activity of the hypothalamic-pituitary-adrenal axis. *European Journal of Pharmacology* 2000; 405(1–3):149–60.

Matthews PM, McQuain J: *The bard on the brain: Understanding the mind through the art of Shakespeare and the science of brain imaging.* Chicago: University of Chicago Press, 2003.

McDermott JF, et al.: Reexamining the concept of adolescence: Differences between adolescent boys and girls in the context of their families. *Annual Progress in Child Psychiatry & Child Development* 1984:155–65.

McLeod JD: Childhood parental loss and adult depression. *Journal of Health & Social Behavior* 1991; 32(3):205–20.

McLeod JD, Kessler RC: Socioeconomic status differences in vulnerability to undesirable life events. *Journal of Health & Social Behavior* 1990; 31(2):162–72.

National Mental Health Association: *American attitudes about clinical depression and its treatment.* Washington, DC: National Mental Health Association, 1996.

Nolen-Hoeksema S, Girgus JS: The emergence of gender differences in depression during adolescence. *Psychological Bulletin* 1994; 115(3):424–43.

Nolen-Hoeksema S, Larson J, Grayson C: Explaining the gender difference in depressive symptoms. *Journal of Personality & Social Psychology* 1999; 77(5):1061–72.

Rubinow DR, Schmidt PJ, Roca CA: Estrogen-serotonin interactions: implications for affective regulation. *Biological Psychiatry* 1998; 44(9):839–50.

Ruble DN, Greulich F, Pomerantz EM, Gochberg B: The role of gender-related processes in the development of sex differences in self-evaluation and depression. *Journal of Affective Disorders* 1993; 29(2–3):97–128.

Seeman MV: Psychopathology in women and men: focus on female hormones. *American Journal of Psychiatry* 1997; 154(12):1641–47.

Simon RW: Parental role strains, salience of parental identity and gender differences in psychological distress. *Journal of Health & Social Behavior* 1992; 33(1):25–35.

Solomon A: *The noonday demon: An atlas of depression.* New York: Scribner, 2001.

Weinstock M: Does prenatal stress impair coping and regulation of hypothalamic-pituitary-adrenal axis? *Neuroscience & Biobehavioral Reviews* 1997; 21(1):1–10.

Weissman MM, Bland R, Joyce PR, Newman S, Wells JE, Wittchen HU: Sex differences in rates of depression: Cross-national perspectives. *Journal of Affective Disorders* 1993; 29(2–3):77–84.

Weissman MM, Klerman G: *Gender and depression.* Formanek, Ruth, 1987.

3. The Ripple Effect: How Depression Affects the Family

Abrams SM, Field T, Scafidi F, Prodromidis M: Newborns of depressed mothers. *Infant Mental Health Journal* 1995; 16(3):233–39.

Alpern L, Lyons-Ruth K: Preschool children at social risk: Chronicity and timing of maternal depressive symptoms and child behavior problems at school and at home. *Development and Psychopathology* 1993; 5(3):371–87.

Armstrong KL, Van Haeringen AR, Dadds MR, Cash R: Sleep deprivation or postnatal depression in later infancy: Separating the chicken from the egg. *Journal of Paediatrics & Child Health* 1998; 34(3):260–62.

Ashman SB, Dawson G, Panagiotides H, Yamada E, Wilkinson CW: Stress hormone levels of children of depressed mothers. *Development & Psychopathology* 2002; 14(2):333–49.

Austin MP, Hadzi-Pavlovic D, Leader L, Saint K, Parker G: Maternal trait anxiety, depression and life event stress in pregnancy: Relationships with infant temperament. *Early Human Development* 2005; 81(2):183–90.

Beardslee WR, Versage EM, Gladstone TR: Children of affectively ill parents: A review of the past 10 years. *Journal of the American Academy of Child & Adolescent Psychiatry* 1998; 37(11):1134–41.

Berle JO, Mykletun A, Daltveit AK, Rasmussen S, Holsten F, Dahl AA: Neonatal outcomes in offspring of women with anxiety and depression during pregnancy. A linkage study from The Nord-Trondelag Health Study (HUNT) and Medical Birth Registry of Norway. *Archives of Women's Mental Health* 2005; 8(3):181–89.

Beck C: The effects of postpartum depression on child development: A meta-analysis. *Archives of Psychiatric Nursing* 1998; 12(1):12–20.

Bonari L, Pinto N, Ahn E, Einarson A, Steiner M, Koren G: Perinatal risks of untreated depression during pregnancy. *Canadian Journal of Psychiatry* 2004; 49(11): 726–35.

Bowlby J: *Secure base: Parent-child attachment and healthy human development.* New York: Basic Books, 1990.

Cicchetti D, Rogosch FA, Toth SL: Maternal depressive disorder and contextual risk: Contributions to the development of attachment insecurity and behavior problems in toddlerhood. *Developmental Psychopathology* 1998; 10(2):283–300.

Clarke GN, Hornbrook M, Lynch F, Polen M, Gale J, Beardslee W, O'Connor E, Seeley J: A randomized trial of a group cognitive intervention for preventing depression in adolescent offspring of depressed parents. *Archives of General Psychiatry* 2001; 58(12):1127–34.

Cogill SR, Caplan HL, Alexandra H, Robson KM, Kumar R: Impact of maternal depression on cognitive development of young children. *British Medical Journal* 1986; 292:1165–67.

Cummings E, Davies P: Maternal deprssion and child development. *Journal of Child Psychology and Psychiatry* 1994; 35:73–112.

Diego MA, Field T, Hernandez-Reif M, Cullen C, Schanberg S, Kuhn C: Prepartum, postpartum, and chronic depression effects on newborns. *Psychiatry* 2004; 67(1):63–80.

Downey G, Coyne J: Children of depressed parents: An integrative review. *Psychological Bulletin* 1990; 108:1–27.

Essex MJ, Klein MH, Cho E, Kalin NH: Maternal stress beginning in infancy may sensitize children to later stress exposure: Effects on cortisol and behavior. *Biological Psychiatry* 2002; 52(8):776–84.

Essex MJ, Klein MH, Cho E, Kraemer HC: Exposure to maternal depression and marital conflict: Gender differences in children's later mental health symptoms. *Journal of the American Academy of Child & Adolescent Psychiatry* 2003; 42(6):728–37.

Essex MJ, Klein MH, Miech R, Smider NA: Timing of initial exposure to maternal major depression and children's mental health symptoms in kindergarten. *British Journal of Psychiatry* 2001; 179:151–56.

Field T: Early interventions for infants of depressed mothers. *Pediatrics* 1305; 102(5 Suppl E):1305–10.

Field T: Maternal depression effects on infants and early interventions. *Preventive Medicine* 1998; 27(2):200–203.

Field T, Diego M, Hernandez-Reif M, Gil K, Vera Y: Prenatal maternal cortisol, fetal activity and growth. *International Journal of Neuroscience* 2005; 115(3):423–29.

Field T, Diego M, Dieter J, Hernandez-Reif M, Schanberg S, Kuhn C, Yando R, Bendell D: Prenatal depression effects on the fetus and the newborn. *Infant Behavior & Development* 2004; 27(2):216–29.

Field T, Diego M, Hernandez-Reif M, Salman F, Schanberg S, Kuhn C, Yando R,

Bendell D: Prenatal anger effects on the fetus and neonate. *Journal of Obstetrics & Gynaecology* 2002; 22(3):260–66.

Field T, Diego M, Hernandez-Reif M, Schanberg S, Kuhn C, Yando R, Bendell D: Pregnancy anxiety and comorbid depression and anger: Effects on the fetus and neonate. *Depression & Anxiety* 2003; 17(3):140–51.

Field T, Grizzle N, Scafidi F, Abrams S, Richardson S, Kuhn C, Schanberg S: Massage therapy for infants of depressed mothers. *Infant Behavior & Development* 1996; 19(1):107–12.

Field T, Healy B, Goldstein S, Perry S, Bendell D, Schanberg S, Zimmerman EA, Kuhn C: Infants of depressed mothers show "depressed" behavior even with nondepressed adults. *Child Development* 1988; 59(6):1569–79.

Goodman SH, Gotlib IH: Risk for psychopathology in the children of depressed mothers: A developmental model for understanding mechanisms of transmission. *Psychological Review* 1999; 106(3):458–90.

Goodman SH, Gotlib IH, eds.: *Children of depressed parents: Mechanisms of risk and implications for treatment.* Washington, DC: American Psychological Association, 2001.

Hammen C, Adrian C, Hiroto D: A longitudinal test of the attributional vulnerability model in children at risk for depression. *British Journal of Clinical Psychology* 1988; 27(Pt. 1):37–46.

Hammen C, Brennan PA: Severity, chronicity, and timing of maternal depression and risk for adolescent offspring diagnoses in a community sample. *Archives of General Psychiatry* 2003; 60(3):253–58.

Hart S, Field T, Roitfarb M: Depressed mothers' assessments of their neonates' behaviors. *Infant Mental Health Journal* 1999; 20(2):200–210.

Hay DF, Pawlby S, Sharp D, Asten P, Mills A, Kumar R: Intellectual problems shown by 11-year-old children whose mothers had postnatal depression. *J Child Psychol Psychiatry* 2001; 42(7):871–89.

Hiscock H, Wake M: Infant sleep problems and postnatal depression: A community-based study. *Pediatrics* 1317; 107(6):1317–22.

Hossain Z, Field T, Gonzalez J, Malphurs J, et al.: Infants of "depressed" mothers interact better with their nondepressed fathers. *Infant Mental Health Journal* 1994; 15(4):348–57.

Jones NA, Field T, Fox NA, Davalos M, Lundy B, Hart S: Newborns of mothers with depressive symptoms are physiologically less developed. *Infant Behavior & Development* 1998; 21(3):537–41.

Katz LF, Gottman JM: Patterns of marital conflict predict children's internalizing and externalizing behaviors. *Developmental Psychology* 1993; 29(6):940–50.

Kerr S, Jowett S: Sleep problems in preschool children: a review of the literature. *Child: Care, Health & Development* 1994; 20(6):379–91.

Kramer RA, Warner V, Olfson M, Ebanks CM, Chaput F, Weissman MM: General medical problems among the offspring of depressed parents: A 10-year follow-up. *Journal of the American Academy of Child & Adolescent Psychiatry* 1998; 37(6):602–11.

Leiferman J: The effect of maternal depressive symptomatology on maternal behaviors associated with child health. *Health Education & Behavior* 2002; 29(5):596–607.

Lesesne CA, Visser SN, White CP: Attention-deficit/hyperactivity disorder in school-aged children: Association with maternal mental health and use of health care resources. *Pediatrics* 1232; 111(5 Part 2):1232–37.

Lundy B, Field T, Pickens J: Newborns of mothers with depressive symptoms are less expressive. *Infant Behavior & Development* 1996; 19(4):419–24.

Lundy BL, Field T, Cuadra A, Nearing G, Cigales M, Hashimoto M: Mothers with depressive symptoms touching newborns. *Early Development & Parenting* 1996; 5(3):129–34.

Lundy BL, Jones NA, Field T, Nearing G, Davalos M, Pietro PA, Schanberg S, Kuhn C: Prenatal depression effects on neonates. *Infant Behavior & Development* 1999; 22(1):119–29.

Luoma I, Tamminen T, Kaukonen P, Laippala P, Puura K, Salmelin R, Almqvist F: Longitudinal study of maternal depressive symptoms and child well-being. *Journal of the American Academy of Child and Adolescent Psychiatry* 2001; 40(12):1367–74.

Lyons-Ruth K, Wolfe R, Lyubchik A: Depression and the parenting of young children: Making the case for early preventive mental health services. *Harvard Review of Psychiatry* 2000; 8(3):148–53.

Maccari S, Darnaudery M, Morley-Fletcher S, Zuena AR, Cinque C, Van Reeth O: Prenatal stress and long-term consequences: Implications of glucocorticoid hormones. *Neuroscience & Biobehavioral Reviews* 2003; 27(1–2):119–27.

Martins C, Gaffan EA: Effects of early maternal depression on patterns of infant-mother attachment: A meta-analytic investigation. *Journal of Child Psychology & Psychiatry & Allied Disciplines* 2000; 41(6):737–46.

Murray L: The impact of postnatal depression on infant development. *Journal of Child Psychology and Psychiatry* 1992; 33:543–61.

Murray L, Cooper P, eds. *Postpartum depression and child development.* New York: Guilford, 1997.

Murray L, Cooper PJ: The impact of postpartum depression on child development. *International Review of Psychiatry* 1996; 8:55–63.

Murray L, Fiori-Cowley A, Hooper R, Cooper P: The impact of postnatal depression and associated adversity on early mother-infant interactions and later infant outcome. *Child Development* 1996; 67(5):2512–26.

Murray L, Hipwell A, Hooper R, Stein A, Cooper P: The cognitive development of 5-year-old children of postnatally depressed mothers. *Journal of Child Psychology & Psychiatry & Allied Disciplines* 1996; 37(8):927–35.

Onozawa K, Glover V, Adams D, et al.: Infant massage improves mother-infant interaction for mothers with postnatal depression. *Journal of Affective Disorders* 2001; 63(1–3):201–7.

Pelaez-Nogueras M, Field TM, Hossain Z, Pickens J: Depressed mothers' touching increases infants' positive affect and attention in still-face interactions. *Child Development* 1780; 67(4):1780–92.

Radke-Yarrow M, Nottelmann E, Martinez P, Fox MB, Belmont B: Young children of affectively ill parents: A longitudinal study of psychosocial development. *Journal of the American Academy of Child & Adolescent Psychiatry* 1992; 31(1):68–77.

Sameroff AJ, Seifer R, Barocas R: Impact of parental psychopathology: Diagnosis, severity, or social status effects. *Infant Mental Health Journal* 1983; 4(3):236–49.

Sameroff AJ, Seifer R, Zax M: Early development of children at risk for emotional disorder. *Monographs of the Society for Research in Child Development* 1982; 47(7):1–82.

Sinclair D, Murray L: Effects of postnatal depression on children's adjustment to school. Teacher's reports. *British Journal of Psychiatry* 1998; 172:58–63.

Stern D: *The interpersonal world of the infant.* New York: Basic Books, 1985.

Teti D, Gelfand D, Messinger D: Maternal depression and the quality of early attachment: An examination of infants, preschoolers, and their mothers. *Developmental Psychology* 1995; 31:364–76.

Turner C, Boyle F, O'Rourke P: Mothers' health post-partum and their patterns of seeking vaccination for their infants. *International Journal of Nursing Practice* 2003; 9(2):120–26.

Warner V, Mufson L, Weissman MM: Offspring at high and low risk for depression and anxiety: mechanisms of psychiatric disorder. *Journal of the American Academy of Child & Adolescent Psychiatry* 1995; 34(6):786–97.

Weinberg M, Tronick E: The impact of maternal psychiatric illness on infant development. *Journal of Clinical Psychiatry* 1998; 59 (suppl. 2):53–61.

Weissman MM, John K, Merikangas KR, Prusoff BA, Wickramaratne P, Gammon GD, Angold A, Warner V: Depressed parents and their children. General health, social, and psychiatric problems. *American Journal of Diseases of Children* 1986; 140(8): 801–5.

Weissman MM, Warner V, Wickramaratne P, Moreau D, Olfson M: Offspring of depressed parents. 10 years later. *Archives of General Psychiatry* 1997; 54(10):932–40.

Wickramaratne PJ, Weissman MM: Onset of psychopathology in offspring by developmental phase and parental depression. *Journal of the American Academy of Child & Adolescent Psychiatry* 1998; 37(9):933–42.

4. Modern Technology Meets Mother Nature: Getting Pregnant

Anderson KM, Sharpe M, Rattray A, Irvine DS: Distress and concerns in couples referred to a specialist infertility clinic. *Journal of Psychosomatic Research* 2003; 54(4): 353–55.

Beaurepaire J, Jones M, Thiering P, Saunders D, Tennant C: Psychosocial adjustment to infertility and its treatment: Male and female responses at different stages of IVF/ET treatment. *Journal of Psychosomatic Research* 1994; 38(3):229–40.

Berghuis JP, Stanton AL: Adjustment to a dyadic stressor: A longitudinal study of coping and depressive symptoms in infertile couples over an insemination attempt. *Journal of Consulting and Clinical Psychology* 2002; 70(2):433–38.

Chen TH, Chang SP, Tsai CF, Juang KD: Prevalence of depressive and anxiety disorders in an assisted reproductive technique clinic. *Human Reproduction* 2004; 19(10):2313–18.

de Klerk C, Hunfeld JA, Duivenvoorden HJ, den Outer MA, Fauser BC, Passchier J, Macklon NS: Effectiveness of a psychosocial counseling intervention for first-time IVF couples: A randomized controlled trial. *Human Reproduction* 1333; 20(5):1333–38.

de Liz TM, Strauss B: Differential efficacy of group and individual/couple psychotherapy with infertile patients. *Human Reproduction* 1324; 20(5):1324–32.

Demyttenaere K, Bonte L, Gheldof M, Vervaeke M, Meuleman C, Vanderschuerem D, D'Hooghe T: Coping style and depression level influence outcome in in-vitro fertilization. *Fertility & Sterility* 1998; 69(6):1026–33.

Demyttenaere K, Nijs P, Evers-Kiebooms G, Koninckx PR: Coping, ineffectiveness of coping and the psychoendocrinological stress responses during in-vitro fertilization. *Journal of Psychosomatic Research* 1991; 35(2–3):231–43.

Demyttenaere K, Nijs P, Evers-Kiebooms G, Koninckx PR: Personality characteristics, psychoendocrinological stress and outcome of IVF depend upon the etiology of infertility. *Gynecological Endocrinology* 1994; 8(4):233–40.

Domar AD: Impact of psychological factors on dropout rates in insured infertility patients. *Fertility & Sterility* 2004; 81(2):271–73.

Domar AD, Broome A, Zuttermeister PC, Seibel M, Friedman R: The prevalence and predictability of depression in infertile women. *Fertility & Sterility* 1158; 58(6): 1158–63.

Domar AD, Clapp D, Slawsby E, Kessel B, Orav J, Freizinger M: The impact of group psychological interventions on distress in infertile women. *Health Psychology* 2000; 19(6):568–75.

Domar AD, Clapp D, Slawsby EA, Dusek J, Kessel B, Freizinger M: Impact of group psychological interventions on pregnancy rates in infertile women. *Fertility & Sterility* 2000; 73(4):805–11.

Domar AD, Seibel MM, Benson H: The mind/body program for infertility: A new behavioral treatment approach for women with infertility. *Fertility & Sterility* 1990; 53(2):246–49.

Domar AD, Zuttermeister PC, Friedman R: The psychological impact of infertility: A comparison with patients with other medical conditions. *Journal of Psychosomatic Obstetrics & Gynecology* 1993; 14:45–52.

Hammarberg K, Astbury J, Baker H: Women's experience of IVF: A follow-up study. *Human Reproduction* 2001; 16(2):374–83.

Hynes GJ, Callan VJ, Terry DJ, Gallois C: The psychological well-being of infertile women after a failed IVF attempt: The effects of coping. *British Journal of Medical Psychology* 1992; 65(3):269–78.

Kemeter P: Studies on psychosomatic implications of infertility—effects of emotional stress on fertilization and implantation in in-vitro fertilization. *Human Reproduction* 1988; 3(3):341–52.

Lapane KL, Zierler S, Lasater TM, Stein M, Barbour MM, Hume AL: Is a history of depressive symptoms associated with an increased risk of infertility in women? *Psychosomatic Medicine* 1995; 57(6):509–13.

Lemmens GM, Vervaeke M, Enzlin P, Bakelants E, Vanderschueren D, D'Hooghe T, Demyttenaere K: Coping with infertility: a body-mind group intervention programme for infertile couples. *Human Reproduction* 1917; 19(8):1917–23.

Lukse MP, Vacc NA: Grief, depression, and coping in women undergoing infertility treatment. *Obstetrics & Gynecology* 1999; 93(2):245–51.

Nonacs R, Cohen L: Approach to the patient with infertility. In *The MGH guide to psychiatry and primary care*, ed. Stern T, Herman J, Slavin P, 289–95. New York: McGraw Hill, 1998.

Olivius C, Friden B, Borg G, Bergh C: Why do couples discontinue in vitro fertilization treatment? A cohort study. *Fertility & Sterility* 2004; 81(2):258–61.

O'Moore MA, Harrison RF: Anxiety and reproductive failure: Experiences from a Dublin fertility clinic. *Irish Journal of Psychology* 1991; 12(2):276–85.

Sanders KA, Bruce NW: Psychosocial stress and treatment outcome following assisted reproductive technology. *Human Reproduction* 1656; 14(6):1656–62.

Shepherd J: Stress management and infertility. *Australian & New Zealand Journal of Obstetrics & Gynecology* 1992; 32(4):353–56.

Smeenk JM, Verhaak CM, Eugster A, van Minnen A, Zielhuis GA, Braat DD: The effect of anxiety and depression on the outcome of in-vitro fertilization. *Human Reproduction* 2001; 16(7):1420–23.

Terzioglu F: Investigation into effectiveness of counseling on assisted reproductive techniques in Turkey. *Journal of Psychosomatic Obstetrics & Gynecology* 2001; 22(3):133–41.

Thiering P, Beaurepaire J, Jones M, Saunders D, Tennant C: Mood state as a predictor of treatment outcome after in vitro fertilization/embryo transfer technology (IVF/ET). *Journal of Psychosomatic Research* 1993; 37(5):481–91.

Verhaak CM, Smeenk JM, van Minnen A, Kremer JA, Kraaimaat FW: A longitudinal, prospective study on emotional adjustment before, during and after consecutive fertility treatment cycles. *Human Reproduction* 2005; 20(8):2253–60.

Wasser SK, Sewall G, Soules MR: Psychosocial stress as a cause of infertility. *Fertility & Sterility* 1993; 59(3):685–89.

Wright J, Allard M, Lecours A, Sabourin S: Psychosocial distress and infertility: A review of controlled research. *International Journal of Fertility* 1989; 34(2):126–42.

Wright J, Duchesne C, Sabourin S, Bissonnette F, Benoit J, Girard Y: Psychosocial distress and infertility: Men and women respond differently. *Fertility & Sterility* 1991; 55(1):100–108.

5. Unexpected Tragedies: Coping with Pregnancy Loss and Other Complications

Armstrong DS: Impact of prior perinatal loss on subsequent pregnancies. *Journal of Obstetric, Gynecologic, & Neonatal Nursing* 2004; 33(6):765–73.

Bradshaw Z, Slade P: The effects of induced abortion on emotional experiences and relationships: A critical review of the literature. *Clinical Psychology Review* 2003; 23(7):929–58.

Craig M, Tata P, Regan L: Psychiatric morbidity among patients with recurrent miscarriage. *Journal of Psychosomatic Obstetrics & Gynecology* 2002; 23(3):157–64.

Davies V, Gledhill J, McFadyen A, Whitlow B, Economides D: Psychological outcome in women undergoing termination of pregnancy for ultrasound-detected fetal anomaly in the first and second trimesters: A pilot study. *Ultrasound in Obstetrics & Gynecology* 2005; 25(4):389–92.

Geller PA, Klier CM, Neugebauer R: Anxiety disorders following miscarriage. *Journal of Clinical Psychiatry* 2001; 62(6):432–38.

Hughes P, Turton P, Hopper E, McGauley GA, Fonagy P: Disorganised attachment behaviour among infants born subsequent to stillbirth. *Journal of Child Psychology & Psychiatry & Allied Disciplines* 2001; 42(6):791–801.

Hughes PM, Turton P, Evans CD: Stillbirth as risk factor for depression and anxiety in the subsequent pregnancy: Cohort study. *British Medical Journal* 1999; 318(7200):1721–24.

Klier CM, Geller PA, Neugebauer R: Minor depressive disorder in the context of miscarriage. *Journal of Affective Disorders* 2000; 59(1):13–21.

Klock SC, Chang G, Hiley A, Hill J: Psychological distress among women with recurrent spontaneous abortion. *Psychosomatics* 1997; 38(5):503–7.

Lobel M, Dias L, Meyer BA: Distress associated with prenatal screening for fetal abnormality. *Journal of Behavioral Medicine* 2005; 28(1):65–76.

McKinney MK, Tuber SB, Downey JI: Multifetal pregnancy reduction: Psychodynamic implications. *Psychiatry* 1996; 59(4):393–407.

Neugebauer R: Depressive symptoms at two months after miscarriage: Interpreting study findings from an epidemiological versus clinical perspective. *Depression & Anxiety* 2003; 17(3):152–61.

Neugebauer R, Kline J, O'Connor P, Shrout P, Johnson J, Skodol A, Wicks J, Susser M: Determinants of depressive symptoms in the early weeks after miscarriage. *American Journal of Public Health* 1992; 82(10):1332–39.

Neugebauer R, Kline J, O'Connor P, Shrout P, Johnson J, Skodol A, Wicks J, Susser M: Depressive symptoms in women in the six months after miscarriage. *American Journal of Obstetrics & Gynecology* 1992; 166(1 Pt. 1):104–9.

Neugebauer R, Kline J, Shrout P, Skodol A, O'Connor P, Geller PA, Stein Z, Susser

M: Major depressive disorder in the 6 months after miscarriage. *JAMA* 1997; 277(5): 383–88.

O'Leary J: Grief and its impact on prenatal attachment in the subsequent pregnancy. *Archives of Women's Mental Health* 2004; 7(1):7–18.

Ritsher JB, Neugebauer R: Perinatal Bereavement Grief Scale: Distinguishing grief from depression following miscarriage. *Assessment* 2002; 9(1):31–40.

Schreiner-Engel P, Walther VN, Mindes J, Lynch L, Berkowitz RL: First-trimester multifetal pregnancy reduction: Acute and persistent psychologic reactions. *American Journal of Obstetrics & Gynecology* 1995; 172(2 Pt. 1):541–47.

Turton P, Hughes P, Evans CD, Fainman D: Incidence, correlates and predictors of posttraumatic stress disorder in the pregnancy after stillbirth. *British Journal of Psychiatry* 2001; 178:556–60.

Turton P, Hughes P, Fonagy P, Fainman D: An investigation into the possible overlap between PTSD and unresolved responses following stillbirth: An absence of linkage with only unresolved status predicting infant disorganization. *Attachment & Human Development* 2004; 6(3):241–53.

6. A Not-So-Rosy Blush: Depression During Pregnancy

Altshuler LL, Hendrick V, Cohen LS: An update on mood and anxiety disorders during pregnancy and the postpartum period. *Primary Care Companion Journal of Clinical Psychiatry* 2000; 2(6):217–22.

Andersson L, Sundstrom-Poromaa I, Bixo M, Wulff M, Bondestam K, Astrom M: Point prevalence of psychiatric disorders during the second trimester of pregnancy: A population-based study. *American Journal of Obstetrics & Gynecology* 2003; 189(1):148–54.

Andersson L, Sundstrom-Poromaa I, Wulff M, Astrom M, Bixo M: Implications of antenatal depression and anxiety for obstetric outcome. *Obstetrics & Gynecology* 2004; 104(3):467–76.

Andersson L, Sundstrom-Poromaa I, Wulff M, Astrom M, Bixo M: Neonatal outcome following maternal antenatal depression and anxiety: A population-based study. *American Journal of Epidemiology* 2004; 159(9):872–81.

Austin MP, Hadzi-Pavlovic D, Leader L, Saint K, Parker G: Maternal trait anxiety, depression and life event stress in pregnancy: Relationships with infant temperament. *Early Human Development* 2005; 81(2):183–90.

Berle JO, Mykletun A, Daltveit AK, Rasmussen S, Holsten F, Dahl AA: Neonatal outcomes in offspring of women with anxiety and depression during pregnancy. A linkage study from the Nord-Trondelag Health Study (HUNT) and Medical Birth Registry of Norway. *Archives of Women's Mental Health* 2005; 8(3):181–89.

Bolton HL, Hughes PM, Turton P, Sedgwick P: Incidence and demographic correlates of depressive symptoms during pregnancy in an inner London population. *Journal of Psychosomatic Obstetrics & Gynecology* 1998; 19(4):202–9.

Bonari L, Pinto N, Ahn E, Einarson A, Steiner M, Koren G: Perinatal risks of untreated depression during pregnancy. *Canadian Journal of Psychiatry* 2004; 49 (11):726–35.

Buist A, Bilszta J, Barnett B, Milgrom J, Ericksen J, Condon J, Hayes B, Brooks J: Recognition and management of perinatal depression in general practice — a survey of GPs and postnatal women. *Australian Family Physician* 2005; 34(9):787–90.

Cohen LS, Altshuler LL, Harlow BL, Nonacs R, et al.: Relapse of major depression during pregnancy in women who maintain or discontinue antidepressant treatment. *JAMA* 2006; 295:499–507.

Cohen LS, Nonacs R, eds.: *Mood and anxiety disorders during pregnancy and post-partum*. Arlington, VA: *American Psychiatric Publishing*, 2005.

Cohen LS, Nonacs RM, Bailey JW, Viguera AC, Reminick AM, Altshuler LL, Stowe ZN, Faraone SV: Relapse of depression during pregnancy following antidepressant discontinuation: A preliminary prospective study. *Archives of Women's Mental Health* 2004; 7(4):217–21.

Collins NL, Dunkel-Schetter C, Lobel M, Scrimshaw SCM: Social support in pregnancy: Psychosocial correlates of birth outcomes and postpartum depression. *Journal of Personality and Social Psychology* 1993; 65(6):1243–58.

Dayan J, Creveuil C, Herlicoviez M, Herbel C, Baranger E, Savoye C, Thouin A: Role of anxiety and depression in the onset of spontaneous preterm labor. *American Journal of Epidemiology* 2002; 155(4):293–301.

Dipietro JA, Millet S, Costigan KA, Gurewitsch E, Caulfield LE: Psychosocial influences on weight gain attitudes and behaviors during pregnancy. *Journal of the American Dietetic Association* 1314; 103(10):1314–19.

Evans J, Heron J, Francomb H, Oke S, Golding J: Cohort study of depressed mood during pregnancy and after childbirth. *British Medical Journal* 2001; 323(7307): 257–60.

Field T, Diego M, Hernandez-Reif M, Gil K, Vera Y: Prenatal maternal cortisol, fetal activity and growth. *International Journal of Neuroscience* 2005; 115(3):423–29.

Geller PA: Pregnancy as a stressful life event. *CNS Spectrums* 2004; 9(3):188–97.

Gotlib IH, Whiffen VE, Mount JH, Milne K, Cordy NI: Prevalence rates and demographic characteristics associated with depression in pregnancy and the postpartum period. *Journal of Consulting and Clinical Psychology* 1989; 57:269–74.

Halbreich U: Prevalence of mood symptoms and depressions during pregnancy: Implications for clinical practice and research. *CNS Spectrums* 2004; 9(3):177–84.

Jesse DE, Seaver W, Wallace DC: Maternal psychosocial risks predict preterm birth in a group of women from Appalachia. *Midwifery* 2003; 19(3):191–202.

Larsson C, Sydsjo G, Josefsson A: Health, sociodemographic data, and pregnancy outcome in women with antepartum depressive symptoms. *Obstetrics & Gynecology* 2004; 104(3):459–66.

Lundy BL, Jones NA, Field T, Nearing G, Davalos M, Pietro PA, Schanberg S, Kuhn C: Prenatal depression effects on neonates. *Infant Behavior & Development* 1999; 22(1):119–29.

Maccari S, Darnaudery M, Morley-Fletcher S, Zuena AR, Cinque C, Van Reeth O: Prenatal stress and long-term consequences: Implications of glucocorticoid hormones. *Neuroscience & Biobehavioral Reviews* 2003; 27(1–2):119–27.

Marcus SM, Flynn HA, Blow F, Barry K: A screening study of antidepressant treatment rates and mood symptoms in pregnancy. *Archives of Women's Mental Health* 2005; 8(1):25–27.

Marcus SM, Flynn HA, Blow FC, Barry KL: Depressive symptoms among pregnant women screened in obstetrics settings. *Journal of Women's Health* 2003; 12(4):373–80.

Nelson DB, McMahon K, Joffe M, Brensinger C: The effect of depressive symptoms and optimism on the risk of spontaneous abortion among innercity women. *Journal of Women's Health* 2003; 12(6):569–76.

Nonacs R, Cohen L: Assessment and treatment of depression during pregnancy: An update. *Psychiatric Clinics of North America*. 2003; 26(3):547–62.

Nonacs R, Viguera A, Cohen L: Psychiatric aspects of pregnancy. In *Women's mental health*, ed. Clayton AH and Kornstein SC. New York: Guilford, 2001.

O'Hara MW: Social support, life events, and depression during pregnancy and the puerperium. *Archives of General Psychiatry* 1986; 43:569–73.

Orr S, James SA, Blackmore Prince C.: Maternal prenatal depressive symptoms and spontaneous preterm births among African-American women in Baltimore, Maryland. *American Journal of Epidemiology* 2002; 156(9):797–802.

Orr S, Miller C: Maternal depressive symptoms and the risk of poor pregnancy outcome. Review of the literature and preliminary findings. *Epidemiologic Reviews* 1995; 17(1):165–71.

Rubertsson C, Wickberg B, Gustavsson P, Radestad I: Depressive symptoms in early pregnancy, two months and one year postpartum—prevalence and psychosocial risk factors in a national Swedish sample. *Archives of Women's Mental Health* 2005; 8(2):97–104.

Sleath B, West S, Tudor G, Perreira K, King V, Morrissey J: Ethnicity and depression treatment preferences of pregnant women. *Journal of Psychosomatic Obstetrics & Gynecology* 2005; 26(2):135–40.

Sondergaard C, Olsen J, Friis-Hasche E, Dirdal M, Thrane N, Sorensen HT: Psychosocial distress during pregnancy and the risk of infantile colic: A follow-up study. *Acta Paediatrica* 2003; 92(7):811–16.

Steer RA, Scholl TO, Hediger ML, Fischer RL: Self-reported depression and negative pregnancy outcomes. *Journal of Clinical Epidemiology* 1992; 45(10):1093–99.

Sugiura-Ogasawara M, Furukawa TA, Nakano Y, Hori S, Aoki K, Kitamura T: Depression as a potential causal factor in subsequent miscarriage in recurrent spontaneous aborters. *Human Reproduction* 2002; 17(10):2580–84.

Thoppil J, Riutcel TL, Nalesnik SW: Early intervention for perinatal depression. *American Journal of Obstetrics & Gynecology* 2005; 192(5):1446–48.

Viguera AC, Nonacs R, Cohen LS, Tondo L, Murray A, Baldessarini RJ: Risk of recurrence of bipolar disorder in pregnant and nonpregnant women after discontinuing lithium maintenance. *American Journal of Psychiatry* 2000; 157(2):179–84.

Viguera AC, Cohen LS, Baldessarini RJ, Nonacs R: Managing bipolar disorder during pregnancy: Weighing the risks and benefits. *Canadian Journal of Psychiatry* 2002; 47:426–36.

Zuckerman B, Bauchner H, Parker S, Cabral H: Maternal depressive symptoms during pregnancy, and newborn irritability. *Journal of Developmental and Behavioral Pediatrics* 1990; 11(4):190–94.

Zuckerman BS, Amaro H, Bauchner H, et al.: Depression during pregnancy: Relationship to prior health behaviors. *American Journal of Obstetrics and Gynecology* 1989; 160:1107–11.

7. Crying for No Good Reason: Baby Blues and the Transition to Motherhood

American Academy of Pediatrics: Ten steps to support parents' choice to breastfeed their baby. American Academy of Pediatrics Work Group on Breastfeeding. *Pediatric Clinics of North America* 2001; 48(2):533–37.

Arpels JC: The female brain hypoestrogenic continuum from the premenstrual syndrome to menopause: A hypothesis and review of supporting data. *Journal of Reproductive Medicine* 1996; 41(9):633–39.

Dinges DF, Pack F, Williams K, Gillen KA, Powell JW, Ott GE, Aptowicz C, Pack AI: Cumulative sleepiness, mood disturbance, and psychomotor vigilance performance decrements during a week of sleep restricted to 4–5 hours per night. *Sleep* 1997; 20(4):267–77.

Feksi A, Harris B, Walker RF, et al.: "Maternity blues" and hormone levels in saliva. *Journal of Affective Disorders* 1984; 6:351.

Fossey L, Papiernik E, Bydlowski M: Postpartum blues: A clinical syndrome and predictor of postnatal depression? *Journal of Psychosomatic Obstetrics & Gynecology* 1997; 18(1):17–21.

Heidrich A, Schleyer M, Spingler H, Albert P, Knoche M, Fritze J, Lanczik M: Postpartum blues: Relationship between not-protein bound steroid in plasma and postpartum mood changes. *Journal of Affective Disorders* 1994; 30:93–98.

Henshaw C: Mood disturbance in the early puerperium: A review. *Archives of Women's Mental Health* 2003; 6 Suppl 2:S33–42.

Henshaw C, Foreman D, Cox J: Postnatal blues: A risk factor for postnatal depression. *Journal of Psychosomatic Obstetrics & Gynecology* 2004; 25(3–4):267–72.

Henshaw C, Foreman D, O'Brien S, Cox JL: Are women with severe blues at increased risk of postpartum depression? *European Psychiatry* 1996; 11(4):288s.

Iles S, Gath D, Kennerley H: Maternity blues: II. A comparison between postoperative women and post-natal women. *British Journal of Psychiatry* 1989; 155:363–66.

Kennerly H, Gath D: Maternity blues: I. Detection and measurement by questionnaire. *British Journal of Psychiatry* 1989; 155:356–62.

Kennerly H, Gath D: Maternity blues: III. Associations with obstetric, psychological, and psychiatric factors. *British Journal of Psychiatry* 1989; 155:367–73.

Nappi RE, Petraglia F, Luisi S, Polatti F, Farina C, Genazzani AR: Serum allopregnanolone in women with postpartum "blues." *Obstetrics & Gynecology* 2001; 97(1):77–80.

O'Hara MW: Postpartum blues, depression, and psychosis: A review. *Journal of Psychosomatic Obstetrics & Gynecology* 1987; 7:205–27.

O'Hara MW, Schlechte JA, Lewis DA, Wright EJ: Prospective study of postpartum blues: Biologic and psychosocial factors. *Archives of General Psychiatry* 1991; 48:801–6.

Pilcher JJ, Huffcutt AI: Effects of sleep deprivation on performance: A meta-analysis. *Sleep* 1996; 19(4):318–26.

Pitt B: Maternity blues. *British Journal of Psychiatry* 1973; 122:431–33.

Ross LE, Murray BJ, Steiner M: Sleep and perinatal mood disorders: A critical review. *Journal of Psychiatry & Neuroscience* 2005; 30(4):247–56.

Swain AM, O'Hara MW, Starr KR, Gorman LL: A prospective study of sleep, mood, and cognitive function in postpartum and nonpostpartum women. *Obstetrics & Gynecology* 1997; 90(3):381–86.

Williamson AM, Feyer AM: Moderate sleep deprivation produces impairments in cognitive and motor performance equivalent to legally prescribed levels of alcohol intoxication. *Occupational & Environmental Medicine* 2000; 57(10):649–55.

Yalom ID, Lunde DT, Moos RH, et al.: "Postpartum blues" syndrome. *Archives of General Psychiatry* 1968; 18:16–27.

Zammit GK, Weiner J, Damato N, Sillup GP, McMillan CA: Quality of life in people with insomnia. *Sleep* 1999; 22(2):1.

8: Beyond the Blues: Postpartum Depression and Anxiety

Abramowitz JS, Schwartz SA, Moore KM, Luenzmann KR: Obsessive-compulsive symptoms in pregnancy and the puerperium: A review of the literature. *Journal of Anxiety Disorders* 2003; 17(4):461–78.

Appleby L: Suicide during pregnancy and in the first postnatal year. *British Medical Journal* 1991; 302(6769):137–40.

Armstrong KL, Van Haeringen AR, Dadds MR, Cash R: Sleep deprivation or postnatal depression in later infancy: Separating the chicken from the egg. *Journal of Paediatrics & Child Health* 1998; 34(3):260–62.

Beck C: A meta-analysis of predictors of postpartum depression. *Nursing Research* 1996; 45(5):297–303.

Beck CT: Predictors of postpartum depression: An update. *Nursing Research* 2001; 50(5):275–85.

Campbell SB, Cohn JF: Prevalence of correlates of postpartum depression in first-time mothers. *Journal of Abnormal Psychology* 1991; 100(4):594–99.

Campbell SB, Cohn JF, Flanagan C, Popper S, Meyers T: Course and correlates of postpartum depression during the transition to parenthood. *Developmental Psychopathology* 1992; 4(1):29–47.

Chaudron LH, Klein MH, Remington P, Palta M, Allen C, Essex MJ: Predictors, prodromes and incidence of postpartum depression. *Journal of Psychosomatic Obstetrics & Gynecology* 2001; 22(2):103–12.

Cooper P, Campbell E, Day A, et al.: Non-psychotic pychiatric disorder after childbirth: A prospective study of prevalence, incidence, course and nature. *British Journal of Psychiatry* 1988; 152:799–806.

Cooper PJ, Murray L: Course and recurrence of postnatal depression. Evidence for the specificity of the diagnostic concept. *British Journal of Psychiatry* 1995; 166(2): 191–95.

Cox JL, Connor Y, Kendell RE: Prospective study of the psychiatric disorders of childbirth. *British Journal of Psychiatry* 1982; 140:111–17.

Cox JL, Holden JM, Sagovsky R: Detection of postnatal depression: Development of the 10-item Edinburgh Postnatal Depression Scale. *British Journal of Psychiatry* 1987; 150:782–86.

Evans J, Heron J, Francomb H, Oke S, Golding J: Cohort study of depressed mood during pregnancy and after childbirth. *British Medical Journal* 2001; 323(7307):257–60.

Evins GG, Theofrastous JP, Galvin SL: Postpartum depression: A comparison of screening and routine clinical evaluation. *American Journal of Obstetrics and Gynecology* 2000; 182(5):1080–82.

Field T, Hernandez-Reif M, Feijo L: Breast-feeding in depressed mother-infant dyads. *Early Child Development and Care* 2002; 172(6):539–45.

Fossey L, Papiernik E, Bydlowski M: Postpartum blues: A clinical syndrome and predictor of postnatal depression? *Journal of Psychosomatic Obstetrics & Gynecology* 1997; 18(1):17–21.

Garfield P, Kent A, Paykel ES, Creighton FJ, Jacobson RR: Outcome of postpartum disorders: A 10-year follow-up of hospital admissions. *Acta Psychiatrica Scandinavica* 2004; 109(6):434–39.

Georgiopoulos AM, Bryan TL, Yawn BP, Houston MS, Rummans TA, Therneau TM: *Population-based screening for postpartum depression. Obstetrics & Gynecology* 1999; 93(5 Pt 1):653–57.

Goodman JH: Postpartum depression beyond the early postpartum period. *Journal of Obstetric, Gynecologic, and Neonatal Nursing* 2004; 33(4):410–20.

Gotlib IH, Whiffen VE, Mount JH, Milne K, Cordy NI: Prevalence rates and demographic characteristics associated with depression in pregnancy and the postpartum period. *Journal of Consulting and Clinical Psychology* 1989; 57:269–74.

Henderson JJ, Evans SF, Straton JA, Priest SR, Hagan R: Impact of postnatal depression on breast-feeding duration. *Birth* 2003; 30(3):175–80.

Hendrick V, Altshuler L, Strouse T, Grosser S: Postpartum and nonpostpartum depression: Differences in presentation and response to pharmacologic treatment. *Depression & Anxiety* 2000; 11(2):66–72.

Hendrick V, Altshuler L, Suri R: Hormonal changes in the postpartum and implications for postpartum depression. *Psychosomatics* 1998; 39:93–101.

Henshaw C: Mood disturbance in the early puerperium: A review. *Archives of Women's Mental Health* 2003; 6 *Suppl* 2:S33–42.

Henshaw C, Foreman D, Cox J: Postnatal blues: A risk factor for postnatal depression. *Journal of Psychosomatic Obstetrics & Gynecology* 2004; 25(3–4):267–72.

Henshaw C, Foreman D, O'Brien S, Cox, JL: Are women with severe blues at increased risk of postpartum depression? *European Psychiatry* 1996; 11(4):288s.

Heron J, O'Connor TG, Evans J, Golding J, Glover V: The course of anxiety and depression through pregnancy and the postpartum in a community sample. *Journal of Affective Disorders* 2004; 80(1):65–73.

Hiscock H, Wake M: Randomised controlled trial of behavioural infant sleep intervention to improve infant sleep and maternal mood. *British Medical Journal* 1062; 324(7345):1062–65.

Hiscock H, Wake M: Infant sleep problems and postnatal depression: A community-based study. *Pediatrics* 1317; 107(6):1317–22.

Lam P, Hiscock H, Wake M: Outcomes of infant sleep problems: A longitudinal study of sleep, behavior, and maternal well-being. *Pediatrics* 2003; 111(3).

Logsdon MC, McBride AB, Birkimer JC: Social support and postpartum depression. *Research in Nursing Health* 1994; 17:449–57.

Nonacs R, Cohen L: Postpartum mood disorders: Diagnosis and treatment guidelines. *Journal of Clinical Psychiatry* 1998; 59 (suppl 2):34–30.

O'Hara MW: *Postpartum depression: Causes and consequences.* New York: Springer-Verlag, 1995.

O'Hara MW, Neunaber DJ, Zekoski EM: A prospective study of postpartum depression: Prevalence, course, and predictive factors. *Journal of Abnormal Psychology* 1984; 93:158.

O'Hara MW, Rehm LP, Campbell SB: Postpartum depression: A role for social network and life stress variables. *Journal of Nervous and Mental Disorders* 1983; 171:336.

O'Hara MW, Swain AM: Rates and risk of postpartum depression—a meta-analysis. *International Review of Psychiatry* 1996; 8:37–54.

Robertson E, Grace S, Wallington T, Stewart DE: Antenatal risk factors for postpartum depression: A synthesis of recent literature. *General Hospital Psychiatry* 2004; 26(4):289–95.

Ross LE, Murray BJ, Steiner M: Sleep and perinatal mood disorders: A critical review. *Journal of Psychiatry & Neuroscience* 2005; 30(4):247–56.

Sichel DA, Cohen LS, Dimmock JA, Rosenbaum JF: Postpartum obsessive-compulsive disorder: A case series. *Journal of Clinical Psychiatry* 1993; 54(4).

Sutter-Dallay AL, Murray L, Glatigny-Dallay E, Verdoux H: Newborn behavior and risk of postnatal depression in the mother. *Infancy* 2003; 4(4):589–602.

Warner R, Appleby L, Whitton A, Faragher B: Demographic and obstetric risk factors for postnatal psychiatric morbidity. *British Journal of Psychiatry* 1996; 168(5):607–11.

Whiffen VE: Is postpartum depression a distinct diagnosis. *Clinical Psychology Review* 1992; 12:485–508.

Williams K, Koran L: Obsessive-compulsive disorder in pregnancy, and the premenstrum. *Journal of Clinical Psychiatry* 1997; 58:330–34.

Wisner KL, Parry BL, Piontek CM: Postpartum depression. *New England Journal of Medicine* 2002; 347(3):194–99.

Wisner KL, Peindl KS, Gigliotti T, Hanusa BH: Obsessions and compulsions in women with postpartum depression. *Journal of Clinical Psychiatry* 1999; 60(3):176–80.

Zelkowitz P, Milet TH: The course of postpartum psychiatric disorders in women and their partners. *Journal of Nervous and Mental Disorders* 2001; 189(9):575–82.

9. No Sense of Reality: Postpartum Psychosis

Ahokas A, Aito M, Rimon R: Positive treatment effect of estradiol in postpartum psychosis: A pilot study. *Journal of Clinical Psychiatry* 2000; 61(3):166–69.

Austin MP. Puerperal affective psychosis: Is there a case for lithium prophylaxis? *British Journal of Psychiatry* 1882; 161:692–94.

Brockington IF, Cernik KF, Schofield EM, et al.: Puerperal psychosis: Phenomena and diagnosis. *Archives of General Psychiatry* 1981; 38:829–33.

Brockington IF, Winokur G, Dean C: Puerperal psychosis. In *Motherhood and mental illness*, ed. Brockington IF, Kumar R, 37–69. London: Academic, 1982.

Chaudron LH, Pies RW: The relationship between postpartum psychosis and bipolar disorder: A review. *Journal of Clinical Psychiatry* 2003; 64(11):1284–92.

Cohen LS, Sichel DA, Robertson LM, Heckscher E, Rosenbaum JF: Postpartum prophylaxis for women with bipolar disorder. *American Journal of Psychiatry* 1995; 152(11):164–65.

Dean C, Williams RJ, Brockington IF: Is puerperal psychosis the same as bipolar manic-depressive disorder? A family study. *Psychological Medicine* 1989; 19:637–47.

D'Orban PT: Women who kill their children. *British Journal of Psychiatry* 1979; 134:570–71.

Kendell RE: Emotional and physical factors in the genesis of puerperal mental disorders. *Journal of Psychosomatic Research* 1985; 29:3.

Kendell RE, Chalmers JC, Platz C: Epidemiology of puerperal psychoses. *British Journal of Psychiatry* 1987; 150:662–73.

Klompenhouwer J, van Hulst A: Classification of postpartum psychosis: A study of 250 mother and baby admissions in the Netherlands. *Acta Psychaitrica Scandinavica* 1991; 84:255–61.

Kumar R, et al.: Neuroendocrine and psychosocial mechanisms in postpartum psychosis. *Progress in Neuro-psychopharmacology & Biological Psychiatry* 1993; 17(4): 570–79.

McNeil TF: A prospective study of postpartum psychosis in a high-risk group: 2. Relationships to demographic and psychiatric history characteristics. *Acta Psychiatrica Scandinavica* 1987; 75:35–43.

O'Hara MW: Postpartum blues, depression, and psychosis: A review. *Journal of Psychosomatic Obstetrics and Gynaecology* 1987; 7:205–27.

Paffenbarger RA: Epidemiological aspects of mental illness associated with childbearing. In *Motherhood and mental illness*, ed. Brockington IF, Kumar R. New York: Grune and Stratton, 1982.

Platz C, Kendell R: A matched-control follow-up and family study of "puerperal psychosis." *British Journal of Psychiatry* 1998; 153:90–94.

Reich T, Winokur G: Postpartum psychosis in patients with manic-depressive disease. *Journal of Nervous and Mental Disorders* 1970; 151:60–68.

Robertson E, Jones I, Haque S, Holder R, Craddock N: Risk of puerperal and nonpuerperal recurrence of illness following bipolar affective puerperal (postpartum) psychosis. *British Journal of Psychiatry* 2005; 186:258–59.

Robling SA, Paykel ES, Dunn VJ, Abbott R, Katona C: Long-term outcome of severe puerperal psychiatric illness: A 23-year follow-up study. *Psychological Medicine* 2000; 30(6):1263–71.

Schopf J, Rust B: Follow-up and family study of postpartum psychoses. Part I: Overview. *European Archives of Psychiatry & Clinical Neuroscience* 1994; 244(2):101–11.

Schopf J, Rust B: Follow-up and family study of postpartum psychoses. Part III: Characteristics of psychoses occurring exclusively in relation to childbirth. *European Archives of Psychiatry & Clinical Neuroscience* 1994; 244(3):138–40.

Spinelli MG: Maternal infanticide associated with mental illness: Prevention and the promise of saved lives. *American Journal of Psychiatry* 2004; 161(9):1548–57.

Stewart DE, Klompenhouwer JL, Kendell RE, van Hulst AM. Prophylactic lithium in puerperal psychosis. The experience of three centres. *British Journal of Psychiatry* 1991; 158:393–97.

Stewart DE: Prophylactic lithium in postpartum affective psychosis. *Journal of Nervous and Mental Disease* 1988; 176(8):485–89.

10. Life After Children: Partners As Parents

Carrere S, Buehlman KT, Gottman JM, Coan JA, Ruckstuhl L: Predicting marital stability and divorce in newlywed couples. *Journal of Family Psychology* 2000; 14(1):42–58.

Cowan C, Cowan P: A *preventative intervention for couples becoming parents.* New Jersey: Ablex, 1987.

Cowan C, Cowan P: *When parents become partners: The big life change for couples.* New York: Basic Books, 1992.

Fincham FD, Bradbury TN: Marital satisfaction, depression, and attributions: A longitudinal analysis. *Journal of Personality & Social Psychology* 1993; 64(3):442–52.

Gottman JM: The roles of conflict engagement, escalation, and avoidance in marital interaction: A longitudinal view of five types of couples. *Journal of Consulting & Clinical Psychology* 1993; 61(1):6–15.

Gottman JM, Krokoff LJ: Marital interaction and satisfaction: A longitudinal view. *Journal of Consulting & Clinical Psychology* 1989; 57(1):47–52.

Hammen C, Brennan PA: Interpersonal dysfunction in depressed women: Impairments independent of depressive symptoms. *Journal of Affective Disorders* 2002; 72(2): 145–56.

Hoover CF, Fitzgerald RG: Marital conflict of manic-depressive patients. *Archives of General Psychiatry* 1981; 38(1):65–67.

Levenson RW, Carstensen LL, Gottman JM: Long-term marriage: Age, gender, and satisfaction. *Psychology & Aging* 1993; 8(2):301–13.

Marchand JF: Husbands' and wives' marital quality: The role of adult attachment orientations, depressive symptoms, and conflict resolution behaviors. *Attachment & Human Development* 2004; 6(1):99–112.

Shapiro AF, Gottman JM, Carrere S: The baby and the marriage: Identifying factors that buffer against decline in marital satisfaction after the first baby arrives. *Journal of Family Psychology* 2000; 14(1):59–70.

Whisman MA, Uebelacker LA, Weinstock LM: Psychopathology and marital satisfaction: The importance of evaluating both partners. *Journal of Consulting & Clinical Psychology* 2004; 72(5):830–38.

11. Helping Yourself: Practical Techniques for Managing Stress and Depression

Armstrong KL, Ván Haeringen AR, Dadds MR, Cash R: Sleep deprivation or postnatal depression in later infancy: Separating the chicken from the egg. *Journal of Paediatrics & Child Health* 1998; 34(3):260–62.

Blumenthal JA, Babyak MA, Moore KA, Craighead WE, Herman S, Khatri P, Waugh R, Napolitano MA, Forman LM, Appelbaum M, Doraiswamy PM, Krishnan KR: Effects of exercise training on older patients with major depression. *Archives of Internal Medicine* 1999; 159(19):2349–56.

Brown GW, Andrews B, Harris T, Adler Z, Bridge L: Social support, self-esteem and depression. *Psychological Medicine* 1986; 16(4):813–31.

Brown GW, Harris TO, Eales MJ: Social factors and comorbidity of depressive and anxiety disorders. *British Journal of Psychiatry Supplementum* 1996; 30:50–57.

Burns, DD: *The feeling good handbook*. New York: Plume, 1999.

Collins NL, Dunkel-Schetter C, Lobel M, Scrimshaw SCM: Social support in pregnancy: Psychosocial correlates of birth outcomes and postpartum depression. *Journal of Personality and Social Psychology* 1993; 65(6):1243–58.

Cutrona CE: Social support and stress in the transition to parenthood. *Journal of Abnormal Psychology* 1984; 93:378–90.

Dinges DF, Pack F, Williams K, Gillen KA, Powell JW, Ott GE, Aptowicz C, Pack AI: Cumulative sleepiness, mood disturbance, and psychomotor vigilance performance decrements during a week of sleep restricted to 4–5 hours per night. *Sleep* 1997; 20(4): 267–77.

Fleming AS, Klein E, Corter C: The effects of a social support group on depression, maternal attitudes and behavior in new mothers. *Journal of Child Psychology and Psychiatry* 1992; 33(4):685–98.

George LK, Blazer DG, Hughes DC, Fowler N: Social support and the outcome of major depression. *British Journal of Psychiatry* 1989; 154:478–85.

Goodwin RD: Association between physical activity and mental disorders among adults in the United States. *Preventive Medicine* 2003; 36(6):698–703.

Hiscock H, Wake M: Infant sleep problems and postnatal depression: A community-based study. *Pediatrics* 1317; 107(6):1317–22.

Lam P, Hiscock H, Wake M: Outcomes of infant sleep problems: A longitudinal study of sleep, behavior, and maternal well-being. *Pediatrics* 2003; 111(3).

Pilcher JJ, Huffcutt AI: Effects of sleep deprivation on performance: A meta-analysis. *Sleep* 1996; 19(4):318–26.

Ross LE, Murray BJ, Steiner M: Sleep and perinatal mood disorders: A critical review. *Journal of Psychiatry & Neuroscience* 2005; 30(4):247–56.

Smit HJ, Gaffan EA, Rogers PJ: Methylxanthines are the psycho-pharmacologically active constituents of chocolate. *Psychopharmacology* 2004; 176(3–4):412–19.

Swain AM, O'Hara MW, Starr KR, Gorman LL: A prospective study of sleep, mood, and cognitive function in postpartum and nonpostpartum women. *Obstetrics & Gynecology* 1997; 90(3):381–86.

Wang TW, Apgar BS: Exercise during pregnancy. *American Family Physician* 1998; 57(8):1846–52.

Williamson AM, Feyer AM: Moderate sleep deprivation produces impairments in cognitive and motor performance equivalent to legally prescribed levels of alcohol intoxication. *Occupational & Environmental Medicine* 2000; 57(10):649–55.

Wolfson AR, Crowley SJ, Anwer U, Bassett JL: Changes in sleep patterns and depressive symptoms in first-time mothers: Last trimester to 1-year postpartum. *Behavioral Sleep Medicine* 2003; 1(1):54–67.

Zammit GK, Weiner J, Damato N, Sillup GP, McMillan CA: Quality of life in people with insomnia. *Sleep* 1999; 22(2):1.

12. Seeking Professional Help: Treatment of Maternal Depression

Alpert JE, Mischoulon D, Nierenberg AA, Fava M: Nutrition and depression: Focus on folate. *Nutrition* 2000; 16(7–8):544–46.

Alpert JE, Papakostas G, Mischoulon D, Worthington JJ, III, Petersen T, Mahal Y, Burns A, Bottiglieri T, Nierenberg AA, Fava M: S-adenosyl-L-methionine (SAMe) as an adjunct for resistant major depressive disorder: An open trial following partial or nonresponse to selective serotonin reuptake inhibitors or venlafaxine. *Journal of Clinical Psychopharmacology* 2004; 24(6):661–64.

Beck AT, Rush AJ, Shaw BF, Emery G: *Cognitive therapy of depression.* New York: Guilford, 1979.

Conover EA: Over-the-counter products: Nonprescription medications, nutraceuticals, and herbal agents. *Clinical Obstetrics & Gynecology* 2002; 45(1):89–98.

De Smet PA: Herbal remedies. *New England Journal of Medicine* 2002; 347 (25):2046–56.

De Smet PA: Health risks of herbal remedies: An update. *Clinical Pharmacology & Therapeutics* 2004; 76(1):1–17.

Dove D, Johnson P: Oral evening primrose oil: Its effect on length of pregnancy and selected intrapartum outcomes in low-risk nulliparous women. *Journal of Nurse Midwifery* 1999; 44(3):320–24.

Eisenberg DM, Davis RB, Ettner SL, Appel S, Wilkey S, Van Rompay M, Kessler RC: Trends in alternative medicine use in the United States, 1990–1997: Results of a follow-up national survey. *JAMA* 1569; 280(18):1569–75.

Ernst E, Rand JI, Barnes J, Stevinson C: Adverse effects profile of the herbal antidepressant St. John's wort (Hypericum perforatum). *European Journal of Clinical Pharmacology* 1998; 54(8):589–94.

Frank E, Kupfer DJ, Perel JM: Three-year outcomes for maintenance therapies in recurrent depression. *Archives of General Psychiatry* 1990; 47:1093–99.

Freeman MP, Helgason C, Hill RA: Selected integrative medicine treatments for depression: Considerations for women. *Journal of the American Medical Womens Association* 2004; 59(3):216–24.

Gallagher SM, Allen JJ, Hitt SK, Schnyer RN, Manber R: Six-month depression relapse rates among women treated with acupuncture. *Complementary Therapies in Medicine* 2001; 9(4):216–18.

Gaster B, Holroyd J: St. John's wort for depression: A systematic review. *Archives of Internal Medicine* 2000; 160(2):152–56.

Geddes JR, Carney SM, Davies C, Furukawa TA, Kupfer DJ, Frank E, Goodwin GM: Relapse prevention with antidepressant drug treatment in depressive disorders: A systematic review. *Lancet* 2003; 361(9358):653–61.

Hypericum Depression Trial Study G: Effect of Hypericum perforatum (St. John's wort) in major depressive disorder: A randomized controlled trial. *JAMA* 2002; 287(14):1807–14.

Jindal RD, Thase ME: Integrating psychotherapy and pharmacotherapy to improve outcomes among patients with mood disorders. *Psychiatric Services* 2003; 54(11): 1484–90.

Keller MB, Klerman GL, Lavori PW, Coryell W, Endicott J: Long-term outcome of episodes of major depression: Clinical and public health significance. *JAMA* 1984; 252:788–92.

Keller MB, Lavori PW, Lewis C, Klerman GL: Predictors of relapse in major depressive disorder. *JAMA* 1983; 250:3299–3309.

Klerman GL, Weissman MM, Rounsaville BJ, et al.: *Interpersonal psychotherapy of depression.* New York: Basic Books, 1984.

Kupfer D, Frank E, Perel J, Cornes C, Mallinger A, Thase M, McEachran A, Grochocinski V: Five-year outcome for maintenance therapies in recurrent depression. *Archives of General Psychiatry* 1992; 49(10):769–73.

Linde K, Berner M, Egger M, Mulrow C: St. John's wort for depression: Meta-analysis of randomised controlled trials. *British Journal of Psychiatry* 2005; 186:99–107.

Manber R, Allen JJ, Morris MM: Alternative treatments for depression: Empirical support and relevance to women. *Journal of Clinical Psychiatry* 2002; 63(7):628–40.

Mischoulon D, Fava M: Role of S-adenosyl-L-methionine in the treatment of depression: A review of the evidence. *American Journal of Clinical Nutrition* 1158; 76(5).

Mischoulon D, Fava M: Docosahexanoic acid and omega-3 fatty acids in depression. *Psychiatric Clinics of North America* 2000; 23(4):785–94.

Mischoulon D, Rosenbaum JF: The use of natural remedies in psychiatry: A commentary. *Harvard Review of Psychiatry* 1999; 6(5):279–83.

Morris MS, Fava M, Jacques PF, Selhub J, Rosenberg IH: Depression and folate status in the U.S. population. *Psychotherapy & Psychosomatics* 2003; 72(2):80–87.

Nemets B, Osher Y, Belmaker RH: Omega-3 fatty acids and augmentation strategies in treating resistant depression. *Essential Psychopharmacology* 2004; 6(1):59–64.

Nemets B, Stahl Z, Belmaker RH: Addition of omega-3 fatty acid to maintenance medication treatment for recurrent unipolar depressive disorder. *American Journal of Psychiatry* 2002; 159(3):477–79.

Papakostas GI, Petersen T, Mischoulon D, Green CH, Nierenberg AA, Bottiglieri T, Rosenbaum JF, Alpert JE, Fava M: Serum folate, vitamin B_{12}, and homocysteine in major depressive disorder, part 2: Predictors of relapse during the continuation phase of pharmacotherapy. *Journal of Clinical Psychiatry* 1096; 65(8):1096–98.

Papakostas GI, Petersen T, Mischoulon D, Ryan JL, Nierenberg AA, Bottiglieri T, Rosenbaum JF, Alpert JE, Fava M: Serum folate, vitamin B_{12}, and homocysteine in major depressive disorder, part 1: Predictors of clinical response in fluoxetine-resistant depression. *Journal of Clinical Psychiatry* 1090; 65(8):1090–95.

Pies R: Adverse neuropsychiatric reactions to herbal and over-the-counter "antidepressants." *Journal of Clinical Psychiatry* 2000; 61(11):815–20.

Roper Reports: *To medicate: What people do for minor health problems.* New York: Roper Organization, 1986, 86–88.

Rosenbaum JF, Arana GW, Hyman SE, Labbate LA, and Fava M: *Handbook of psychiatric drug therapy.* Hagerstown, MD: Williams & Wilkins, 2005.

Severus WE, Littman AB, Stoll AL: Omega-3 fatty acids, homocysteine, and the increased risk of cardiovascular mortality in major depressive disorder. *Harvard Review of Psychiatry* 2001; 9(6):280–93.

Shelton RC, Keller MB, Gelenberg A, Dunner DL, Hirschfeld R, Thase ME, Russell J, Lydiard RB, Crits-Cristoph P, Gallop R, Todd L, Hellerstein D, Goodnick P, Keitner G, Stahl SM, Halbreich U: Effectiveness of St. John's wort in major depression: A randomized controlled trial. *JAMA* 1978; 285(15):1978–86.

Stoll AL, Severus WE, Freeman MP, Rueter S, Zboyan HA, Diamond E, Cress KK,

Marangell LB: Omega-3 fatty acids in bipolar disorder: A preliminary double-blind, placebo-controlled trial. *Archives of General Psychiatry* 1999; 56(5):407–12.

Su KP, Huang SY, Chiu CC, Shen WW: Omega-3 fatty acids in major depressive disorder: A preliminary double-blind, placebo-controlled trial. Erratum appears in *European Neuropsychopharmacology* 2004; 14(2):173; *European Neuropsychopharmacology* 2003; 13(4):267–71.

Thase ME: Relapse and recurrence in unipolar major depression: Short-term and long-term approaches. *Journal of Clinical Psychiatry* 1990; 51:51–57.

Thase ME: Integrating psychotherapy and pharmacotherapy for treatment of major depressive disorder: Current status and future considerations. *Journal of Psychotherapy Practice & Research* 1997; 6(4):300–306.

Thase ME, Greenhouse JB, Frank E, Reynolds CF, III, Pilkonis PA, Hurley K, Grochocinski V, Kupfer DJ: Treatment of major depression with psychotherapy or psychotherapy-pharmacotherapy combinations. *Archives of General Psychiatry* 1997; 54(11):1009–15.

Tiemeier H, van Tuijl HR, Hofman A, Meijer J, Kiliaan AJ, Breteler MM: Vitamin B_{12}, folate, and homocysteine in depression: The Rotterdam study. *American Journal of Psychiatry* 2002; 159(12):2099–101.

Vaughan SC: *The talking cure: The science behind psychotherapy.* New York: Putnam, 1997.

13. Understanding Your Options: Treating Depression During Pregnancy and the Postpartum Period

Addis A, Koren G: Safety of fluoxetine during the first trimester of pregnancy: A meta-analytical review of epidemiological studies. *Psychological Medicine* 2000; 30(1):89–94.

Altshuler L, Cohen L, Moline M, Kahn D, Carpenter D, Docherty J: Expert Consensus Guideline Series: Treatment of depression in women. *Postgraduate Medicine Special Report* 2001:1–116.

Altshuler LL, Cohen LS, Szuba MP, Burt VK, Gitlin M, Mintz J: Pharmacologic management of psychiatric illness in pregnancy: Dilemmas and guidelines. *American Journal of Psychiatry* 1996; 153:592–606.

Appleby L, Warner R, Whitton A, Faragher B: A controlled study of fluoxetine and cognitive-behavioral counselling in the treatment of postnatal depression. *British Medical Journal* 1997; 314(7085):932–36.

Birnbaum CS, Cohen LS, Bailey JW, Grush LR, Robertson LM, Stowe ZN: Serum concentrations of antidepressants and benzodiazepines in nursing infants: A case series. *Pediatrics* 1999; 104(1):e11.

Bromiker R, Kaplan M: Apparent intrauterine fetal withdrawal from clomipramine hydrochloride. *JAMA* 1994; 272(22):1722–23.

Briggs GG, Freeman RK, and Yaffe SJ: *Drugs in pregnancy and lactation*, 7th ed. New York: Lippincott Williams & Wilkins, 2005.

Burt VK, Rasgon N: Special considerations in treating bipolar disorder in women. *Bipolar Disorders* 2004; 6(1):2–13.

Burt VK, Suri R, Altshuler L, Stowe Z, Hendrick VC, Muntean E: The use of psychotropic medications during breast-feeding. *American Journal of Psychiatry* 2001; 158(7):1001–9.

Casper RC, et al.: Follow-up of children of depressed mothers exposed or not exposed to antidepressant drugs during pregnancy. *Journal of Pediatrics* 2003; 142: 402–8.

Chambers C, Johnson K, Dick L, Felix R, Jones KL: Birth outcomes in pregnant women taking fluoxetine. *New England Journal of Medicine* 1996; 335(14):1010–15.

Chaudron LH, Jefferson JW: Mood stabilizers during breast-feeding: A review. *Journal of Clinical Psychiatry* 2000; 61(2):79–90.

Chaudron LH, Schoenecker CJ: Bupropion and breastfeeding: A case of a possible infant seizure. Journal of Clinical Psychiatry 2004; 65:881–82.

Cohen L, Altshuler L: Pharmacologic management of psychiatric illness during pregnancy and the postpartum period. In *The Psychiatric Clinics of North America Annual of Drug Therapy*, eds. Dunner D, Rosenbaum J., 21–60, Philadelphia: WB Saunders Company, 1997.

Cohen LS, Friedman JM, Jefferson JW, Johnson EM, Weiner ML: A reevaluation of risk of in utero exposure to lithium. *JAMA* 1994; 271(2):146–50.

Cohen LS, Heller VL, Bailey JW, Grush L, Ablon JS, Bouffard SM: Birth outcomes following prenatal exposure to fluoxetine. *Biological Psychiatry* 2000; 48(10):996–1000.

Cohen L, Nonacs R, eds.: *Mood and anxiety disorders during pregnancy and postpartum.* Arlington, VA: American Psychiatric Publishing, 2005.

Cohen LS, Nonacs RM, Bailey JW, Viguera AC, Reminick AM, Altshuler LL, Stowe ZN, Faraone SV: Relapse of depression during pregnancy following antidepressant discontinuation: A preliminary prospective study. *Archives of Women's Mental Health* 2004; 7(4):217–21.

Cohen LS, Nonacs R, Viguera AC, Reminick A: Diagnosis and treatment of depression during pregnancy. *CNS Spectrums* 2004; 9(3):209–16.

Cohen LS, Rosenbaum JF: Psychotropic drug use during pregnancy: Weighing the risks. *Journal of Clinical Psychiatry* 1998; 59(suppl 2): 18–28.

Cohen LS, Sichel DA, Robertson LM, Heckscher E, Rosenbaum JF: Postpartum prophylaxis for women with bipolar disorder. *American Journal of Psychiatry* 1995; 152:1641–45.

Cohen LS, Viguera AC, Bouffard SM, Nonacs RM, Morabito C, Collins MH, Ablon JS: Venlafaxine in the treatment of postpartum depression. *Journal of Clinical Psychiatry* 2001; 62(8):592–96.

Corral M, Kuan A, Kostaras D: Bright light therapy's effect on postpartum depression. *American Journal of Psychiatry* 2000; 157(2):303–4.

Cowe L, Lloyd D, Dawling S: Neonatal convulsions caused by withdrawal from maternal clomipramine. *British Medical Journal* 1982; 284:1837–38.

Dennis C: Can we identify mothers at risk for postpartum depression in the immediate postpartum period using the Edinburgh Postnatal Depression Scale? *Journal of Affective Disorders* 2004; 78(2):163–69.

Dennis CL: The effect of peer support on postpartum depression: A pilot randomized controlled trial. *Canadian Journal of Psychiatry* 2003; 48(2):115–24.

Dennis CL: Treatment of postpartum depression, part 2: A critical review of nonbiological interventions. *Journal of Clinical Psychiatry* 2004; 65(9):1252–65.

Dennis CL, Stewart DE: Treatment of postpartum depression, part 1: A critical review of biological interventions. *Journal of Clinical Psychiatry* 2004; 65(9):1242–51.

Diav-Citrin O, Shechtman S, Ornoy S, Arnon J, Schaefer C, Garbis H, Clementi M, Ornoy A: Safety of haloperidol and penfluridol in pregnancy: a multicenter, prospective, controlled study. *Journal of Clinical Psychiatry* 2005; 66(3):317–22.

Dolovich L, Antonio A, Vaillancourt JR, Power JB, Koren G, Einarson T: Benziodiazepine use in pregnancy and major malformations or oral cleft: Meta-analysis of cohort and case-control studies. *British Medical Journal* 1998; 317:839–43.

Eggermont E: Withdrawal symptoms in neonates associated with maternal imipramine therapy. *Lancet* 1973; 2:680.

Einarson A, Bonari L, Voyer-Lavigne S, Addis A, Matsui D, Johnson Y, Koren G: A multicentre prospective controlled study to determine the safety of trazodone and nefazodone use during pregnancy. *Canadian Journal of Psychiatry* 2003; 48(2):106–10.

Einarson A, Fatoye B, Sarkar M, Lavigne SV, Brochu J, Chambers C, Mastroiacovo P, Addis A, Matsui D, Schuler L Einarson TR, Koren G: Pregnancy outcome following gestational exposure to venlafaxine: A multicenter prospective controlled study. *American Journal of Psychiatry* 2001; 158(10):1728–30.

Einarson TR, Einarson A: Newer antidepressants in pregnancy and rates of major malformations: A meta-analysis of prospective comparative studies. *Pharmacoepidemiology and Drug Safety* 2005; 14(12):823–27.

Elliott SA, Leverton TJ, Sanjack M, Turner H, Cowmeadow P, Hopkins J, Bushnell D: Promoting mental health after childbirth: A controlled trial of primary prevention of postnatal depression. *British Journal of Clinical Psychology* 2000; 39(Pt. 3):223–41.

Epperson CN, Anderson GM, McDougle CJ: Sertraline and breast-feeding. *New England Journal of Medicine* 1997; 336(16):1189–90.

Ericson A KB, Wilhom B: Delivery outcome after the use of antidepressants in early pregnancy. *European Journal of Clinical Psychopharmacology* 1999; 55(7):503–8.

Ernst CL, Goldberg JF: The reproductive safety profile of mood stabilizers, atypical antipsychotics, and broad-spectrum psychotropics. *Journal of Clinical Psychiatry* 2002; 4:42–55.

Gentile S: Clinical utilization of atypical antipsychotics in pregnancy and lactation. *Annals of Pharmacotherapy* 1265; 38(7–8):1265–71.

Goldstein DJ: Effects of third trimester fluoxetine exposure on the newborn. *Clinical Psychopharmacology* 1995; 15:417–20.

Goldstein DJ, Fung MC: Olanzapine-exposed pregnancies and lactation: Early experience. *Journal of Clinical Psychopharmacology* 2000; 20:399–403.

Goldstein DJ, Sundell KL, Corbin LA: Birth outcomes in pregnant women taking fluoxetine. *New England Journal of Medicine* 1997; 336(12):872–73.

Goldstein DJ, Williams ML, Pearson DK: Fluoxetine-exposed pregnancies. *Clinical Research* 1991; 39(3):768A.

Gracious BL, Wisner KL: Phenelzine use throughout pregnancy and the puerperium: Case report, review of the literature, and management recommendations. *Depression & Anxiety* 1997; 6(3):124–28.

Hallberg P, et al.: The use of selective serotonin reuptake inhibitors during pregnancy and breast-feeding: A review and clinical aspects. *Journal of Clinical Psychopharmacology* 2005; 25:59–73.

Hemels ME, Einarson A, Koren G, Lanctot KL, Einarson TR: Antidepressant use during pregnancy and the rates of spontaneous abortions: A meta-analysis. *Annals of Pharmacotherapy* 2005; 39(5):803–9.

Hendrick V. Alternative treatments for postpartum depression. *Psychiatric Times* 2003; 20(8).

Hendrick V, Fukuchi A, Altshuler L, et al.: Use of sertraline, paroxetine and fluvoxamine by nursing women. *British Journal of Psychiatry* 2001; 179:163–66.

Hendrick V, Smith LM, Suri R, Hwang S, Haynes D, Altshuler L: Birth outcomes after prenatal exposure to antidepressant medication. *American Journal of Obstetrics and Gynecology* 2003; 188(3):812–15.

Hendrick V, Smith LM, Hwang S, Altshuler LL, Haynes D: Weight gain in breast-fed infants of mothers taking antidepressant medications. *Journal of Clinical Psychiatry* 2003; 64(4):410–12.

Hendrick V, Stowe ZN, Altshuler LL, Hostetter A, Fukuchi A: Paroxetine use during breast-feeding. *Journal of Clinical Psychopharmacology* 2000; 20(5):587–89.

Hendrick V, Stowe ZN, Altshuler LL, Mintz J, Hwang S, Hostetter A, Suri R, Leight K, Fukuchi A: Fluoxetine and norfluoxetine concentrations in nursing infants and breast milk. *Biological Psychiatry* 2001; 50(10):775–82.

Hibbeln JR: Seafood consumption, the DHA content of mothers' milk and prevalence rates of postpartum depression: A cross-national, ecological analysis. *Journal of Affective Disorders* 2002; 69(1–3):15–29.

Holmes LB: The teratogenicity of anticonvulsant drugs: A progress report. *Journal of Medical Genetics* 2002; 39(4):245–47.

Holmes LB, Harvey EA, Coull BA, Huntington KB, Khoshbin S, et al.: The teratogenicity of anticonvulsant drugs. *New England Journal of Medicine* 2001; 344(15): 1132–38.

Hostetter A, Ritchie JC, Stowe ZN: Amniotic fluid and umbilical cord blood concentrations of antidepressants in three women. *Biological Psychiatry* 2000; 48(10):1032–34.

Hostetter A, Stowe ZN, Strader JR, Jr., McLaughlin E, Llewellyn A: Dose of selective serotonin uptake inhibitors across pregnancy: Clinical implications. *Depression & Anxiety* 2000; 11(2):51–57.

Inman W, Kobotu K, Pearce G, et al.: Prescription event monitoring of paroxetine. *PEM Reports* 1993; PXL 1206:1–44.

Iqbal MM, Sobhan T, Ryals T: Effects of commonly used benzodiazepines on the fetus, the neonate, and the nursing infant. *Psychiatric Services* 2002; 53(1):39–49.

Kallen B. Neonate characteristics after maternal use of antidepressants in late pregnancy. *Archives of Pediatric and Adolescent Medicine* 2004; 158:312–16.

Klier CM, Schafer MR, Schmid-Siegel B, et al.: St. John's wort (Hypericum perforate): Is it safe during breast-feeding? *Pharmacopsychiatry* 2002; 35(1):29–30.

Kozma C: Valproic acid embryopathy: Report of two siblings with further expansion of the phenotypic abnormalities and a review of the literature. *American Journal of Medical Genetics* 2001; 98(2):168–75.

Kulin N, Pastuszak A, Sage S, et al.: Pregnancy outcome following maternal use of the new selective serotonin reuptake inhibitors: A prospective controlled multicenter study. *JAMA* 1998; 279:609–10.

Laine K, Heikkinen T, Ekblad U, Kero P: Effects of exposure to selective serotonin reuptake inhibitors during pregnancy on serotonergic symptoms in newborns and cord blood monoamine and prolactin concentrations. *Archives of General Psychiatry* 2003; 60(7):720–26.

Lee A, Minhas R, Matsuda N, Lam M, Ito S: The safety of St. John's wort (Hypericum perforatum) during breast-feeding. *Journal of Clinical Psychiatry* 2003; 64(8): 966–68.

Leibenluft E: Issues in the treatment of women with bipolar illness. *Journal of Clinical Psychiatry* 1997; 58 Suppl 15:5–11.

Lin AE, Peller AJ, Westgate MN, Houde K, Franz A, Holmes LB: Clonazepam use in pregnancy and the risk of malformations. *Birth Defects Research* 2004; 70(8):534–36.

Llewellyn A, Stowe Z: Psychotropic medications in lactation. *Journal of Clinical Psychiatry* 1998; 59 (suppl 2):41–52.

Llewellyn A, Stowe ZN, James R, Strader J: The use of lithium and management of women with bipolar disorder during pregnancy and lactation. *Journal of Clinical Psychiatry* 1998; 59(suppl 6):57–64.

Llorente AM, Jensen CL, Voigt RG, Fraley JK, Berretta MC, Heird WC: Effect of maternal docosahexaenoic acid supplementation on postpartum depression and information processing. *American Journal of Obstetrics & Gynecology* 1348; 188(5):1348–53.

Loebstein R, Koren G: Pregnancy outcome and neurodevelopment of children exposed in utero to psychoactive drugs: The Motherisk experience. *Journal of Psychiatry and Neuroscience* 1997; 22(3):192–96.

McElhatton P, Garbis H, Elefant E, Vial T, Bellemin B, Mastroiacovo P, Arnon J, Rodriguez-Pinella E, Schaefer C, Pexieder T, Merlob P, Verme SD: The outcome of pregnancy in 689 women exposed to theraputic doses of antidepressants. A collaborative study of the European Network of Teratology Information Services (ENTIS). *Reproductive Toxicology* 1996; 10(4):285–94.

McKenna K, Koren G, Tetelbaum M, Wilton L, Shakir S, Diav-Citrin O, Levinson A, Zipursky RB, Einarson A: Pregnancy outcome of women using atypical antipsychotic drugs: A prospective comparative study. *Journal of Clinical Psychiatry* 2005; 66(4):444–49.

Miller LJ: Use of electroconvulsive therapy during pregnancy. *Hospital and Community Psychiatry* 1994; 45(5):444–50.

Misri S, Kostaras X: Benefits and risks to mother and infant of drug treatment for postnatal depression. *Drug Safety* 2002; 25(13):903–11.

Misri S, Oberlander TF, Fairbrother N, Carter D, Ryan D, Kuan AJ, Reebye P: Relation between prenatal maternal mood and anxiety and neonatal health. *Canadian Journal of Psychiatry* 2004; 49: 684–89.

Misri S, Sivertz K: Tricyclic drugs in pregnancy and lactation: A preliminary report. *International Journal of Psychiatry in Medicine* 1991; 21(2):157–71.

Moore K: *The developing human: Clinically oriented embryology*. Philadelphia: W. B. Saunders, 1993.

Newport DJ, Hostetter A, Arnold A, Stowe ZN: The treatment of postpartum depression: Minimizing infant exposures. *Journal of Clinical Psychiatry* 2002; 7:31–44.

Newport JD, Viguera AC, Beach AJ, et al.: Lithium placental passage and obstetrical outcome: Implications for clinical management during late pregnancy. *American Journal of Psychiatry* 2005; 162:2162–70.

Nonacs R, Cohen L: Postpartum mood disorders: Diagnosis and treatment guidelines. *Journal of Clinical Psychiatry* 1998; 59 (suppl. 2):34–30.

Nonacs R, Cohen L: Assessment and treatment of depression during pregnancy: An update. *Psychiatric Clinics of North America*. 2003; 26(3):547–62.

Nonacs RM, Soares CN, Viguera AC, Pearson K, Poitras JR, Cohen LS: Bupropion SR for the treatment of postpartum depression: A pilot study. *International Journal of Neuropsychopharmacology* 2005: 8(3):445–49.

Nulman I, Koren G: The safety of fluoxetine during pregnancy and lactation. *Teratology* 1996; 53:304–8.

Nulman I, Rovet J, Stewart D, Wolpin J, Gardner HA, Theis JG, Kulin N, Koren G: Neurodevelopment of children exposed in utero to antidepressant drugs. *New England Journal of Medicine* 1997; 336:258–62.

Nulman I, Rovet J, Stewart DE, Wolpin J, Pace-Asciak P, Shuhaiber S, Koren G: Child development following exposure to tricyclic antidepressants or fluoxetine throughout fetal life: A prospective, controlled study. *American Journal of Psychiatry* 2002; 159(11):1889–95.

Oberlander TF, Misri S, Fitzgerald C, Kostaras X, Rurak D, Riggs W: Pharmacologic factors associated with transient neonatal symptoms following prenatal psychotropic medication exposure. *Journal of Clinical Psychiatry* 2004; 65:230–37.

O'Hara MW, Stuart S, Gorman LL, Wenzel A: Efficacy of interpersonal psychotherapy for postpartum depression. *Archives of General Psychiatry* 2000; 57(11):1039–45.

Oren DA, Wisner KL, Spineli M, et al.: An open trial of morning light therapy for treatment of antepartum depression. *American Journal of Psychiatry* 2002; 159(4):666–69.

Ornoy A, Arnon J, Shechtman S, Moerman L, Lukashova I: Is benzodiazepine use during pregnancy really teratogenic? *Reproductive Toxicology* 1998; 12(5):511–15.

Pastuszak A, Schick-Boschetto B, Zuber C, Feldkamp M, Pinelli M, Sihn S, Donnenfeld A, McCormack M, Leen-Mitchell M, Woodland C, Gardner A, Hom M, Koren G: Pregnancy outcome following first-trimester exposure to fluoxetine (Prozac). *JAMA* 1993; 269(17):2246–48.

Patton SW, Misri S, Corral MR, Perry KF, Kuan AJ: Antipsychotic medication during pregnancy and lactation in women with schizophrenia: Evaluating the risk. *Canadian Journal of Psychiatry* 2002; 47(10):959–65.

Perucca E: Birth defects after prenatal exposure to antiepileptic drugs. *Lancet Neurology* 2005; 4(11):781–86.

Repke JT, Berger NG: Electroconvulsive therapy in pregnancy. *Obstetrics and Gynecology* 1984; 63(suppl.):39S–40S.

Rosenberg L, Mitchell AA, Parsells JL, Pashayan H, Louik C, Shapiro S: Lack of relation of oral clefts to diazepam use during pregnancy. *New England Journal of Medicine* 1983; 309:1282–85.

Sabers A, Dam M, A-Rogvi-Hansen B, Boas J, Sidenius P, Laue Friis M, Alving J, Dahl M, Ankerhus J, Mouritzen Dam A: Epilepsy and pregnancy: Lamotrigine as main drug used. *Acta Neurologica Scandinavica* 2004; 109(1):9–13.

Schimmel M, Katz E, Shaag Y, Pastuszak A, Koren G: Toxic neonatal effects following maternal clomipramine therapy. *Clinical Toxicology* 1991; 29:479–84.

Sherer DM, D'Amico LD, Warshal DP, Stern RA, Grunert HF, Abramowicz JS: Recurrent mild abruption placentae occurring immediately after repeated electroconvulsive therapy in pregnancy. *American Journal of Obstetrics and Gynecology* 1991; 165:652–53.

Simon GE, Davis RL: Outcomes of prenatal antidepressant exposure. *American Journal of Psychiatry* 2002; 159(12):2055–61.

Spinelli M: Interpersonal psychotherapy for depressed antepartum women: A pilot study. *American Journal of Psychiatry* 1997; 154:1028–30.

Stowe ZN, Casarella J, Landrey J, Nemeroff CB: Sertraline in the treatment of women with postpartum major depression. *Depression* 1995; 3:49–55.

Stowe ZN, Cohen LS, Hostetter A, Ritchie JC, Owens MJ, Nemeroff CB: Paroxetine in human breast milk and nursing infants. *American Journal of Psychiatry* 2000; 157(2):185–89.

Stowe ZN, Owens MJ, Landry JC, Kilts CD, Ely T, Llewellyn A, Nemeroff CB: Sertraline and desmethylsertraline in human breast milk and nursing infants. *American Journal of Psychiatry* 1997; 154:1255–60.

Suri R, Altshuler L, Burt V, Hendrick V: Managing psychiatric medications in the breast-feeding woman. *Medscape Women's Health* 1998; 3(1).

Suri R, Altshuler L, Hendrick V, Rasgon N, Lee E, Mintz J: The impact of depression and fluoxetine treatment on obstetrical outcome. *Archives of Women's Mental Health* 2004; 7(3):193–200.

Suri R, Burt VK, Altshuler LL, Zuckerbrow-Miller J, Fairbanks L: Fluvoxamine for postpartum depression. *American Journal of Psychiatry* 2001; 158(10):1739–40.

Tennis P, Eldridge RR; International Lamotrigine Pregnancy Registry Scientific Advisory Committee: Preliminary results on pregnancy outcome in women using lamotrigine. *Epilepsia* 2002; 43(10):1161–67.

van Gent EM, Verhoeven WMA: Bipolar illness, lithium prophylaxis, and pregnancy. *Pharmacopsychiatry* 1992; 25:187–91.

Viguera AC, Cohen LS, Baldessarini RJ, Nonacs R: Managing bipolar disorder during pregnancy: Weighing the risks and benefits. *Canadian Journal of Psychiatry* 2002; 47:426–36.

Viguera AC, Cohen LS, Bouffard S, Whitfield TH, Baldessarini RJ: Reproductive decisions by women with bipolar disorder after prepregnancy psychiatric consultation. *American Journal of Psychiatry* 2002; 159(12):2102–4.

Viguera AC, Nonacs R, Cohen LS, Tondo L, Murray A, Baldessarini RJ: Risk of recurrence of bipolar disorder in pregnant and nonpregnant women after discontinuing lithium maintenance. *American Journal of Psychiatry* 2000; 157(2):179–84.

Webb RT, Howard L, Abel KM: Antipsychotic drugs for non-affective psychosis during pregnancy and postpartum. *Cochrane Database of Systematic Reviews* 2004; 2.

Webster PAC: Withdrawal symptoms in neonates associated with maternal antidepressant therapy. *Lancet* 1973; 2:318–19.

Weinstock L, Cohen LS, Bailey JW, Blatman R, Rosenbaum JF: Obstetrical and neonatal outcome following clonazepam use during pregnancy: A case series. *Psychotherapy & Psychosomatics* 2001; 3:158–62.

Weissman AM, Levy BT, Hartz AJ, Bentler S, Donohue M, Ellingrod VL, Wisner KL: Pooled analysis of antidepressant levels in lactating mothers, breast milk, and nursing infants. *American Journal of Psychiatry* 2004; 161(6):1066–78.

Wise MG, Ward SC, Townsend-Parchman W, Giltrap LC, III, Hauth JC: Case report of ECT during high-risk pregnancy. *American Journal of Psychiatry* 1984; 141:99–101.

Wisner KL, Gelenberg AJ, Leonard H, Zarin D, Frank E: Pharmacologic treatment of depression during pregnancy. *JAMA* 1999; 282(13):1264–69.

Wisner KL, Parry BL, Piontek CM: Clinical practice: Postpartum depression. *New England Journal of Medicine* 2002; 347(3):194–99.

Wisner K, Perel J, Blumer J: Serum sertraline and N-desmethylsertraline levels in breast-feeding mother-infant pairs. *American Journal of Psychiatry* 1998; 155:690–92.

Wisner K, Perel J, Findling R, Hinnes R: Nortriptyline and its hydroxymetabolites in breast-feeding mothers and newborns. *Psychopharmacology Bulletin* 1997; 33 (2):249–51.

Wisner K, Perel J, Wheeler S: Tricyclic dose requirements across pregnancy. *American Journal of Psychiatry* 1993; 150:1541–42.

Wisner KL, Perel JM: Serum nortriptyline levels in nursing mothers and their infants. *American Journal of Psychiatry* 1991; 148:1234–36.

Wisner KL, Perel JM: Nortriptyline treatment of breast-feeding women (letter). *American Journal of Psychiatry* 1996; 153:295.

Wisner KL, Perel JM, Findling RL. Antidepressant treatment during breast-feeding. *American Journal of Psychiatry* 1996; 153:1132–37.

Wisner KL, Perel JM, Foglia JP: Serum clomipramine and metabolite levels in four nursing mother-infant pairs. *Journal of Clinical Psychiatry* 1995; 56(1):17–20.

Wisner KL, Perel JM, Peindl KS, Hanusa BH, Piontek CM, Findling RL: Prevention of postpartum depression: A pilot randomized clinical trial. *American Journal of Psychiatry* 2004; 161(7):1290–92.

Wisner KL, Wheeler SB: Prevention of recurrent postpartum major depression. *Hospital and Community Psychiatry* 1994; 45(12):1191–96.

Wisner P: Prevention of recurrent postpartum depression: a randomized clinical trial. *Journal of Clinical Psychiatry* 2001; 62(2):82–86.

Yapp P, Ilett KF, Kristensen JH, Hackett LP, Paech MJ, Rampono J: Drowsiness and poor feeding in a breast-fed infant: Association with nefazodone and its metabolites. *Annals of Pharmacotherapy* 2000; 34(11):1269–72.

Yonkers K, Little B, March D: Lithium during pregnancy: Drug effects and their therapeutic implications. *CNS Drugs* 1998; 4:261–69.

Yonkers KA, Wisner KL, Stowe Z, Leibenluft E, Cohen L, Miller L, Manber R, Viguera A, Suppes T, Altshuler L: Management of bipolar disorder during pregnancy and the postpartum period. *American Journal of Psychiatry* 2004; 161(4):608–20.

Zeskind P, Stephens L: Maternal selective serotonin reuptake inhibitor use during pregnancy and newborn neurobehavior. *Pediatrics* 2004; 113(2):368–75.

Index